Imaging of Salivary Glands

Editor

AHMED ABDEL KHALEK ABDEL RAZEK

NEUROIMAGING CLINICS OF NORTH AMERICA

www.neuroimaging.theclinics.com

Consulting Editor
SURESH K. MUKHERJI

May 2018 • Volume 28 • Number 2

ELSEVIER

1600 John F. Kennedy Boulevard • Suite 1800 • Philadelphia, Pennsylvania, 19103-2899

http://www.neuroimaging.theclinics.com

NEUROIMAGING CLINICS OF NORTH AMERICA Volume 28, Number 2
May 2018 ISSN 1052-5149, ISBN 13: 978-0-323-58366-4

Editor: John Vassallo (j.vassallo@elsevier.com)
Developmental Editor: Casey Potter

Neuroimaging Clinics of North America (ISSN 1052-5149) is published quarterly by Elsevier Inc., 360 Park Avenue South, New York, NY 10010-1710. Months of issue are February, May, August, and November. Business and editorial offices: 1600 John F. Kennedy Blvd., Suite 1800, Philadelphia, PA 19103-2899. Business and editorial offices: 6277 Sea Harbor Drive, Orlando, FL 32887-4800. Periodicals postage paid at New York, NY, and additional mailing offices. Subscription prices are USD 387 per year for US individuals, USD 622 per year for US institutions, USD 100 per year for US students and residents, USD 440 per year for Canadian individuals, USD 791 per year for Canadian institutions, USD 525 per year for international individuals, USD 791 per year for international institutions and USD 260 per year for Canadian and foreign students and residents. To receive student/resident rate, orders must be accompanied by name of affiliated institution, date of term, and the *signature* of program/residency coordinator on institution letterhead. Orders will be billed at individual rate until proof of status is received. Foreign air speed delivery is included in all *Clinics* subscription prices. All prices are subject to change without notice. POSTMASTER: Send address changes to *Neuroimaging Clinics of North America*, Elsevier Health Sciences Division, Subscription **Customer Service, 3251 Riverport Lane, Maryland Heights, MO 63043. Telephone: 1-800-654-2452 (U.S. and Canada); 314-447-8871 (outside U.S. and Canada). Fax: 314-447-8029. E-mail: journalscustomer service-usa@elsevier.com (for print support); journalsonlinesupport-usa@elsevier.com (for online support)**.

Reprints. For copies of 100 or more of articles in this publication, please contact the Commercial Reprints Department, Elsevier Inc., 360 Park Avenue South, New York, NY 10010-1710. Tel.: 212-633-3874; Fax: 212-633-3820; E-mail: reprints@elsevier.com.

Neuroimaging Clinics of North America is covered by *Excerpta Medica/EMBASE,* the RSNA Index of Imaging Literature, *MEDLINE/PubMed (Index Medicus),* MEDLINE/MEDLARS, SciSearch, Research Alert, and Neuroscience Citation Index.

Printed in the United States of America.

PROGRAM OBJECTIVE

The goal of *Neuroimaging Clinics of North America* is to keep practicing radiologists and radiology residents up to date with current clinical practice in radiology by providing timely articles reviewing the state of the art in patient care.

TARGET AUDIENCE

Practicing radiologists, radiology residents, and other healthcare professionals who utilize neuroimaging findings to provide patient care.

LEARNING OBJECTIVES

Upon completion of this activity, participants will be able to:
1. Review normal anatomy of the salivary glands and imaging techniques
2. Discuss ultrasound and diffusion imaging modules of the salivary glands
3. Recognize state of art imaging and post treatment of salivary gland tumors

ACCREDITATION

The Elsevier Office of Continuing Medical Education (EOCME) is accredited by the Accreditation Council for Continuing Medical Education (ACCME) to provide continuing medical education for physicians.

The EOCME designates this enduring material for a maximum of 15 *AMA PRA Category 1 Credit*(s)™. Physicians should claim only the credit commensurate with the extent of their participation in the activity.

All other healthcare professionals requesting continuing education credit for this enduring material will be issued a certificate of participation.

DISCLOSURE OF CONFLICTS OF INTEREST

The EOCME assesses conflict of interest with its instructors, faculty, planners, and other individuals who are in a position to control the content of CME activities. All relevant conflicts of interest that are identified are thoroughly vetted by EOCME for fair balance, scientific objectivity, and patient care recommendations. EOCME is committed to providing its learners with CME activities that promote improvements or quality in healthcare and not a specific proprietary business or a commercial interest.

The planning committee, staff, authors and editors listed below have identified no financial relationships or relationships to products or devices they or their spouse/life partner have with commercial interest related to the content of this CME activity:

Ahmed Abdel Khalek Abdel Razek, MD; Amit K. Agarwal, MD; Christopher Atkinson, MD; Asim K. Bag, MD; Kunwar Suryaveer Singh Bhatia, B Med Sci, MBBS, MRCS, DLO, FRCR; Philip R. Chapman, MD; Joel K. Curé, MD; Yuk-Ling Dai, MBBS, MRes (Med), FRCR; Elliott Friedman, MD; Akifumi Fujita, MD, PhD; Joseph Fuller III, MD; Daniel Thomas Ginat, MD, MS; Atif Wasim Haneef Mohamed, MD; Jeffrey Hawk, MD; Benjamin Huang, MD, MPH; Sangam G. Kanekar, MD; Alison Kemp; Remy Lobo, MD; Suresh K. Mukherji, MD, MBA, FACR; Maria Olga Patiño, MD; Aparna Singhal, MD; Ashok Srinivasan, MBBS, MD; Karthik Subramaniam; Unni K. Udayasankar, MD; John Vassallo.

UNAPPROVED/OFF-LABEL USE DISCLOSURE

The EOCME requires CME faculty to disclose to the participants:
1. When products or procedures being discussed are off-label, unlabelled, experimental, and/or investigational (not US Food and Drug Administration [FDA] approved); and
2. Any limitations on the information presented, such as data that are preliminary or that represent ongoing research, interim analyses, and/or unsupported opinions. Faculty may discuss information about pharmaceutical agents that is outside of FDA-approved labelling. This information is intended solely for CME and is not intended to promote off-label use of these medications. If you have any questions, contact the medical affairs department of the manufacturer for the most recent prescribing information.

TO ENROLL

To enroll in the *Neuroimaging Clinics of North America* Continuing Medical Education program, call customer service at 1-800-654-2452 or sign up online at http://www.theclinics.com/home/cme. The CME program is available to subscribers for an additional annual fee of USD 244.40.

METHOD OF PARTICIPATION

In order to claim credit, participants must complete the following:
1. Complete enrolment as indicated above.
2. Read the activity.
3. Complete the CME Test and Evaluation. Participants must achieve a score of 70% on the test. All CME Tests and Evaluations must be completed online.

CME INQUIRIES/SPECIAL NEEDS

For all CME inquiries or special needs, please contact elsevierCME@elsevier.com.

NEUROIMAGING CLINICS OF NORTH AMERICA

Contributors

CONSULTING EDITOR

SURESH K. MUKHERJI, MD, MBA, FACR
Professor and Chairman, Walter F. Patenge
Endowed Chair, Department of Radiology,
Michigan State University, Chief Medical
Officer and Director of Health Care Delivery,
Michigan State University Health Team, East
Lansing, Michigan, USA

EDITOR

**AHMED ABDEL KHALEK ABDEL RAZEK,
MD**
Professor and Head, Department of Diagnostic
Radiology, Faculty of Medicine, Mansoura
University, Mansoura, Egypt

AUTHORS

**AHMED ABDEL KHALEK ABDEL RAZEK,
MD**
Professor and Head, Department of Diagnostic
Radiology, Faculty of Medicine, Mansoura
University, Mansoura, Egypt

AMIT K. AGARWAL, MD
Associate Professor of Radiology, The
University of Texas Southwestern Medical
Center, Dallas, Texas, USA

CHRISTOPHER ATKINSON, MD
Department of Radiology, The University of
North Carolina at Chapel Hill, Chapel Hill, North
Carolina, USA

ASIM K. BAG, MD
Associate Professor, Department of Radiology,
The University of Alabama at Birmingham,
Birmingham, Alabama, USA

**KUNWAR SURYAVEER SINGH BHATIA,
B Med Sci, MBBS, MRCS, DLO, FRCR**
Imaging Department, Imperial College
Healthcare NHS Trust, St Mary's Hospital,
London, United Kingdom

PHILIP R. CHAPMAN, MD
Associate Professor, Department of Radiology,
The University of Alabama at Birmingham,
Birmingham, Alabama, USA

JOEL K. CURÉ, MD
Professor, Department of Radiology, The
University of Alabama at Birmingham,
Birmingham, Alabama, USA

YUK-LING DAI, MBBS, MRes (Med), FRCR
Department of Imaging and Interventional
Radiology, Prince of Wales Hospital, The
Chinese University of Hong Kong, Sha Tin,
Hong Kong

ELLIOTT FRIEDMAN, MD
Associate Professor, Department of Diagnostic
and Interventional Imaging, The University of
Texas Health Science Center at Houston,
McGovern Medical School, Houston, Texas,
USA

AKIFUMI FUJITA, MD, PhD
Associate Professor, Department of Radiology,
Jichi Medical University School of Medicine,
Shimotsuke, Tochigi, Japan

JOSEPH FULLER III, MD
Department of Radiology, The University of North Carolina at Chapel Hill, Chapel Hill, North Carolina, USA

DANIEL THOMAS GINAT, MD, MS
Department of Radiology, The University of Chicago, Pritzker School of Medicine, Chicago, Illinois, USA

ATIF WASIM HANEEF MOHAMED, MD
Instructor, Department of Radiology, The University of Alabama at Birmingham, Birmingham, Alabama, USA

JEFFREY HAWK, MD
Department of Neuroradiology, University of Michigan, Ann Arbor, Michigan, USA

BENJAMIN HUANG, MD, MPH
Department of Radiology, The University of North Carolina at Chapel Hill, Chapel Hill, North Carolina, USA

SANGAM G. KANEKAR, MD
Professor of Radiology and Neurology, The Pennsylvania State University, Hershey, Pennsylvania, USA

REMY LOBO, MD
Department of Neuroradiology, University of Michigan, Ann Arbor, Michigan, USA

SURESH K. MUKHERJI, MD, MBA, FACR
Professor and Chairman, Walter F. Patenge Endowed Chair, Department of Radiology, Michigan State University, Chief Medical Officer and Director of Health Care Delivery, Michigan State University Health Team, East Lansing, Michigan, USA

MARIA OLGA PATIÑO, MD
Assistant Professor, Department of Diagnostic and Interventional Imaging, The University of Texas Health Science Center at Houston, McGovern Medical School, Houston, Texas, USA

APARNA SINGHAL, MD
Assistant Professor, Department of Radiology, The University of Alabama at Birmingham, Birmingham, Alabama, USA

ASHOK SRINIVASAN, MBBS, MD
Professor and Director, Department of Neuroradiology, University of Michigan, Ann Arbor, Michigan, USA

UNNI K. UDAYASANKAR, MD
Associate Professor, Department of Medical Imaging, University of Arizona College of Medicine–Tucson, Tucson, Arizona, USA

Contents

The salivary glands play an important role in digestion and oral hygiene and give rise to a variety of benign and malignant pathologies. In suspected pathology, the goal of imaging is to confirm a lesion as being of salivary gland origin, narrow the list of differential considerations, define the extent of disease, and guide further management decisions. This article outlines the function, embryologic development, anatomy, and normal imaging features of the major salivary glands. The article also discusses imaging indications, the general approach to imaging the salivary glands, and the commonly used cross-sectional techniques used for evaluating the salivary gland.

This article reviews the multimodality diagnostic imaging features of benign neoplastic and nonneoplastic tumors associated with the major salivary glands. Examples of neoplastic conditions that are depicted and discussed include pleomorphic adenoma, Warthin tumor, oncocytoma, peripheral nerve sheath tumors, lipoma, and hemangiomas or hemangioendotheliomas. Examples of nonneoplastic conditions that are depicted and discussed include ranulas, benign lymphoepithelial lesions, Kimura disease, and vascular malformations. Specific imaging and clinical features of these conditions are emphasized in this article.

Major and minor salivary gland malignancies come in various shapes and sizes. They can present as palpable masses or can be detected incidentally when imaging patients for other indications. A complete evaluation of salivary gland malignancies requires knowledge of the anatomy and various routes of spread of neoplasias. Computed tomography (CT) and MR imaging are complementary tools in this respect and offer useful information to the proceduralist. Advanced imaging (diffusion-weighted imaging and PET-CT) and other modalities (eg, ultrasound) help with characterization, although biopsy or excision is often needed for definitive tissue diagnosis.

The salivary glands are commonly affected in systemic autoimmune disease and diseases of unknown pathogenesis. Sjögren syndrome (SjS) can be affected by other systemic diseases. Immunoglobulin G4-related disease (IgG4-RD) commonly affects salivary glands. Imaging findings are usually nonspecific; however, radiologists should be familiar with the manifestations to avoid diagnostic delay. Findings of early-stage SjS are difficult to identify on routine computed tomography or MR imaging. Chronic SjS can be diagnosed from MR imaging and sialographic findings. Multiglandular and localized involvement of IgG4-RD is difficult to differentiate from malignant lymphoma for multiglandular disease and salivary gland carcinoma for localized disease.

Sialadenitis is among the most common conditions that affect the salivary glands. Inflammation of the salivary glands occurs as the end result of a variety of pathologic conditions, including infectious, autoimmune, and idiopathic causes. Clinically, inflammation of the salivary gland causes pain and localized swelling. The presentation may be acute or chronic and can be recurrent. Because there is significant overlap of underlying disease mechanisms and clinical presentations, radiologic examination often plays a significant role in evaluation. This article is a brief review of sialadenitis, including disease mechanisms, causes, and the practical imaging of the salivary glands.

 Video content accompanies this article at http://www.neuroimaging.theclinics.com/.

Ultrasound is the preferred initial imaging modality in Europe and Asia for assessing the major salivary glands. In experienced hands, it is sensitive for a range of salivary pathologies, often diagnostic, and also a safe, cost-effective gatekeeper for further investigations as well as image-guided diagnostic biopsies and aspirations. This article reviews the scanning technique and normal sonographic anatomy of major salivary glands and overviews typical sonographic appearances of salivary pathologies, including infective and inflammatory conditions, sialolithiasis, and neoplasms. Limitations of ultrasound imaging and the current evidence for advanced techniques, including contrast-enhanced ultrasound imaging and ultrasound elastography, are also discussed.

Neoplastic and nonneoplastic lesions may involve the minor salivary glands. Tumors of minor salivary glands are commonly seen in the oral cavity. Malignant tumors are more common than benign minor salivary gland tumors. The most common malignant tumors are adenoid cystic carcinoma and mucoepidermoid carcinoma, and the most common benign tumor is pleomorphic adenoma. Nonneoplastic lesions may involve minor salivary glands, such as Sjögren disease, immunoglobulin G4–related disease, necrotizing sialometaplasia, and subacute necrotizing sialadenitis. Contrast MR imaging and computed tomography are adequate for the localization and extension of neoplastic and nonneoplastic lesions of minor salivary glands.

MR imaging is the modality of choice in the evaluation of salivary gland tumors. Postcontrast MR imaging is adequate for the exact localization and extension of salivary gland tumors, and multiparametric of diffusion-weighted and dynamic contrast-enhanced MR imaging helps in the characterization of benign and malignant salivary gland tumors. Imaging is important for preoperative localization, characterization of salivary gland tumors, and locoregional extension, perineural spread, and nodal and distant staging of malignant salivary gland tumors. Imaging has a role in detection of tumor recurrence, monitoring patients after therapy, prediction of malignant transformation of benign tumors, and differentiation of salivary gland tumors from simulating inflammatory and autoimmune disorders.

Foreword
Imaging of Salivary Glands

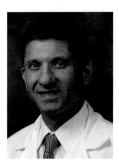

Suresh K. Mukherji, MD, MBA, FACR
Consulting Editor

The salivary glands can be considered a "forgotten" organ! Seriously...how many readers can recite the difference between a "major" and "minor" salivary tumor at a moment's notice. In this wonderful issue, Dr Abdel Razek comprehensively reviews the anatomy, pathology, and various techniques to image the salivary glands. This issue covers pathology involving both children and adults and also provides an intuitive approach for arriving at different types of salivary gland pathology.

I want to thank all of the article authors for their outstanding contributions. The contributions are truly superb. I also want to thank my colleague and friend, Dr Abdel Razek, MD. His passion and energy for Head and Neck imaging is unmatched and is one of my inspirations for continuing to push the scientific borders of our field. Ahmed... thank you for all you have and continue to accomplish!

Suresh K. Mukherji, MD, MBA, FACR
Department of Radiology
Michigan State University
Michigan State University Health Team
846 Service Road
East Lansing, MI 48824, USA

E-mail address:
mukherji@rad.msu.edu

Neuroimag Clin N Am 28 (2018) xi
https://doi.org/10.1016/j.nic.2018.02.002
1052-5149/18/© 2018 Published by Elsevier Inc.

Preface
State-of-the-Art Imaging of Salivary Glands Disorders

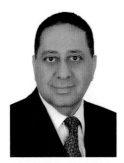

Ahmed Abdel Khalek Abdel Razek, MD
Editor

The salivary glands are affected by a spectrum of disorders that the physician and surgeon may face that require imaging. In this issue, I attempt to comprehensively cover state-of-the-art imaging modalities of salivary gland disorders. First, I wish to express my gratitude to the consulting editor, Dr Suresh K. Mukherji, for the opportunity to be guest editor for this issue of *Neuroimaging Clinics* and to share in writing and providing excellent images for some articles in this issue. All the authors of this issue of *Neuroimaging Clinics* are authoritative figures on the topic, and the readers get a wonderful review of updated imaging of the salivary glands.

This issue offers a comprehensive review of the state-of-the-art of the basic and advanced imaging approach for tumoral and nontumoral disorders of the salivary glands and an overview of basic background and imaging appearance of the common disorders of the salivary glands. The first four articles provide a detailed overview of normal anatomy and clinical applications of routine and advanced imaging modalities, including MR imaging, ultrasound, and CT scans, in evaluation of the salivary glands. In the next three articles, the reader faces a step-by-step journey over imaging of benign, malignant, and posttreatment of salivary gland tumors with state-of-the-art ultrasound and MR imaging. Later, we discuss imaging appearance of the spectrum of inflammatory and autoimmune disorders of the salivary glands. Last, we review disorders affecting the minor and submandibular salivary glands as well as salivary gland disorders of children. This issue of *Neuroimaging Clinics* shows many high-quality images of different disorders of the salivary gland and includes an extensive list of references in each article of the issue.

I would like to sincerely thank all of the expert international authors of this issue for accepting my invitation and for their invaluable contributions. I would also like to thank the series editor, John Vassallo, and developmental editor, Casey Potter, at Elsevier, for their guidance and support during the preparation of this issue.

Ahmed Abdel Khalek Abdel Razek, MD
Department of Diagnostic Radiology
Mansoura University
Elgomheryia Street
Mansoura 35512, Egypt

E-mail address:
arazek@mans.edu.eg

Neuroimag Clin N Am 28 (2018) xiii
https://doi.org/10.1016/j.nic.2018.02.001
1052-5149/18/© 2018 Published by Elsevier Inc.

Cross-Sectional Imaging Techniques and Normal Anatomy of the Salivary Glands

Christopher Atkinson, MD, Joseph Fuller III, MD, Benjamin Huang, MD, MPH*

KEYWORDS

- Salivary glands • Salivary gland anatomy • Parotid gland • Submandibular gland • Sublingual gland
- Salivary gland imaging

KEY POINTS

- The salivary glands include the 3 paired major salivary glands and 1000 minor salivary glands scattered throughout the aerodigestive tract.
- The goal of imaging is to confirm a lesion as being of salivary gland origin, narrow the list of differential considerations, define the extent of disease, and guide management decisions.
- Inflammatory lesions are often first evaluated with computed tomography; MR sialography may be a useful adjunct in further evaluating duct anatomy in chronic inflammatory conditions.
- MR imaging is the modality of choice for characterizing neoplastic lesions, and should be performed when there is concern for extraglandular or perineural tumor spread of malignancy.
- Diffusion-weighted imaging and advanced MR imaging techniques may be useful adjunct modalities in distinguishing benign and malignant salivary gland tumors.

INTRODUCTION

The salivary glands, which include the paired major salivary glands and as well as numerous minor salivary glands, play several important functions in normal digestion and oral hygiene. Any of these glands can be affected by a variety of pathologies, including benign and malignant neoplasms, inflammatory and infectious processes, congenital lesions, autoimmune disorders, and dysfunction owing to various iatrogenic causes. Although most of these processes are not unique to any of the individual salivary glands, each gland has unique characteristics that may influence the specific diseases which may be more likely to affect it.

Imaging is often warranted in patients with suspected salivary gland disease to help distinguish inflammatory from neoplastic processes and to help confirm the salivary gland as the origin of the process. In certain instances, imaging can be helpful in differentiating benign from malignant neoplasms; however, it is important to keep in mind that conventional imaging features of parotid tumors are often nonspecific. Many low-grade malignancies can be difficult or impossible to differentiate from benign entities by imaging alone, and in these cases imaging is not necessarily done to provide a definitive histologic diagnosis, but rather to narrow the list of diagnostic considerations, define the anatomic extent of abnormality (including possible perineural spread), help guide workup and management, and aid in biopsy and surgical planning.

Disclosure: The authors have nothing to disclose.
Department of Radiology, University of North Carolina, 101 Manning Drive, CB#7510, Chapel Hill, NC 27599, USA
* Corresponding author.
E-mail address: bhuang@med.unc.edu

Neuroimag Clin N Am 28 (2018) 137–158
https://doi.org/10.1016/j.nic.2018.01.001

Cross-sectional techniques, including computed tomography (CT) and MR imaging are often the first modalities for salivary gland imaging. Regardless of the indication for imaging or the type of imaging performed, providing quality interpretation relies not only on knowing the diseases that may affect the glands, but also on understanding the anatomy of the glands and of the structures that reside within or beside them, because the diseases of a gland can easily spread to involve these structures or vice versa. In addition, one's ability to identify pathology in a gland requires familiarity with the normal appearances of each gland on the different imaging modalities.

This article reviews the function, embryologic development, anatomy, and normal imaging features of the major salivary glands. Additional topics covered include common indications for salivary gland imaging, the general approach to imaging salivary gland pathology, and commonly used cross-sectional techniques used for salivary evaluation—namely CT, MR imaging, and PET/CT scanning—as well as more specialized salivary imaging techniques such as MR sialography and diffusion-weighted imaging (DWI). Newer investigational techniques for characterization of salivary tumors including CT perfusion scanning, dynamic susceptibility contrast perfusion MR imaging, and dynamic contrast-enhanced MR imaging are also briefly discussed.

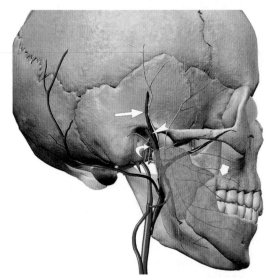

Fig. 1. Normal parotid anatomy. Three-dimensional rendered model demonstrating the anatomic relationships between the parotid gland, parotid duct (*fat arrow*, shaded in *green*), branches of the facial nerve (*curved arrow*, shaded in *yellow*), and neighboring arterial (*red*) and venous (*blue*) structures. The *long arrow* indicates the superficial temporal artery and the *arrowhead* indicates the retromandibular vein.

SALIVARY GLAND FUNCTION

The salivary glands are exocrine glands that are responsible for the production of saliva, a watery substance that contributes to the process of digestion during mastication. There are 3 pairs of major salivary glands that produce most of the saliva in humans: the parotid glands, submandibular glands, and sublingual glands (**Figs. 1** and **2**). In addition to the major salivary glands, there are approximately 1000 minor salivary glands that line and moisten the mucosa of the aerodigestive tract.[1,2]

In normal circumstances, the salivary glands produce approximately 1.0 to 1.5 L of saliva per day. The composition of saliva produced by each gland is slightly different, with the parotid glands producing the most serous fluid, the sublingual glands producing slightly more viscous fluid, and the submandibular glands producing the most viscous and mucinous saliva. Saliva serves several important functions in digestion, including facilitating the tasting of food, moistening food, and initiating the breakdown of fat and starches through the actions of salivary amylase and lipase during mastication.[3–5]

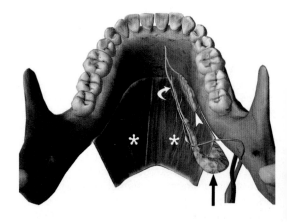

Fig. 2. Normal submandibular and sublingual gland anatomy. (*A*) Three-dimensional rendered model demonstrating the anatomic relationships between the mandible, myelohyoid muscle, submandibular gland (*arrow*), and sublingual gland (*arrowhead*). The myelohyoid muscle (*asterisks*) forms the floor of the sublingual space. The lingual nerve (shaded *yellow*) is shown along the medial margin of the mandible and Wharton's duct (*curved arrow*) courses anteriorly. The anterior facial vein and facial artery (shaded in *blue* and *red*, respectively) can be see along the lateral aspect of the submandibular gland.

Saliva also plays an important role in maintaining oral hygiene and health by acting to protect the mucosa and teeth from minor trauma and infection. Immunoglobulin A, enzymes, and the glycoproteins contained in saliva serve as one of the first lines of defense against infection. In addition, saliva contains numerous electrolytes, including bicarbonate, potassium, and sodium, which help to buffer acids produced by bacteria. Conditions that result in salivary hypofunction, such head and neck radiation and systemic autoimmune disorders such as Sjogren's syndrome, may result in the development of recurrent mucosal ulcers and irritation, fungal overgrowth, multiple dental caries, or gum disease.[3,6]

SALIVARY GLAND EMBRYOLOGY

The embryologic development of the major salivary glands is a complex process linked to the development of the other head and neck structures and begins during weeks 6 to 8 of gestation.[3,5,7,8] The parotid glands develop from the oral ectodermal lining near the angles of the stomodeum in the first and second branchial arches, whereas the submandibular and sublingual glands are believed to develop from oral endoderm (although there is some controversy surrounding their tissue of origin).[3,5,7,8] The primitive glandular tissue interacts with the adjacent mesenchyme, and through multiple signaling pathways, these interactions influence the growth and differentiation of the salivary gland tissue. As each gland develops, the epithelial bud grows and branching ducts form, resulting in terminal buds and acini by around 14 weeks of gestation. Finally, the parotid and submandibular glands are encapsulated in a connective tissue layer.

The parotid gland is the first to begin developing (appearing early in the sixth week), but is the last to become fully encapsulated. This delay allows the developing lymphatic tissue to become entrapped in the parotid gland, explaining why it is the only major salivary gland to contain lymphatic tissue.[3,5,7,8] The submandibular glands appear late in the sixth week of gestation, and the sublingual glands appear during the eighth week.

Functional sympathetic and parasympathetic innervation is necessary for the proper growth and maintenance of gland structure. Disruption of the interaction between the developing glandular epithelium and mesenchyme, disruption of autonomic nervous system innervation, or abnormalities in head and neck development can all lead to salivary gland aplasia.[4–6,8] Craniofacial abnormalities such as cleft palate, skeletal dysplasias, branchial cleft anomalies, and several other syndromes including Treacher-Collins syndrome and syndromes in the oculoauriculovertebral spectrum (eg, Goldenhar syndrome and hemifacial macrosomia) are associated with salivary gland aplasia or the formation of ectopic salivary tissues.[2,7,9–12]

CROSS-SECTIONAL IMAGING TECHNIQUES, INDICATIONS, AND GENERAL APPROACH TO SALIVARY GLAND IMAGING

The most common presenting signs of salivary gland disease are those of obstruction, inflammation, suspected glandular mass, or diffuse gland enlargement.[13] Frequently, nonspecific clinical examination findings highlight the essential role of imaging in the diagnosis of salivary gland disease. State of the art salivary gland imaging has evolved considerably over the last several decades, and CT scanning and MR imaging have become the preferred tools for characterization and localization of salivary gland pathologies. Because of the emergence of sialendoscopy as a primary treatment tool of ductal abnormalities, plain radiography and conventional sialography have largely been abandoned in mainstream clinical practice.[14,15]

According to the American College of Radiology Appropriateness Criteria, both CT scanning and MR imaging are considered to be complementary diagnostic modalities for characterizing febrile and nonfebrile neck masses and adenopathy owing to their overall accuracy in diagnosing inflammation and tumors of the head and neck.[16] They are invaluable in defining disease location, extension into deep spaces of the neck, and invasion of adjacent structures by tumor. The following sections discuss specific cross-sectional imaging techniques and their potential applications in salivary imaging.

Computed Tomography Scanning

CT scanning is the most ordered study for evaluation of the sublingual, submandibular, and parotid spaces. It is the preferred initial modality in the workup of suspected calcification and inflammatory conditions owing to its high sensitivity and spatial resolution (**Fig. 3**). This trend is due to the relatively high frequency of infectious and inflammatory pathologies that affect the salivary glands as well as by the relative speed and ubiquity CT scanners in emergency departments.

Noncontrast CT scanning can be useful in the setting of suspected uncomplicated sialolithiasis.[17] Symptomatology in these cases is related to that of ductal obstruction, namely, postprandial pain and episodic swelling. Iodinated contrast is

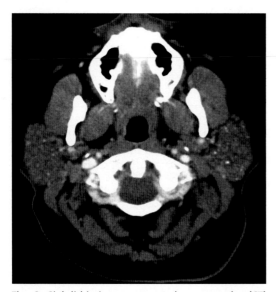

Fig. 3. Sialolithiasis on computed tomography (CT) scanning. Axial contrast-enhanced CT image demonstrating multiple bilateral, high-density, nonobstructing parotid sialoliths in a patient with Sjogren syndrome. Note also how both parotid glands are enlarged and heterogeneous, with innumerable small hypodense regions presumably representing microcysts typical of Sjogren syndrome.

often indicated, particularly if there is a concern for the development of sialadenitis or a parotid or submandibular abscess complicating sialolithiasis. The administration of contrast media generally does not limit the detectability of a ductal calculus. Barring the presence of an iodinated contrast allergy, we believe that intravenous contrast should be administered for most cases of suspected calculus, inflammation, or infection, because its addition provides improved anatomic detail of the gland and adjacent soft tissues, localizes the site of infection, and distinguishes the presence of abscess from phlegmon or cellulitis.

Although it is an excellent diagnostic tool, CT scanning can be of limited usefulness in the setting of extensive streak artifact caused by a dental amalgam or maxillofacial fixation hardware. Angled gantry acquisition can be used to avoid scanning through the regions causing artifact. Image degradation can also be mitigated in certain instances by the application of dual energy CT scans.[17–20]

Imaging the salivary glands can be optimally performed using a standard neck CT protocol. The main goal is to allow sufficient time after contrast administration to achieve optimal tissue enhancement, while also maintaining vascular enhancement. A standard venous phase scan of the neck should extend from the circle of Willis to the aortic arch with intravenous injection of approximately 80 to 100 mL of nonionic isomolar contrast media at a constant rate of 2 to 3 mL/s. We advocate complete neck imaging over limited facial extent to assess for the presence of regional adenopathy both in the setting of tumor and infection. A typical fixed delay time of 60 seconds is usually adequate to achieve optimal tissue and vascular enhancement. Some institutions try to further optimize scan parameters with a split bolus technique where scanning is performed after a 120-second delay. One-half of the contrast dose is given at time zero followed by a second contrast bolus containing the remainder of the contrast at 90 seconds. In this way, an effective 30-second delay of the second injection is achieved to more fully opacify the vessels. Scanning can be performed either during quiet respiration or during breath hold to minimize motion artifact. Using a pitch of less than 1 can provide better image quality and minimize artifacts.

Additional scans with head tilt or angled gantry can be performed if streak artifact is identified. Multiple gantry angles may be necessary to achieve satisfactory images. Image reconstructions should aim for a display of no more than 3 mm thick contiguous slices. It is useful to also have comparatively thin overlapping dataset in the range of 0.75 to 1.5 mm in thickness for troubleshooting. Axial, sagittal, and coronal reformations should be considered standard practice using both soft tissue smoothing and edge enhancement bone kernels.[21]

PET/Computed Tomography

PET/CT scanning is widely used in head and neck oncology for the staging and follow-up of malignant tumors, including those of the salivary glands. In normal circumstances, fluorine-18-fluorodeoxy-D-glucose (FDG) is taken up by the salivary glands and secreted in the saliva. Mild to moderate symmetric physiologic FDG uptake is, therefore, normally seen in the parotid and submandibular glands (**Fig. 4**).[22] Several benign, nonneoplastic processes, including infections, sarcoidosis, and radiation-induced sialadenitis, can produce increased FDG uptake on PET/CT scans, whereas asymmetric gland uptake can be seen in patients after surgical removal of 1 gland or unilateral neck radiation.[23]

For most malignant salivary tumors, the standardized uptake values on PET/CT scans are significantly higher than those of benign tumors, and high-grade salivary malignancies also tend to show higher maximum standardized uptake values compared with many low-grade

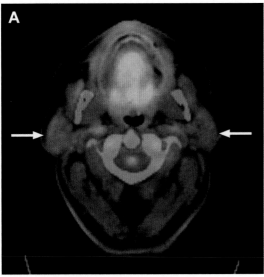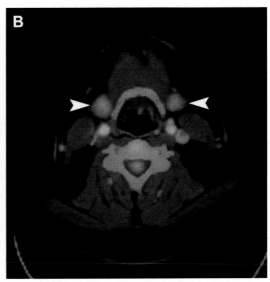

Fig. 4. Normal parotid and submandibular glands on PET with computed tomography (CT) scanning. Axial fused PET CT image of (A) the parotid glands (arrows) and (B) the submandibular glands (arrowheads) demonstrating normal mild physiologic fluorine-18-fluorodeoxy-ᴅ-glucose radiotracer salivary gland uptake.

malignancies.[23] However, some benign tumors (including pleomorphic adenomas and Warthin tumors) can also show very high FDG uptake, and some malignancies such as adenoid cystic carcinoma and low-grade mucoepidermoid carcinoma may show little FDG avidity.[23–25] The usefulness of PET/CT scanning for the discrimination of benign from malignant salivary gland processes is, therefore, hindered by unacceptably high rates of false-positive and false-negative results. As such, any FDG-avid mass in the parotid or submandibular glands should undergo tissue sampling for definitive diagnosis. Despite these limitations, PET/ CT scanning remains a useful complementary technique to conventional imaging for regional and distant staging of malignant salivary gland tumors and for the follow-up and restaging of treated tumors.

Advanced Computed Tomography Techniques

CT perfusion imaging is an advanced method of evaluation that can be performed quantitatively to evaluate tumor vascularity. Dynamic CT images are obtained before, during, and after a bolus of intravenous contrast and the imaging data is post processed to calculate imaging biomarkers such as blood flow, blood volume, mean transit time, and permeability surface area. These imaging biomarkers can help to differentiate between malignant and benign etiologies, with malignancy generally displaying increased blood flow, blood volume, and permeability, with a decreased mean transit time compared with normal tissue.[26]

The advantages of CT perfusion are that it has widespread availability, is rapidly obtained, and is inexpensive compared with MR imaging. The disadvantages of CT perfusion are exposure to ionizing radiation, especially over serial examinations, and limited volume of coverage/evaluation. Although there is some overlap in these parameters, CT perfusion may have a role in the evaluation and management of patients with salivary gland neoplasia.

MR Imaging

MR imaging is the preferred modality in the evaluation of salivary gland tumors. Like CT scanning, MR imaging has the ability to localize a lesion and assess its extent. MR imaging has the advantages of requiring no ionizing radiation exposure, an ability to image patients with iodinated contrast allergies, improved soft tissue contrast, and more accurate assessment of deep tissue planes. MR imaging is the preferred imaging modality for the assessment of parotid tumors, particularly when there is concern for extraglandular or perineural spread. In such cases, MR imaging with contrast should be considered standard. The disadvantages of MR imaging include any contraindications to magnetic field exposure, such as many pacemakers or neural stimulators, metallic susceptibility artifact from adjacent dental amalgam, and relatively long scan times, which may increase the likelihood of motion or necessitate the use of sedation in claustrophobic patients.

A general neck protocol is often adequate for successful imaging of the salivary glands. At both 1.5T and 3T, a suitable protocol should incorporate at minimum the following sequences—coronal short tau inversion recovery, axial T2-weighted, axial T2-weighted with fat saturation, precontrast axial, sagittal and coronal T1-weighted without fat saturation, as well as postcontrast axial, and coronal T1-weighted images, ideally with fat saturation. A field of view no more than 250 × 250 mm and slice thickness of 5 mm or less is desirable. When there is concern for perineural tumor spread in the setting of a malignant salivary gland lesion, performing a dedicated skull base protocol using isotropic T2-weighted balanced steady-state free precession based sequence, such as constructive interference in the steady-state or fast imaging employing steady-state acquisition and thin section 3-dimensional (3D) precontrast and postcontrast fat-suppressed T1-weighted sequences should be considered. When there is specific concern for duct obstruction, ductal pathology, or when evaluation of ductal anatomy is needed, the addition of MR sialography may be helpful.

MR Sialography

MR sialography was developed as a noninvasive method for evaluating the salivary ducts. The development of the first MR sialographic sequence, heavily T2-weighted rapid acquisition with relaxation enhancement, was formulated from MR cholangiopancreatography to take advantage of the intrinsically high T2 signal intensity of stationary fluids.[27] This technique necessitates heavily T2-weighted sequences and extremely long echo times.

MR sialography offers several advantages compared with conventional sialography, including a lack of ionizing radiation, a lack of a need for contrast media, and noninvasiveness. It is also excellent for the preoperative evaluation of ductal anatomy before attempted sialendoscopy.[28] As such, MR sialography is gaining wider use as a supplementary tool for ductal salivary gland disease, and its usefulness has been shown in numerous clinical scenarios, including evaluation of sialolithiasis, sialadenitis, ductal stenosis, xerostomia, Sjögren syndrome, and juvenile recurrent parotitis.[29–32] Imaging may be indicated to assess the sequelae of these conditions such as fistulae, strictures, diverticula, and cysts. MR sialography has been shown to visualize salivary duct wall damage well, and is useful in evaluating for suspected sialocele.[28,33]

Over the years, the development of newer imaging techniques has resulted in improved image quality, allowing for higher spatial resolution and 3D isotropic volumetric acquisitions with improved diagnostic accuracy.[34,35] Resolution has improved from detecting only 10% of tertiary ductal branches to up to 80% of tertiary branches over the last decade.[36,37] Many sequences have shown good ability to achieve heavily T2-weighted sialographic images including but not limited to 3D constructive interference in the steady state,[38] 3D-driven equilibrium pulse/fast recovery fast spin echo, fast imaging with steady state precession, half-Fourier acquisition single-shot turbo spin echo sequences, extended-phase conjugate-symmetry rapid spin-echo, and 2-dimensional and 3D fast asymmetric spin echo.[39–44]

To augment visualization of the salivary ducts, the administration of a secretagogue has been advocated. This state is typically achieved by oral administration of a citric acid–based agent. Authors have described the use of citric acid drops, lemon wedges, lemon juice, or citrus-flavored candies.[32,38] The concept behind this is similar to that of giving secretin during MR cholangiopancreatography, where the administration of the agent is thought to achieve increased secretions and, therefore, result in better distention of the ductal system.[44] Passive ductal occlusion with gauze is also advocated by some investigators.[36] Before imaging, patients should be questioned about a history of obstructive gland disease, because sialadenitis and ductal obstruction may render patients sensitive to pain induced by administration of the sialogogue.[36]

Sialography technique

After careful instructions to the patient to keep still, they are then placed head-first and supine into the bore using a standard head coil. Once the 3-plane localizer has been used to properly position a patient, standard axial noncontrast T1-weighted spin echo, axial noncontrast T2 half-Fourier acquisition single-shot turbo spin echo and coronal short tau inversion recovery sequences are obtained with an adequate field of view, covering the entire area of interest. A safe approach is to scan from the top of the mastoids to the vocal cords so as to achieve adequate coverage.

Subsequently, the secretagogue is administered by moving the patient out of the bore, removing the head coil, and administering the solution into the patient's mouth. They are then instructed to hold the solution in their mouth for 30 seconds before clearing the liquid by swallowing. The patient should then be instructed not to swallow during sequence acquisition.

The gland of interest is then selected for high-resolution image acquisition. The parotid gland is imaged using an oblique sagittal thick slab localizer that parallels the zygomatic arch in the axial plane and parallels the zygomatic arch/mental protuberance on coronal plane. If one is imaging the submandibular gland, it is best visualized on the oblique sagittal thick slab localizer that parallels the body of the mandible in the axial plane and similarly parallels the zygomatic arch and mental protuberance in the coronal plane. Next, separate 20 mm thick axial and coronal oblique T2 half-Fourier acquisition single-shot turbo spin echo or T2 FSE inversion recovery slabs are acquired (**Fig. 5**). Our final sequence is a 3D constructive interference in the steady-state acquired in an axial oblique plane using the same localizer positioning and field of view as the thick slab T2-weighted sequences (**Fig. 6**). A 3D SPACE (Sampling Perfection with Application optimized Contrasts using different flip angle Evolution) acquisition should achieve comparable image quality. It is important to use a wide enough field of view to cover the entire gland of interest with enough overcoverage and oversampling to minimize aliasing, but also small enough so as to achieve high in-plane resolution.

Many technical challenges still exist, including artifacts from patient motion and metallic susceptibility from adjacent dental amalgam or fixation hardware. An important practical point is

that patients should be instructed to not to swallow during image acquisition, which can introduce motion and significantly limit image quality. This caution is especially true after sialogogue administration and when imaging the submandibular gland owing to proximity to the tongue.[44]

The visualization of small salivary stones is limited by the lower limit of spatial resolution and efforts to improve on this are offset by the need for a relatively high signal-to-noise ratio of such a heavily T2-weighted technique.[42] Therefore, CT scanning may be helpful if small stones are suspected.

Diffusion-Weighted Imaging

Distinguishing between benign and malignant salivary gland tumors is frequently a challenge owing to the nonspecific nature of their appearance on conventional MR imaging. There has been great interest in using DWI as an advanced tool to characterize salivary gland lesions. Many studies have shown that pleomorphic adenomas have higher apparent diffusion coefficient (ADC) values than Warthin tumors and malignant tumors[45–52] (**Fig. 7**). Quantitative ADC mapping has also demonstrated that areas of high ADC values are rare in cases of malignant tumors and can be a reliable distinguishing factor for the diagnosis of pleomorphic adenoma when using a threshold of 1.8×10^3 mm^2 to define a high ADC value.[45,53,54] However, a significant drawback to the applicability of ADC mapping is the fact that both malignant tumors and benign tumors such as Warthin tumors exhibited areas with low or extremely low ADC values, averaging up to 60% and 72% of the tumor area, respectively. Therefore, low or extremely low ADC value criterion may not yield a good result in differentiating between benign and malignant tumors.[45,53,54]

Although useful for distinguishing between pleomorphic adenoma and malignancy, a diagnosis of benign versus malignant tumors should not be based solely on ADC values. Instead the use of a combined approach with other MR-based parameters has been recommended.[54]

A significant drawback of quantitative ADC mapping is its susceptibility to dental amalgam artifacts, movement during swallowing, and tongue movements. This finding is especially true of sublingual and submandibular lesions. ADC values are also influenced by the chosen b-values used to acquire the diffusion sequence.[55] Therefore, interscanner and interinstitutional variation may limit the interpretability of results between major centers.

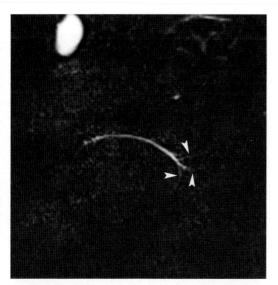

Fig. 5. MR sialography in a normal individual. A 20-mm-thick T2 turbo spin echo inversion recovery image of the right parotid duct in a normal individual. The entirety of Wharton's duct is well-visualized, and several first-order branches (*arrowheads*) can also be seen, although in this case, there is poor visualization of higher order ductal branches.

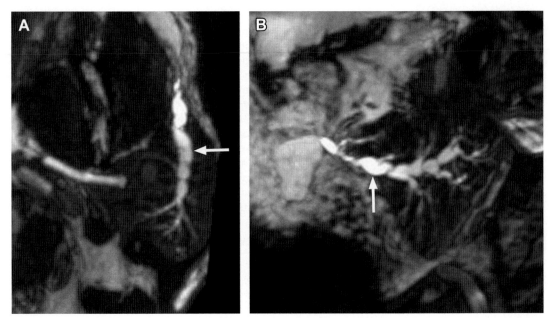

Fig. 6. MR sialography in a patient with chronic recurrent sialadenitis. (*A*) Axial and (*B*) sagittal oblique maximum intensity projection images from a 3-dimensional balanced steady-state free precession acquisition (constructive interference in steady state in this case) demonstrating an abnormal main parotid duct (*arrows*) with alternating areas of stricture and dilatation, along with dilated intraparotid ducts in a patient with chronic recurrent sialadenitis. The high resolution afforded by the sequence allows improved visualization of secondary and tertiary duct branches.

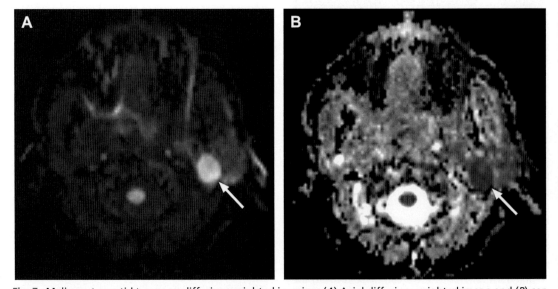

Fig. 7. Malignant parotid tumor on diffusion-weighted imaging. (*A*) Axial diffusion-weighted image and (*B*) corresponding apparent diffusion coefficient (ADC) map demonstrating diffusion restriction of a pathology proven acinic cell carcinoma of deep lobe of the left parotid (*arrows*). Diffusion-weighted imaging has been demonstrated to be helpful in differentiating pleomorphic adenomas from malignant tumors; however, some benign masses such as Warthin tumors may also demonstrate low ADC values.

Advanced MR Imaging Techniques

DWI with quantitative ADC has been shown to improve diagnostic accuracy when combined with perfusion MR imaging using a multiparametric approach to better differentiate benign and malignant salivary neoplasms.[53,56–60]

Perfusion MR imaging can be performed using dynamic contrast-enhanced MR imaging, a T1-weighted technique, or dynamic susceptibility contrast-enhanced MR imaging, a T2*-weighted technique. Dynamic contrast-enhanced MR imaging and dynamic susceptibility contrast MR imaging are similar in that they are modalities obtained before, during, and after a bolus of intravenous contrast and the imaging data is post processed to calculate a time signal intensity curve to evaluate tumor vascularity and hemodynamic kinetics. Imaging biomarkers such as blood flow, blood volume, mean transit time, and permeability surface area can be calculated and may be useful in distinguishing between malignant and benign etiologies. The advantages of these MR imaging perfusion techniques are that they may increase diagnostic accuracy; however, the disadvantages such as expense, need for time-consuming and computationally demanding post processing of data, and a lack of widespread experience limit incorporation into daily clinical practice.[61] Other advanced techniques such as intravoxel incoherent motion MR imaging are also being investigated and show promise in further characterization of malignant and benign salivary gland tumors; however, these modalities are beyond the scope of this paper.[56,62]

Another advanced MR imaging technique that has been investigated in head and neck imaging is proton MR spectroscopy. This technique allows for the measurement of metabolite concentrations in tissues of interest and can be used to evaluate for metabolic changes associated with malignancy. It has been suggested that these metabolic characteristics may be useful in predicting tumor malignancy and monitoring treatment response.[63] Specifically, elevation of choline to creatine ratios is consistently demonstrated in head and neck malignancies, such as squamous cell carcinoma and lymphoma. Unfortunately, some benign neoplasms, including neurogenic tumors and Warthin tumors, as well as inflammatory processes, can also demonstrate high choline levels. These overlapping metabolite characteristics between benign and malignant diseases on proton MR spectroscopy thus far limit its applicability in general clinical imaging.

Ultrasound Imaging

Ultrasound (US) imaging is the initial modality of choice in the evaluation of the pediatric patient owing to its favorable radiation safety profile,[64] and is also frequently used at some centers in adult patients. US imaging is a useful adjunctive diagnostic modality when used in combination with other modalities, and is an excellent tool for differentiating solid from cystic lesions and for characterizing lesion vascularity.[65–67] When indicated, US-guided fine needle aspiration can be helpful in guiding surgical management. US imaging of the salivary glands will not be discussed in further in this article because it is discussed in greater detail in this issue in a subsequent review.

SALIVARY ANATOMY ON CROSS-SECTIONAL IMAGING

Parotid Gland

The parotid gland is the largest salivary gland and is normally situated along the posterior angle of the mandible, anterior to the external auditory canal and mastoid process of the temporal bone. The parotid is palpable just below the subcutaneous fat, and the majority of the gland is superficial to the masseter muscle. The gland extends from the mastoid tip to the sternocleidomastoid muscle, just below the angle of the mandible. A small parotid tail projects off the inferior margin of the gland and is separated from the submandibular space by the stylomandibular ligament. Occasionally, a pedunculated lesion in the parotid tail can be confused with lymphadenopathy or other neck masses.[68]

The parotid gland is encased in a dense capsule formed from the superficial layer of deep cervical fascia, which splits into a thick superficial and thin deep layer to encase the gland. The superficial layer continues superiorly where it attaches to the root of the zygoma, whereas the deep layer extends to the styloid process and the stylomandibular ligament. The masticator space forms the anterior border of the gland and is often separated by a readily visible interposing fat plane.

In adults, the normal parotid gland demonstrates slight hypoattenuation on unenhanced CT scanning relative to muscle and higher attenuation than subcutaneous fat, primarily owing to the presence of adipose tissue interposed with glandular tissue. The parotid glands enhance avidly after contrast administration, and one may observe a lacelike network of interstitial tissues throughout the gland. Intravascular enhancement within the retromandibular vein and external carotid artery are seen on contrast-enhanced imaging. Gland density varies with patient age and tends to become less dense as the patient ages secondary to a slow increase in the relative proportion of intraglandular fat (**Fig. 8**). The normal range of

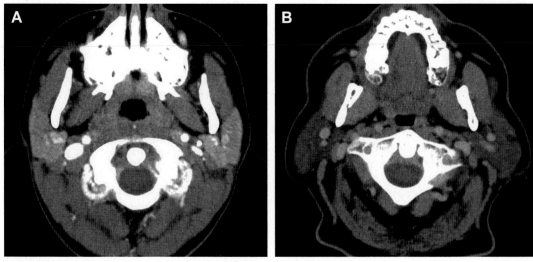

Fig. 8. Normal differences in the appearance of the parotid glands on computed tomography (CT) scanning with age. Axial contrast-enhanced CT images through the level of the parotid glands demonstrating the differences in attenuation of the gland between (*A*) a normal 15-year-old and (*B*) a normal 70-year-old. Note the global decrease in density with age owing to normal fatty replacement of glandular elements.

measured CT density ranges between 15 to 30 Hounsfield units in the adult population.[3,69] Pediatric patients have less glandular fat than adults and have a gland density that is usually isodense to muscle.[70] This factor has the potential to reduce the sensitivity for lesion detection by masking small intraglandular lesions and may necessitate the use of other modalities such as MR imaging or US examination. Elderly patients have a higher glandular fat resulting in s lower average glandular density.

On MR imaging, the normal adult parotid gland demonstrates slightly hyperintense T1- and T2-weighted signal compared with muscle, based primarily on the amount of intraglandular fat content (**Fig. 9**). The gland signal will be more hypointense on T1- and T2-weighted images in pediatric patients.[2,69,70]

The deep and superficial parotid lobes

Although there is not a true anatomic division within the parotid gland, the parotid gland is traditionally divided into superficial and deep lobes, which are demarcated by the plane of the facial nerve surgically. The superficial lobe corresponds with the portion of the gland that is palpable by surgeons and accounts for roughly 80% of the total gland volume, whereas the deep lobe makes up a very small portion of the gland and is not generally evaluable clinically.

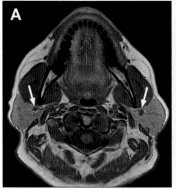
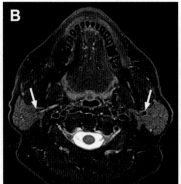
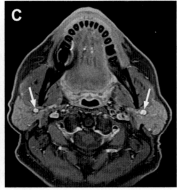

Fig. 9. Normal parotid MR image. (*A*) An axial T1-weighted, (*B*) an axial fat-suppressed T2-weighted image, and (*C*) an axial fat-suppressed, postcontrast T1-weighted image demonstrate the signal characteristics of normal parotid glands, which are typically slightly hyperintense relative to muscle. The *arrows* indicate the retromandibular veins.

Determining whether a lesion originates in the deep or superficial lobe has practical significance in surgical planning, because lesions in the superficial compartment can be treated with partial parotidectomy, whereas lesions in the deep compartment most often require total parotidectomy.

The deep lobe of the parotid gland extends medially, posterior to the mandible through the stylomandibular tunnel into the prestyloid parapharyngeal space (**Fig. 10**). The stylomandibular tunnel represents the space located between the ascending mandibular ramus, the styloid process, and the stylomandibular ligament. Because the capsule along the deep margin of the parotid is thinner and occasionally deficient, parotid tissue or masses arising in the deep lobe of the parotid can herniate through a defect in the cervical fascia, separating it from the parapharyngeal space and can present as a parapharyngeal mass. In these instances, the fat of the parapharyngeal space will typically be displaced anteromedially. Additionally, deep parotid lesions can grow asymptomatically and may develop a characteristic "dumbbell" appearance if they extend toward the superficial aspect of the gland through the stylomandibular tunnel[4] (**Fig. 11**). Lesions in the deep prestyloid parapharyngeal space also characteristically deviate the carotid sheath posterolaterally when they become large.

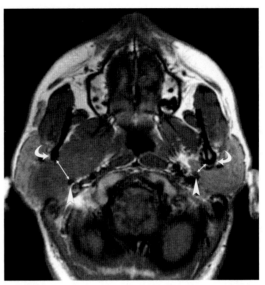

Fig. 11. Typical parotid dumbbell lesion. Axial T1-weighted image demonstrating a large left parotid mass growing through and widening the stylomandibular tunnel. Masses passing through the tunnel frequently take on a "dumbbell" appearance with a waist where the lesion passes through stylomandibular tunnel. The stylomandibular tunnels are indicated by the *double-sided arrows* bilaterally, and the mandibular rami are indicated by the *curved arrows* and the styloid processes by the *arrowheads*.

The parotid tail

The most inferior portion of the superficial parotid lobe is frequently referred to as the parotid tail. Many surgeons consider the parotid tail to include the retromandibular portion of the parotid gland situated inferior to the main trunk of the facial nerve. An accepted imaging landmark to demarcate the upper boundary of the parotid tail is not described, however, so some authors have defined the tail as representing the inferior 2.0 cm of the superficial lobe.[68]

On axial images, the parotid tail is identifiable as a triangular-shaped region of the parotid gland deep to the platysma muscle, posterolateral to the posterior belly of the digastric, and anterolateral to the sternocleidomastoid muscle (**Fig. 12**). Lesions arising from the parotid tail, particularly those that are pedunculated, can be mistaken for an enlarged jugulodigastric lymph node and vice versa. In these situations, scrutinizing coronal images usually helps to clarify the origin of a mass in the region. Common benign lesions arising from the parotid tail include a pleomorphic adenoma (see **Fig. 12**), Warthin tumor (**Fig. 13**), reactive intraparotid lymph nodes, and vascular malformations, whereas non-Hodgkin lymphoma, metastatic disease, and primary salivary gland

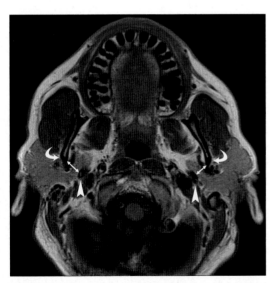

Fig. 10. Location of the stylomandibular tunnel. Axial T1-weighted image demonstrating the location of the stylomandibular tunnels (*double-sided arrows*), which are bordered anterolaterally by the posterior cortices of the mandibular rami (*curved arrows*) and posteromedially by the styloid processes (*arrowheads*).

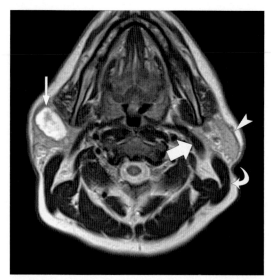

Fig. 12. Parotid tail lesion on MR imaging. Axial T2-weighted image demonstrating the normal parotid tail on the left side as the triangular shaped space deep to the platysma (*arrowhead*), posterolateral to the posterior belly of the digastric muscle (*thick arrow*), and anterolateral to the sternocleidomastoid muscle (*curved arrow*). On the right side there is a large, T2-hyperintense mass (*thin arrow*) in the parotid tail that was biopsy proven to be a pleomorphic adenoma.

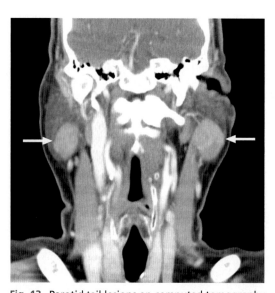

Fig. 13. Parotid tail lesions on computed tomography (CT) scan. Coronal contrast-enhanced CT image demonstrating bilateral pedunculated enhancing parotid tail masses that were biopsy proven to be Warthin tumors (*arrows*). The coronal image nicely demonstrates how the inferior location of these pedunculated lesions may be confused with jugulodigastric adenopathy.

malignancies are the most common malignant lesions to arise there.[68]

Stensen's duct

Saliva produced by the parotid gland empties into the main parotid duct (Stensen's duct), which originates along the anterior aspect of the gland and runs anteriorly, superficial to the masseter muscle. After passing anterior to the masseter muscle, the duct turns medially to penetrate the buccinator muscle at the level of the second maxillary molar, where it empties into the oral cavity. Most symptomatic parotid stones occur in Stensen's duct (**Fig. 14**).

The facial nerve

The facial nerve is a vital structure to identify for the surgeon, because injury to the nerve during surgery can lead to facial paralysis, resulting in significant functional and cosmetic complications for the patient. However, because the nerve is not reliably seen on conventional imaging unless involved by perineural tumor spread (**Fig. 15**), surrogate landmarks are typically used to infer the location of the nerve. Because a large portion of the intraparotid course of the facial nerve is adjacent to the retromandibular vein, this structure is often used to ascertain the location of the facial nerve, although there is some variability with surgical concordance.[71,72] One of the most common imaging surrogates used to estimate the course of the facial nerve is the plane containing the retromandibular vein and stylomastoid foramen (**Fig. 16**). This plane can then be used to separate deep and superficial parotid lobes.[1,4,69] Additional methods exist to predict the location of the nerve, such as Utrecht's line, Conn's arc, and the facial nerve line, and these techniques have been studied with variable success and reliability, but are outside the scope of this review.[73] Other conventions in which the mandible is used as the reference point are also frequently used, with parotid tissue external to the mandible being referred to superficial and tissue deep to the mandible being referred to as retromandibular or deep parotid tissue.[1,2,4,74]

In reality, the course of the facial nerve is complex. The nerve exits the mastoid portion of the temporal bone at the stylomastoid foramen lateral to the styloid process and superficial to the posterior belly of the digastric muscle. The nerve then enters the posterior aspect of the parotid gland and travels within the gland along the superficial aspect of the retromandibular vein before splitting into upper (temporofacial) and lower (cervicofacial) branches. The branching pattern is variable, but the nerve usually ends in 5 terminal branches:

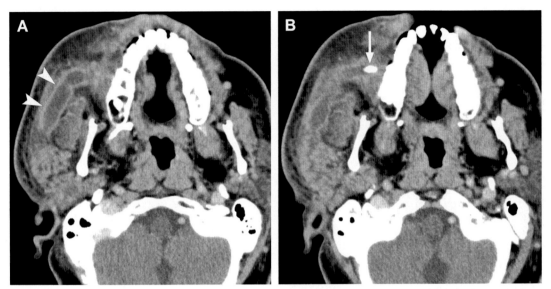

Fig. 14. Normal course of Stenson duct. (*A, B*) Axial contrast-enhanced computed tomography images in a patient with a large obstructing sialolith (*arrow in B*) nicely demonstrate the course of the main parotid duct, also known as Stenson's duct (*arrowheads*), which is markedly dilated in this case. The duct normally courses anteriorly, superficial to the masseter muscle, before turning medially to empty into the oral cavity via a papilla located at the level of the second maxillary muscle.

the temporal, zygomatic, buccal, marginal mandibular, and cervical branches.[4,75]

Although the true intraparotid course of the facial nerve has traditionally been considered difficult or impossible to visualize using conventional imaging methods, several investigators have reported success in localizing the nerve with newer MR imaging techniques. Li and colleagues[76] were able to identify the main facial nerve trunk in 93.5% of patients and the upper and lower divisions of the facial nerve

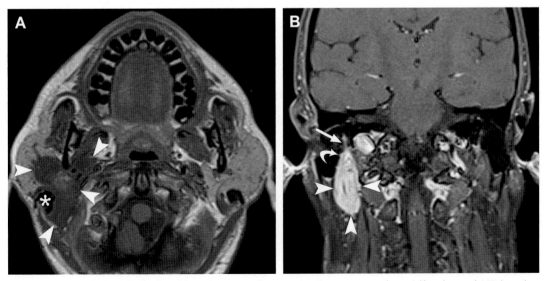

Fig. 15. Perineural spread of adenoid cystic cancer demonstrated on contrast (*asterisk*) enhanced MR imaging. (*A*) Axial T1 precontrast and (*B*) coronal fat-suppressed, postcontrast images demonstrate infiltrative mass of the right parotid gland (*arrowheads*), which is hypointense compared with normal parotid tissue (compare with the gland on the *left*) and enhances homogeneously. On the coronal image (*B*), the tumor invades the right stylomastoid foramen (*curved arrow*) and is spreading along the mastoid segment of the right facial nerve, which is thickened and asymmetrically enhancing (*arrow*).

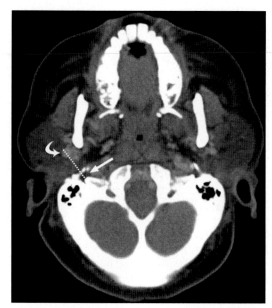

Fig. 16. Estimation of the facial nerve plane. Although the facial nerve cannot be visualized directly in most cases, its intraparotid course can be inferred to lie in the plane (indicated by the *dotted line*) containing the retromandibular vein (*curved arrow*) and the stylomastoid foramen (*arrow*). This plane can be used to divide the parotid gland into superficial and deep portions, with the superficial portion lying lateral to the plane.

in 83.9% of patients with benign parotid tumors using a 3D fast imaging employing steady-state acquisition sequence. In their study, the facial nerve was visible as a low signal intensity structure within the gland, which could be traced back to the stylomastoid foramen. In a more recent study,

Attye and colleagues[77] demonstrated the feasibility of using diffusion tensor imaging–based MR tractography to visualize the main facial nerve trunk and the upper and lower divisions in patients with surgically resected parotid tumors, with tractography being able to identify the main facial nerve trunk and the upper and lower divisions with 100% sensitivity.

The auriculotemporal nerve

There is another important nerve running through the parotid gland that connects the facial nerve to the mandibular (CNV3) branch of the trigeminal nerve called the auriculotemporal nerve. The auriculotemporal nerve is a small branch of CNV3 that runs parallel to the superficial temporal artery and vein and extends posteriorly around the mandibular condyle and laterally toward the periauricular area, carrying postganglionic parasympathetic innervation from the otic ganglion to the parotid gland. When this nerve is injured during surgery, the autonomic innervation to the parotid gland can be interrupted. In some cases, inappropriate neural regeneration produces aberrant innervation of the skin, resulting in the phenomenon of gustatory sweating (Frey's syndrome).[2–5] In patients with parotid tumors, the auriculotemporal nerve is also important because peritumoral spread of malignancy originating in the parotid gland can propagate from the facial nerve to the auriculotemporal nerve to CNV3 and then travel intracranially through foramen ovale[3–5] (**Fig. 17**).

Intraparotid lymph nodes

As mentioned, the parotid gland is the only salivary gland to contain lymphoid tissue. The

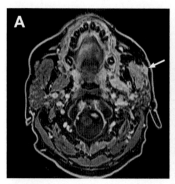
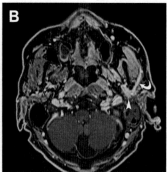
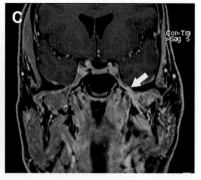

Fig. 17. Perineural spread of tumor along the auriculotemporal nerve. Axial (*A, B*) and coronal (*C*) fat-suppressed contrast-enhanced T1-weighted images demonstrate a small enhancing tumor in the anterior portion of the parotid gland (*thin arrow* in *A*) with evidence of perineural spread extending along a buccal branch of the facial nerve (*curved arrow* in *B*) to involve the auriculotemporal nerve (*arrowhead* in *B*). The auriculotemporal nerve normally courses around the posterior aspect of the mandibular condyle to join with cranial nerve V3. On the coronal image, there is thickening and enhancement of V3 indicating further perineural spread with extension through foramen ovale (*thick arrow*).

intraparotid nodes are a drainage site for the skin of the scalp and are a common site of metastasis from temporal or auricular skin cancers, which can present as a parotid mass. The morphologic features of a normal lymph node such as reniform shape and fatty hilum can help to distinguish a normal lymph node from pathologic parotid adenopathy or a primary parotid mass.

Blood supply to the parotid gland

The external carotid artery enters the inferior aspect of the parotid gland and courses superiorly in the deep aspect of the parotid, typically along the posterior aspect of the mandible. The external carotid artery forms 2 terminal branches in the parotid space, the maxillary artery and the superficial temporal artery. Blood supply to the parotid gland is derived from the transverse facial artery, which is a branch of the superficial temporal artery before it exits the superficial gland.[2–4]

Normal anatomic variants

Approximately 20% of individuals have accessory parotid tissue along the anterior masseter muscle[1] (Fig. 18). Normal accessory tissue can occasionally be confused with a mass, especially because normal parotid gland tissue has some PET avidity;

however, it may also rarely be subject to any pathology that can affect the parotid gland, including neoplasms.[1,4] Accessory parotid tissue should follow the signal of the normal parotid glands on all pulse sequences. Other anatomic variants include unilateral or bilateral parotid aplasia, parotid duct duplication, as well as parotid duct fistulas that can be associated with branchial cleft anomalies.[9,12,78–81]

Submandibular Gland

The second largest major salivary gland is the submandibular gland, which is normally about one-half the weight of the parotid gland. The submandibular gland is located inferior to the mandible between the anterior and posterior bellies of the digastric muscle and along the inferior surface of the mylohyoid muscle. Posteriorly, the submandibular gland is separated from the parotid gland by the stylomandibular ligament. The posterior aspect of the submandibular gland forms a C-shaped structure around the dorsal free margin of the mylohyoid muscle, which divides the submandibular gland into superficial and deep lobes. The posterior submandibular space also communicates freely with the sublingual space and the inferior parapharyngeal space, which can allow for the spread of infection or malignancy between these spaces.[2,74]

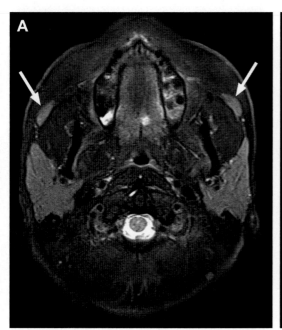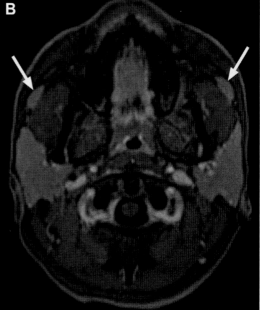

Fig. 18. Accessory parotid tissue. (A) Axial fat-suppressed T2-weighted image and (B) axial fat-suppressed, contrast-enhanced T1-weighted image demonstrating bilateral accessory parotid tissue (arrows), in a typical location superficial to the masseter muscles and ventral to the normal parotid glands. Note how the signal intensity of the accessory tissue is identical to that of the parotid glands on both sequences.

The submandibular gland is encapsulated and covered by the superficial layer of the deep cervical fascia.[2,74]

The submandibular gland is more homogenous in appearance than the parotid gland, with less fatty parenchyma, making it slightly greater in density than the parotid but still slightly less dense than muscle (approximately 25–40 Hounsfield units) on unenhanced CT images. The submandibular glands enhance avidly after contrast administration (**Fig. 19**). On MR imaging, the submandibular gland is slightly T1 hypointense, and slightly T2 hyperintense compared with the parotid gland.[82–84] The normal submandibular glands should be bilaterally symmetric in size, density, and enhancement.

Wharton's duct

The submandibular duct (Wharton's duct) drains the submandibular gland, exiting the medial surface of the gland in the posterior sublingual space and running below the floor of the mouth between the mylohyoid (lateral) and the hyoglossus (medial) muscles, before emptying into the anterior floor of

mouth beneath the tongue at the sublingual caruncle, located just lateral to the lingual frenulum (**Fig. 20**). The lumen of Wharton's duct is larger than the papilla, and it is common for a sialolith to develop within the duct and to be too large to exit the duct.[1,2] Occasionally, mucoid secretions can be identified in the hilum of the gland and submandibular duct, and if seen should not raise concern for obstruction unless other findings to suggest obstruction are present.[2]

Blood supply and innervation

The facial artery courses along the posterolateral aspect of the submandibular gland between the gland and the mandible, before making a superior turn around the mandibular body. The submandibular gland is usually supplied by the submental branch of the facial artery or branches of the external maxillary artery. Venous drainage is provided by the anterior facial vein, which courses along the superficial margin of the gland, and is a useful landmark to determine if a mass arises within or adjacent to the submandibular gland.[84] The submandibular vein may be interposed between a lesion that arises outside the gland, but a lesion arising from the submandibular gland should not be separated from the gland by the vein[1,9,72] (**Fig. 21**).

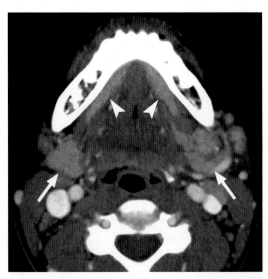

Fig. 19. Normal appearance of the submandibular and sublingual glands on computed tomography (CT) scanning. Axial contrast-enhanced CT image demonstrating the normal location and appearance of the submandibular glands (*arrows*) and sublingual glands (*arrowheads*). The submandibular glands are located inferior to the mandible between the anterior and posterior bellies of the digastric muscle and along the inferior surface of the mylohyoid muscle. The sublingual glands lie along the floor of mouth between the mandible, mylohyoid muscle, and the muscles of the root of the tongue (genioglossus and geniohyoid muscles). Both glands normally enhance avidly after contrast administration.

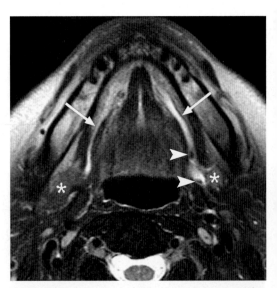

Fig. 20. Normal course of Wharton's ducts. Axial fat-suppressed T2-weighted image through the sublingual region demonstrates the course of Wharton's ducts (*arrows*), which pass anteriomedially through the sublingual space, medial to the myelohyoid muscles and sublingual glands, and lateral to the hyoglossus muscles. In this patient, there are hypointense stones (*arrowheads*) in the duct on the left, which is mildly dilated. The asterisks mark the submandibular glands.

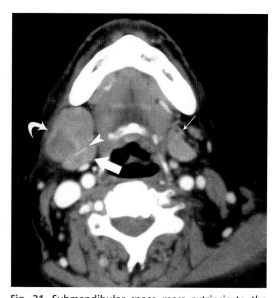

Fig. 21. Submandibular space mass extrinsic to the submandibular gland. Axial (*A*) contrast-enhanced computed tomography (CT) image of the neck demonstrate an enlarged lymph node (*curved arrow*) in the right submandibular space abutting the submandibular gland (*thick arrow*). In some cases, it can be difficult to determine whether the lesion arises within or is separate from the gland. However, in this case, the observation that the anterior facial vein (*arrowhead*) courses between the gland and the lesion suggests that the lesion is extraglandular in origin. A branch of the normal anterior facial vein on the left is indicated by the *small arrow*.

The lingual nerve and submandibular ganglion are located along the lateral margin of the gland. The lingual nerve wraps around Wharton's duct, starting lateral and ending medial to the duct.[1,3] Deep to the submandibular gland are the hypoglossal nerve and vein.[1,74] Postganglionic parasympathetic innervation to the submandibular gland is primarily from the submandibular ganglion, which lies along the lateral aspect of the gland adjacent to the lingual nerve. Sympathetic innervation is from the superior cervical ganglion.[5]

Normal anatomic variants

Accessory submandibular glands have been described, but are rare and can be seen either anterior or posterior to the normal gland. Submandibular duct duplication and gland aplasia have also been described[82,85] (**Fig. 22**). Another rare anatomic variant is intraosseous extension of the submandibular tissue into the medial mandibular body known as a Stafne defect or Stafne cyst.[86]

Sublingual Gland

The sublingual gland is the smallest of the major salivary glands and measures slightly more than 1 cm in adults. The sublingual gland lies along the floor of mouth between the mandible, mylohyoid muscle, and the muscles of the root of the tongue (genioglossus and geniohyoid muscles). The anatomic relationship of sublingual and submandibular lesions to critical floor of the mouth

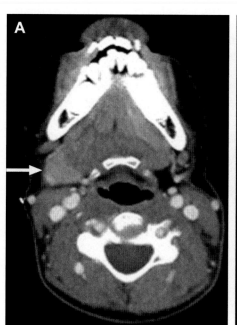
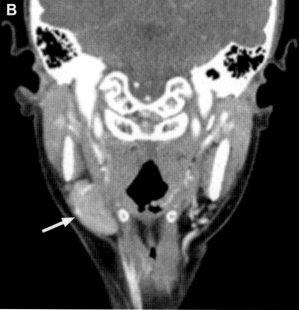

Fig. 22. Submandibular gland aplasia. Contrast-enhanced axial (*A*) and coronal (*B*) computed tomography images demonstrate normal right submandibular gland (*arrow*) and congenital absence of the left submandibular gland.

structures such as the mylohyoid muscle sling is usually nicely depicted in the coronal plane on both CT scanning and MR imaging. The superior contrast resolution of MR imaging can be particularly useful when staging oral cavity malignancies that involve the floor of the mouth and offsets its generally lower spatial resolution compared with CT scanning.

The sublingual gland is more homogenous in appearance than the parotid gland, with less fatty parenchyma, similar in appearance to the submandibular gland. The sublingual gland is slightly greater in density than the parotid on unenhanced CT scanning, is slightly less dense than muscle (approximately 25–40 Hounsfield units), and enhances avidly after contrast administration (see **Fig. 19**). Like the submandibular gland, the sublingual gland is slightly T1 hypointense and slightly T2 hyperintense relative to the parotid gland.[1,2,83] Compared with muscle, the sublingual gland is usually hyperintense on both T1- and T2-weighted sequences and enhances homogeneously (**Fig. 23**).

Sublingual drainage

The sublingual gland does not have a true fascial capsule and lacks a dominant duct, being drained instead by multiple small ducts called the ducts of Rivinus. Some anatomic variation exists, however, and occasionally multiple sublingual ducts may merge to form into the common Bartholin duct, which usually empties into the main submandibular duct.[1,3]

The submandibular duct and lingual nerve pass between the sublingual gland and the genioglossus muscle.[2,74] The sublingual space also contains the lingual artery, and the glossopharyngeal and hypoglossal nerves.[2,74]

Blood supply and innervation of the sublingual gland

Postganglionic parasympathetic innervation to the sublingual gland is from the submandibular ganglion, which lies along the lateral aspect of the gland adjacent to the lingual nerve. Sympathetic innervation is from the superior cervical ganglion.[5,8] Blood supply to the sublingual gland is from the sublingual branch of the nearby lingual artery, and venous drainage is through the submental branch of the facial vein.

Normal anatomic variants

A defect in the anterior mylohyoid muscle can allow the sublingual gland or fat to herniate from the sublingual space into the submandibular space resulting in the boutonnière deformity, which can occasionally be confused with a mass on imaging or physical examination[87] (**Fig. 24**). Sublingual gland aplasia has been described, but is rare.[3,6]

Minor Salivary Glands

There are more than 1000 minor salivary glands throughout the aerodigestive tract, with the majority concentrated in the buccal, labial, palatal, and lingual regions. The minor salivary glands are simple exocrine glands that lack draining ducts, and each minor gland has its own simple duct. These glands are not typically seen on imaging studies; however, salivary tumors can arise anywhere these glands are located. Neoplasms of the minor salivary glands are statistically more likely to be malignant than those of the major salivary glands. The autonomic secretory innervation of the minor salivary glands is provided by the sphenopalatine ganglion, otic ganglion, submandibular ganglion, and by the pharyngeal plexus, depending on their location as well as from the superior cervical ganglion.

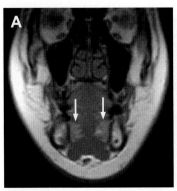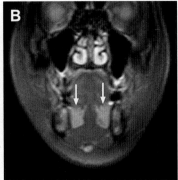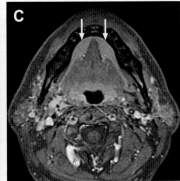

Fig. 23. Normal sublingual gland on MR imaging. Coronal T1-weighted image (*A*), coronal fat-suppressed T2-weighted image (*B*), and contrast-enhanced axial fat-suppressed T1-weighted image (*C*) demonstrating the normal appearance of the sublingual glands (*arrows*), which are hyperintense to muscle on T1- and T2-weighted imaging and enhance homogeneously with contrast.

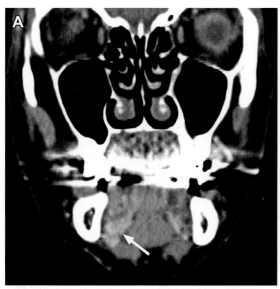
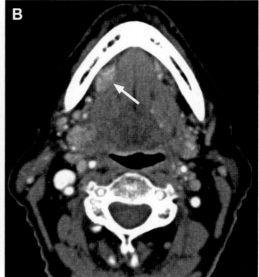

Fig. 24. Boutonniere defect. (*A*) Coronal and (*B*) axial contrast enhanced computed tomography images demonstrate a boutonnière deformity of the right sublingual gland (*arrows*), which represents herniation of the sublingual gland through a defect in the myelohyoid muscle into the submandibular space. This normal variant can occasionally be confused for a mass.

SUMMARY

Cross-sectional imaging with CT scanning and MR imaging are the preferred salivary gland imaging modalities and are often complimentary in evaluation of the salivary glands. These modalities are clinically useful because they can accurately define normal anatomy, delineate the extent of disease, confirm a lesion as being of salivary gland origin, help to narrow the list of differential considerations, and are essential in guiding workup and management, as well as aiding in biopsy and surgical planning. In general, acute inflammatory conditions and suspected sialolithiasis can be adequately characterized with contrast-enhanced CT scans, whereas MR sialography may be useful in evaluation of chronic inflammatory conditions affecting the salivary ducts. MR imaging is the imaging modality of choice for evaluating salivary neoplasms, particularly in instances in which there is suspected extraglandular and perineural spread. Furthermore, adjuvant techniques, including DWI and perfusion imaging, either alone or in combination, may be helpful for differentiating malignant and benign tumors.

REFERENCES

1. Abdullah A, Rivas FF, Srinivasan A. Imaging of the salivary glands. Semin Roentgenol 2013;48(1): 65–74.
2. Som P, Brandwein-Gensler M. Anatomy and pathology of the salivary glands. In: Som PM, Curtin H, editors. Head and Neck Imaging, Volume 2. 5th edition. Missouri: Mosby; 2011. p. 2449–610.
3. Holmberg KV, Hoffman MP. Anatomy, biogenesis and regeneration of salivary glands. Monogr Oral Sci 2014;24:1–13.
4. Kochhar A, Larian B, Azizzadeh B. Facial nerve and parotid gland anatomy. Otolaryngol Clin North Am 2016;49(2):273–84.
5. Proctor GB, Carpenter GH. Regulation of salivary gland function by autonomic nerves. Auton Neurosci 2007;133(1):3–18.
6. Knosp WM, Knox SM, Hoffman MP. Salivary gland organogenesis. Wiley Interdiscip Rev Dev Biol 2012;1(1):69–82.
7. Patel VN, Rebustini IT, Hoffman MP. Salivary gland branching morphogenesis. Differentiation 2006; 74(7):349–64.
8. Tucker AS. Salivary gland development. Semin Cell Dev Biol 2007;18(2):237–44.
9. Almadori G, Ottaviani F, Del Ninno M, et al. Monolateral aplasia of the parotid gland. Ann Otol Rhinol Laryngol 1997;106(6):522–5.
10. Beleza-Meireles A, Clayton-Smith J, Saraiva JM, et al. Oculo-auriculo-vertebral spectrum: a review of the literature and genetic update. J Med Genet 2014;51(10):635–45.
11. Taybi H, Lachman R. Taybi and Lachman's radiology of syndromes, metabolic disorders and skeletal dysplasias. 5th edition. St Louis: Mosby; 2006.
12. Villanueva O, Atkinson DS, Lambert SR. Trigeminal nerve hypoplasia and aplasia in children with Goldenhar syndrome and corneal hypoesthesia. J AAPOS 2005;9(2):202–4.

13. Kane WJ, McCaffrey TV, Olsen KD, et al. Primary parotid malignancies. A clinical and pathologic review. Arch Otolaryngol Head Neck Surg 1991;117(3): 307–15.

14. Marchal F, Dulguerov P. Sialolithiasis management: the state of the art. Arch Otolaryngol Head Neck Surg 2003;129(9):951–6.

15. Ugga L, Ravanelli M, Pallottino AA, et al. Diagnostic work-up in obstructive and inflammatory salivary gland disorders. Acta Otorhinolaryngol Ital 2017; 37(2):83–93.

16. American College of Radiology, Task Force on Appropriateness Criteria. Appropriateness criteria for neck mass/adenopathy. Reston (VA): American College of Radiology; 2009.

17. Stolzmann P, Winklhofer S, Schwendener N, et al. Monoenergetic computed tomography reconstructions reduce beam hardening artifacts from dental restorations. Forensic Sci Med Pathol 2013;9(3):327–32.

18. Johnson TR. Dual-energy CT: general principles. AJR Am J Roentgenol 2012;199(5 Suppl):S3–8.

19. Kuchenbecker S, Faby S, Sawall S, et al. Dual energy CT: how well can pseudo-monochromatic imaging reduce metal artifacts? Med Phys 2015; 42(2):1023–36.

20. Tanaka R, Hayashi T, Ike M, et al. Reduction of dark-band-like metal artifacts caused by dental implant bodies using hypothetical monoenergetic imaging after dual-energy computed tomography. Oral Surg Oral Med Oral Pathol Oral Radiol 2013;115(6): 833–8.

21. American College of Radiology, American Society of Neuroradiology, Society for Pediatric Radiology. ACR-ASNR-SPR practice parameter for the performance of computed tomography (CT) of the extracranial head and neck. Reston (VA): American College of Radiology; 2017.

22. Purohit BS, Ailianou A, Dulguerov N, et al. FDG-PET/CT pitfalls in oncological head and neck imaging. Insights Imaging 2014;5(5):585–602.

23. Roh JL, Ryu CH, Choi SH, et al. Clinical utility of 18F-FDG PET for patients with salivary gland malignancies. J Nucl Med 2007;48(2):240–6.

24. Blodgett TM, Fukui MB, Snyderman CH, et al. Combined PET-CT in the head and neck: part 1. Physiologic, altered physiologic, and artifactual FDG uptake. Radiographics 2005;25(4):897–912.

25. Basu S, Houseni M, Alavi A. Significance of incidental fluorodeoxyglucose uptake in the parotid glands and its impact on patient management. Nucl Med Commun 2008;29(4):367–73.

26. Razek AA, Tawfik AM, Elsorogy LG, et al. Perfusion CT of head and neck cancer. Eur J Radiol 2014; 83(3):537–44.

27. Lomas DJ, Carroll NR, Johnson G, et al. MR sialography. Work in progress. Radiology 1996;200(1): 129–33.

28. Gadodia A, Bhalla AS, Sharma R, et al. MR sialography of iatrogenic sialocele: comparison with conventional sialography. Dentomaxillofac Radiol 2011; 40(3):147–53.

29. Gadodia A, Seith A, Sharma R, et al. MRI and MR sialography of juvenile recurrent parotitis. Pediatr Radiol 2010;40(8):1405–10.

30. Capaccio P, Canzi P, Gaffuri M, et al. Modern management of paediatric obstructive salivary disorders: long-term clinical experience. Acta Otorhinolaryngol Ital 2017;37(2):160–7.

31. Izumi M, Eguchi K, Ohki M, et al. MR imaging of the parotid gland in Sjogren's syndrome: a proposal for new diagnostic criteria. AJR Am J Roentgenol 1996; 166(6):1483–7.

32. Capaccio P, Cuccarini V, Ottaviani F, et al. Comparative ultrasonographic, magnetic resonance sialographic, and videoendoscopic assessment of salivary duct disorders. Ann Otol Rhinol Laryngol 2008;117(4):245–52.

33. Capaccio P, Paglia M, Minorati D, et al. Diagnosis and therapeutic management of iatrogenic parotid sialocele. Ann Otol Rhinol Laryngol 2004;113(7): 562–4.

34. Gadodia A, Seith A, Sharma R, et al. Magnetic resonance sialography using CISS and HASTE sequences in inflammatory salivary gland diseases: comparison with digital sialography. Acta Radiol 2010;51(2):156–63.

35. Kalinowski M, Heverhagen JT, Rehberg E, et al. Comparative study of MR sialography and digital subtraction sialography for benign salivary gland disorders. AJNR Am J Neuroradiol 2002;23(9): 1485–92.

36. Hugill J, Sala E, Hollingsworth KG, et al. MR sialography: the effect of a sialogogue and ductal occlusion in volunteers. Br J Radiol 2008;81(967): 583–6.

37. Karaca Erdogan N, Altay C, Ozenler N, et al. Magnetic resonance sialography findings of submandibular ducts imaging. Biomed Res Int 2013;2013: 417052.

38. Jager L, Menauer F, Holzknecht N, et al. Sialolithiasis: MR sialography of the submandibular duct–an alternative to conventional sialography and US? Radiology 2000;216(3):665–71.

39. Becker M, Marchal F, Becker CD, et al. Sialolithiasis and salivary ductal stenosis: diagnostic accuracy of MR sialography with a three-dimensional extended-phase conjugate-symmetry rapid spin-echo sequence. Radiology 2000;217(2):347–58.

40. Morimoto Y, Tanaka T, Kito S, et al. Utility of three dimension fast asymmetric spin-echo (3D-FASE) sequences in MR sialographic sequences: model and volunteer studies. Oral Dis 2005;11(1):35–43.

41. Murakami R, Baba Y, Nishimura R, et al. MR sialography using half-Fourier acquisition single-shot

turbo spin-echo (HASTE) sequences. AJNR Am J Neuroradiol 1998;19(5):959–61.

42. Niemela RK, Paakko E, Suramo I, et al. Magnetic resonance imaging and magnetic resonance sialography of parotid glands in primary Sjogren's syndrome. Arthritis Rheum 2001;45(6):512–8.

43. Ren YD, Li XR, Zhang J, et al. Conventional MRI techniques combined with MR sialography on T2-3D-DRIVE in Sjogren syndrome. Int J Clin Exp Med 2015;8(3):3974–82.

44. Tanaka T, Ono K, Ansai T, et al. Dynamic magnetic resonance sialography for patients with xerostomia. Oral Surg Oral Med Oral Pathol Oral Radiol Endod 2008;106(1):115–23.

45. Eida S, Sumi M, Sakihama N, et al. Apparent diffusion coefficient mapping of salivary gland tumors: prediction of the benignancy and malignancy. AJNR Am J Neuroradiol 2007;28(1):116–21.

46. Jungehulsing M, Fischbach R, Schroder U, et al. Magnetic resonance sialography. Otolaryngol Head Neck Surg 1999;121(4):488–94.

47. Milad P, Elbegiermy M, Shokry T, et al. The added value of pretreatment DW MRI in characterization of salivary glands pathologies. Am J Otolaryngol 2017;38(1):13–20.

48. Motoori K, Iida Y, Nagai Y, et al. MR imaging of salivary duct carcinoma. AJNR Am J Neuroradiol 2005; 26(5):1201–6.

49. Schlakman BN, Yousem DM. MR of intraparotid masses. AJNR Am J Neuroradiol 1993;14(5): 1173–80.

50. Sharafuddin MJ, Diemer DP, Levine RS, et al. A comparison of MR sequences for lesions of the parotid gland. AJNR Am J Neuroradiol 1995;16(9): 1895–902.

51. Takashima S, Sone S, Takayama F, et al. Assessment of parotid masses: which MR pulse sequences are optimal? Eur J Radiol 1997;24(3):206–15.

52. Thoeny HC, De Keyzer F. Extracranial applications of diffusion-weighted magnetic resonance imaging. Eur Radiol 2007;17(6):1385–93.

53. Celebi I, Mahmutoglu AS, Ucgul A, et al. Quantitative diffusion-weighted magnetic resonance imaging in the evaluation of parotid gland masses: a study with histopathological correlation. Clin Imaging 2013;37(2):232–8.

54. Habermann CR, Gossrau P, Graessner J, et al. Diffusion-weighted echo-planar MRI: a valuable tool for differentiating primary parotid gland tumors? Rofo 2005;177(7):940–5.

55. Kitamoto E, Chikui T, Kawano S, et al. The application of dynamic contrast-enhanced MRI and diffusion-weighted MRI in patients with maxillofacial tumors. Acad Radiol 2015;22(2):210–6.

56. Sumi M, Van Cauteren M, Sumi T, et al. Salivary gland tumors: use of intravoxel incoherent motion MR imaging for assessment of diffusion and perfusion for the differentiation of benign from malignant tumors. Radiology 2012;263(3):770–7.

57. Eida S, Sumi M, Nakamura T. Multiparametric magnetic resonance imaging for the differentiation between benign and malignant salivary gland tumors. J Magn Reson Imaging 2010;31(3):673–9.

58. Sumi M, Nakamura T. Extranodal spread in the neck: MRI detection on the basis of pixel-based time-signal intensity curve analysis. J Magn Reson Imaging 2011;33(4):830–8.

59. Abdel Razek AA, Samir S, Ashmalla GA. Characterization of parotid tumors with dynamic susceptibility contrast perfusion-weighted magnetic resonance imaging and diffusion-weighted MR imaging. J Comput Assist Tomogr 2017;41(1):131–6.

60. Yabuuchi H, Matsuo Y, Kamitani T, et al. Parotid gland tumors: can addition of diffusion-weighted MR imaging to dynamic contrast-enhanced MR imaging improve diagnostic accuracy in characterization? Radiology 2008;249(3):909–16.

61. Attye A, Tropres I, Rouchy RC, et al. Diffusion MRI: literature review in salivary gland tumors. Oral Dis 2017;23(5):572–5.

62. Iima M, Le Bihan D. Clinical intravoxel incoherent motion and diffusion MR imaging: past, present, and future. Radiology 2016;278(1):13–32.

63. Abdel Razek AA, Poptani H. MR spectroscopy of head and neck cancer. Eur J Radiol 2013;82(6): 982–9.

64. Tanaka T, Morimoto Y, Takano H, et al. Three-dimensional identification of hemangiomas and feeding arteries in the head and neck region using combined phase-contrast MR angiography and fast asymmetric spin-echo sequences. Oral Surg Oral Med Oral Pathol Oral Radiol Endod 2005;100(5):609–13.

65. Bialek EJ, Jakubowski W, Zajkowski P, et al. US of the major salivary glands: anatomy and spatial relationships, pathologic conditions, and pitfalls. Radiographics 2006;26(3):745–63.

66. Scholbach T, Scholbach J, Krombach GA, et al. New method of dynamic color doppler signal quantification in metastatic lymph nodes compared to direct polarographic measurements of tissue oxygenation. Int J Cancer 2005;114(6):957–62.

67. Zengel P, Schrotzlmair F, Reichel C, et al. Sonography: the leading diagnostic tool for diseases of the salivary glands. Semin Ultrasound CT MR 2013; 34(3):196–203.

68. Hamilton BE, Salzman KL, Wiggins RH 3rd, et al. Earring lesions of the parotid tail. AJNR Am J Neuroradiol 2003;24(9):1757–64.

69. Prasad RS. Parotid gland imaging. Otolaryngol Clin North Am 2016;49(2):285–312.

70. Lowe LH, Stokes LS, Johnson JE, et al. Swelling at the angle of the mandible: imaging of the pediatric parotid gland and periparotid region. Radiographics 2001;21(5):1211–27.

71. Imaizumi A, Kuribayashi A, Okochi K, et al. Differentiation between superficial and deep lobe parotid tumors by magnetic resonance imaging: usefulness of the parotid duct criterion. Acta Radiol 2009;50(7): 806–11.

72. Vaiman M, Luckman J, Sigal T, et al. Correlation between preoperative predictions and surgical findings in the parotid surgery for tumors. Head Face Med 2016;12:4.

73. Kim JY, Yang HC, Lee S, et al. Effectiveness of anatomic criteria for predicting parotid tumour location. Clin Otolaryngol 2016;41(2):154–9.

74. Netter F. Anatomy of the nervous system. In: The CIBA collection of medical illustrations, vol. 1. Ardsley (New York): CIBA-GEIGY Corp; 1953. p. 80–7.

75. Ho ML, Juliano A, Eisenberg RL, et al. Anatomy and pathology of the facial nerve. AJR Am J Roentgenol 2015;204(6):W612–9.

76. Li C, Li Y, Zhang D, et al. 3D-FIESTA MRI at 3 T demonstrating branches of the intraparotid facial nerve, parotid ducts and relation with benign parotid tumours. Clin Radiol 2012;67(11):1078–82.

77. Attye A, Karkas A, Tropres I, et al. Parotid gland tumours: MR tractography to assess contact with the facial nerve. Eur Radiol 2016;26(7):2233–41.

78. Benson MT, Dalen K, Mancuso AA, et al. Congenital anomalies of the branchial apparatus: embryology and pathologic anatomy. Radiographics 1992; 12(5):943–60.

79. Moon WK, Han MH, Kim IO, et al. Congenital fistula from ectopic accessory parotid gland: diagnosis with CT sialography and CT fistulography. AJNR Am J Neuroradiol 1995;16(4 Suppl):997–9.

80. Sun L, Sun Z, Ma X. Partial duplication of the mandible, parotid aplasia and facial cleft: a rare developmental disorder. Oral Surg Oral Med Oral Pathol Oral Radiol 2013;116(3):e202–9.

81. Teymoortash A, Hoch S. Congenital unilateral agenesis of the parotid gland: a case report and review of the literature. Case Rep Dent 2016;2016:2672496.

82. Gadodia A, Seith A, Neyaz Z, et al. Magnetic resonance identification of an accessory submandibular duct and gland: an unusual variant. J Laryngol Otol 2007;121(9):e18.

83. Tabor EK, Curtin HD. MR of the salivary glands. Radiol Clin North Am 1989;27(2):379–92.

84. Weissman JL, Carrau RL. Anterior facial vein and submandibular gland together: predicting the histology of submandibular masses with CT or MR imaging. Radiology 1998;208(2):441–6.

85. Pownell PH, Brown OE, Pransky SM, et al. Congenital abnormalities of the submandibular duct. Int J Pediatr Otorhinolaryngol 1992;24(2):161–9.

86. Branstetter BF, Weissman JL, Kaplan SB. Imaging of a Stafne bone cavity: what MR adds and why a new name is needed. AJNR Am J Neuroradiol 1999; 20(4):587–9.

87. White DK, Davidson HC, Harnsberger HR, et al. Accessory salivary tissue in the mylohyoid boutonniere: a clinical and radiologic pseudolesion of the oral cavity. AJNR Am J Neuroradiol 2001;22(2): 406–12.

Imaging of Benign Neoplastic and Nonneoplastic Salivary Gland Tumors

Daniel Thomas Ginat, MD, MS

KEYWORDS

• Salivary gland • Tumor • Benign • Imaging

KEY POINTS

- The role of imaging is mainly to delineate the location and extent of salivary tumors and to assess for benign features or in some cases to suggest a specific diagnosis.
- Pleomorphic adenomas are the most common benign parotid neoplasms in adults and classically appear as well-defined, multilobulated, T2 hyperintense tumors with nodular enhancement and a T2 dark rim.
- Warthin tumors are associated with smoking, are typically located in the parotid tail, are often multiple and/or bilateral, can be cystic and/or solid, and are typically very hypermetabolic on 18-fluorodeoxyglucose ([18]FDG)-PET, which can mimic malignancy.
- Oncocytomas tend to be inconspicuous on fat-suppressed T2 and postcontrast T1-weighted MR imaging and are, therefore, known as vanishing tumors.
- Certain non-neoplastic lesions that may present as salivary gland tumors can have rather characteristic clinicoradiologic features, such as vascular malformations and ranulas.

INTRODUCTION

Diagnostic imaging plays an important role in the evaluation of patients with suspected salivary gland tumors.[1,2] In particular, imaging serves to delineate the location and extent of tumors and assess the features of the tumor, such as cystic versus solid and well-defined versus ill-defined margins, which are relevant considerations for surgical planning. Several imaging modalities are suitable for characterizing salivary tumors, mainly including ultrasound, computed tomography (CT) scan, MR imaging, and sialography, as discussed in Christopher Atkinson and colleagues' article, "Cross-Sectional Imaging Techniques and Normal Anatomy of the Salivary Glands," in this issue.

Numerous benign neoplastic and nonneoplastic lesions can present clinically as salivary tumors (**Table 1**). Differentiating benign from malignant salivary tumors is relevant to clinical management because benign lesions can often be treated less invasively or aggressively than their malignant counterparts. In general, imaging features that suggest that a tumor is benign include well-defined margins, a high T2 signal, and completely cystic contents.[3] Furthermore, advanced MR imaging techniques, including dynamic susceptibility contrast-enhanced perfusion-weighted MR imaging and diffusion-weighted MR imaging, may also aid in the differentiation of malignant from benign parotid

Disclosures: None.
Department of Radiology, University of Chicago, Pritzker School of Medicine, 5841 South Maryland Avenue, Chicago, IL 60637, USA
E-mail address: dtg1@uchicago.edu

Neuroimag Clin N Am 28 (2018) 159–169
https://doi.org/10.1016/j.nic.2018.01.002

Table 1	
Types of benign salivary tumors and tumor-like conditions	
Category	**Examples**
Neoplastic	Epithelial: pleomorphic adenoma (benign mixed tumor), Warthin tumor (papillary cystadenoma lymphomatosum), oncocytoma, myoepithelioma, basal cell adenoma, lymphadenoma, sialadenoma papilliferum, ductal papillomas, sebaceous adenoma, canalicular adenoma, and other ductal adenomas Nonepithelial: lipoma or sialolipoma, peripheral nerve sheath tumors, hemangioma or hemangioendothelioma
Nonneoplastic	Sialolithiasis, chronic sclerosing sialadenitis (Kuttner tumor), granulomatous sialadenitis, lymphoepithelial sialadenitis, ranula or mucocele, sialectasis, abscess, epidermoid, benign lymphoepithelial lesions, lymphoid hyperplasia (both infectious and inflammatory conditions; eg, Kimura disease), sclerosing polycystic adenosis, nodular oncocytic hyperplasia, intercalated duct hyperplasia, posttraumatic or postinfectious cyst, sialocele, vascular malformations

tumors and for characterization of some benign parotid tumors.[4,5]

Certain findings on imaging can help render a fairly specific diagnosis for some tumors, such as most pleomorphic adenomas on MR imaging. On the other hand, the imaging appearance of some benign entities can mimic malignancies, such as infiltrative fibromatosis and hypermetabolism of Warthin tumors on 18-fluorodeoxyglucose ([18]FDG)-PET. The imaging features of selected benign tumors and tumor-like lesions are discussed and depicted in this article. (See discussion of additional information related to this topic, in this issue.)

DISCUSSION
Neoplastic Tumors

Pleomorphic adenoma
Pleomorphic adenomas, also known as benign mixed tumors, are the most common benign parotid tumors. The tumors are composed of epithelial and myoepithelial cells with variable myxoid, hyaline, cartilaginous, or osseous differentiation.[6] Thus, it is not uncommon for pleomorphic adenomas to contain calcified or ossified components, which are most conspicuous on CT (**Fig. 1**). On ultrasound, pleomorphic adenomas are usually hypoechoic, well-defined, lobulated lesions with posterior acoustic enhancement (**Fig. 2**) and tend to be hypovascular centrally on Doppler.[7] Pleomorphic adenomas classically appear as well-defined, multilobulated or bosselated, T2 hyperintense tumors with heterogeneous nodular

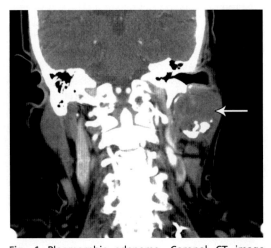

Fig. 1. Pleomorphic adenoma. Coronal CT image shows a low attenuation mass (*arrow*) in the left parotid gland with calcification inferiorly. Pathologic evaluation revealed 2 distinct nodules within the mass: a stroma-predominant myxochondroid nodule with areas of degenerative change and infarction and a cellular nodule with tubuloductal structures and sheets of myoepithelial cells.

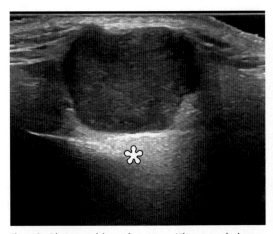

Fig. 2. Pleomorphic adenoma. Ultrasound image shows a multilobulated hypoechoic mass with posterior acoustic enhancement (*asterisk*).

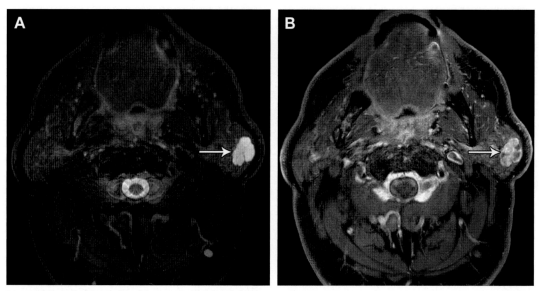

Fig. 3. Pleomorphic adenoma. Axial fat-suppressed T2-weighted (*A*) and fat-suppressed postcontrast T1-weighted (*B*) MR images show a T2 hyperintense, heterogeneously enhancing bossellated mass in the left parotid gland (*arrows*).

enhancement and a T2 dark rim on MR imaging (**Fig. 3**).[6,8] The presence of all these MR imaging features is 95% specific for pleomorphic adenoma.[8]

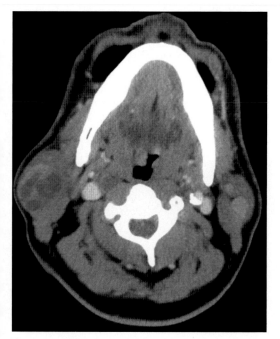

Fig. 4. Warthin tumor. Axial CT image shows a partly cystic right parotid tail tumor and a more solid left parotid tail tumor.

Warthin tumor

Warthin tumors, formerly known as papillary cystadenoma lymphomatosum, are the second most common benign parotid neoplasms and are typically located in the parotid tail, often bilaterally (earing lesions).[1] These tumors are adenomas composed of bilayered columnar and basaloid oncocytic epithelium that form multiple cysts with numerous papillae, as well as a proliferation of follicle-containing lymphoid tissue.[9] Smoking is a risk factor for the development of Warthin tumors.[10] The classic patient history and location of the tumors, which can be cystic and/or solid, can suggest the diagnosis even on a CT scan (**Fig. 4**). Warthin tumors are usually hypoechoic and hypervascularized; however, there may also be anechoic areas that correspond to cystic components (**Fig. 5**).[7] On MR imaging, the presence of hypointense areas on short tau inversion recovery (STIR) and T2-weighted images and hyperintense areas on T1-weighted images is suggestive of Warthin tumors (**Fig. 6**).[11] Warthin tumors can resemble other less common benign neoplasms that can also contain cystic components, such as myoepitheliomas and basal cell adenomas, which tend to involve the superficial lobe of the parotid gland.[12,13] Conversely, Warthin tumors are very hypermetabolic and can mimic malignant neoplasms on [18]FDG-PET (**Fig. 7**).[14] Likewise, Warthin tumors tend to have high uptake on technetium-99m (^{99m}Tc) pertechnetate radionuclide scans if sufficiently large and solid.[14]

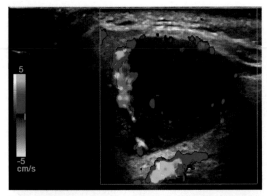

Fig. 5. Warthin tumor. Doppler ultrasound image shows a heterogeneous mass with cystic components with frond-like projections and hypervascular solid components.

Oncocytoma

Oncocytomas are uncommon neoplasms composed of mitochondria-rich oncocytes that mainly involve the parotid glands.[15] Oncocytomas tend to appear as well-defined and solid, enhancing masses on a CT scan (**Fig. 8**).[16] On MR imaging, the tumors are typically the most conspicuous T1-weighted sequences due to a relatively low T1 signal with respect to the normal gland but are isointense to the normal parotid tissue on fat-suppressed T2-weighted and post-contrast T1-weighted sequences (**Fig. 9**). Based on these MR imaging characteristics, oncocytomas have been referred to as vanishing tumors. Similar to Warthin tumors, oncocytomas display high uptake on ^{99m}Tc pertechnetate radionuclide scans.[14]

Peripheral nerve sheath tumors

Schwannomas and neurofibromas are the most common benign peripheral nerve sheath tumors.

Intraparotid neurofibromas can be associated with neurofibromatosis type 1 and schwannomas can be associated with neurofibromatosis type 2; however, these tumors can also arise in patients without these syndromes. When intraparotid peripheral nerve sheath tumors occur in the setting of neurofibromatosis, the diagnosis is usually relatively straightforward. However, in sporadic cases, particularly when facial nerve function is intact, the clinical diagnosis can be elusive.[17,18] The presence of a fusiform tumor with extension into the intratemporal facial nerve canal on diagnostic imaging can be a helpful distinguishing feature, although this can mimic perineural spread associated with malignant neoplasms. Otherwise, the target and fascicular signs are fairly characteristic features of peripheral nerve sheath tumors on MR imaging and ultrasound.[19,20] In particular, the target sign refers to the appearance of central T2 hypointensity and enhancement and peripheral T2 hyperintensity and nonenhancement (**Fig. 10**), whereas the fascicular sign corresponds to multiple ring-like T2 hypointense foci within a relatively T2 hyperintense and enhancing background (**Fig. 11**). Peripheral nerve sheath tumors often appear as hypoechoic tumors with anechoic areas and posterior acoustic enhancement on ultrasound.[7]

Lipoma or sialolipoma

Lipomas are neoplasms composed of mature adipose tissue associated and can be intraglandular or extraglandular with respect to the salivary gland involved. The tumors are readily recognized on a CT scan with diffuse fat attenuation of around −100 HU (**Fig. 12**).[1] Likewise, the use of fat-suppression on MR imaging is also useful for depicting lipomas of the salivary glands (**Fig. 13**). The tumors sometimes engulf vessels, may contain septations, and tend to be

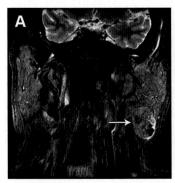
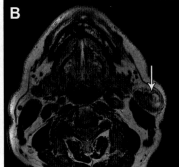
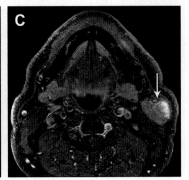

Fig. 6. Warthin tumor. Coronal STIR MR image (*A*) and axial T1-weighted (*B*) and fat-suppressed postcontrast T1-weighted (*C*) MR images show a well-defined but heterogeneous mass in the let parotid tail with areas of very low T2 signal, areas of high T1 signal, and partial enhancement (*arrows*).

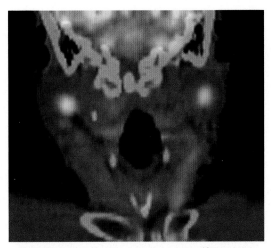

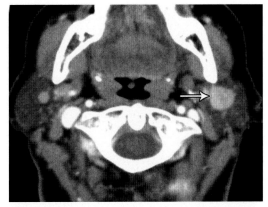

Fig. 8. Oncocytoma. Axial CT image shows an enhancing mass in the right parotid gland (*arrow*).

Fig. 7. Warthin tumor. Fused coronal ¹⁸FDG-PET/CT image shows hypermetabolic parotid tail tumors bilaterally.

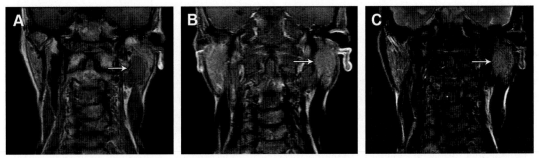

Fig. 9. Oncocytoma. Coronal T1-weighted (*A*), T2-weighted (*B*), and postcontrast T1-weighted (*C*) MR image shows that the mass (*arrows*) is virtually inconspicuous on the T2-weighted sequence and after contrast.

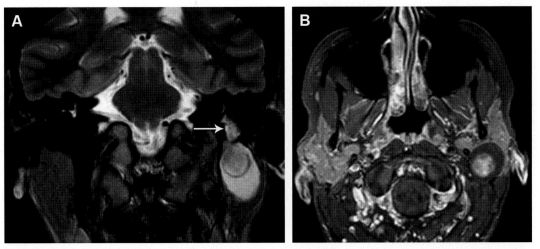

Fig. 10. Schwannoma. Coronal fat-suppressed T2-weighted (*A*) and postcontrast axial T1-weighted (*B*) MR images demonstrate a well-defined mass in the left parotid gland with target sign appearance due to the presence of a peripheral cystic component and a central solid, enhancing component. The tumor also extends into the mastoid segment of the facial nerve canal via the stylomastoid foramen (*arrow*).

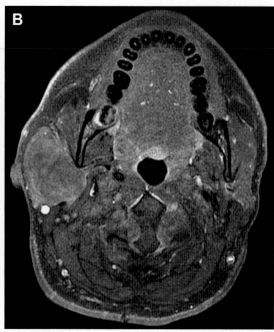

Fig. 11. Neurofibroma. Axial fat-suppressed T2-weighted (*A*) and postcontrast T1-weighted (*B*) MR images show a heterogeneously enhancing mass with areas suggestive of the fascicular sign in the right parotid gland, as well as numerous other spine and neck soft tissue tumors in this patient with neurofibromatosis type 1.

hypoechoic on ultrasound relative to the rest of the gland.[7,21] Sialolipomas are rare variants of lipomas that are composed of neoplastic mature adipose tissue and nonneoplastic salivary gland elements.[22] Thus, these tumors tend to appear heterogeneous with soft tissue components that correspond to salivary gland tissue in addition to fat but are encapsulated.

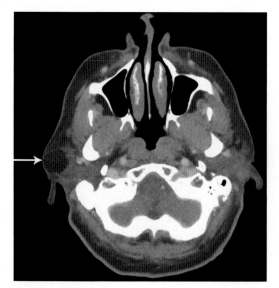

Fig. 12. Lipoma. Axial CT image shows a homogeneous, well-defined fat-attenuation mass in the right parotid space (*arrow*).

Hemangioma or hemangioendothelioma

Hemangiomas or hemangioendotheliomas are the most common neoplasms in infants.[23] Doppler ultrasound imaging can demonstrate the highly vascular nature of these tumors, as evidenced by the present of multiple prominent vessels (**Fig. 14**) but can be confounded with vascular malformations on this modality.[23] Alternatively, MR imaging characteristically demonstrates homogeneously T2 hyperintense and avidly enhancing tumors with prominent flow voids (**Fig. 15**). The tumors often involve the entire gland and can be multiple, with additional lesions present elsewhere in the head and neck and beyond. The tumors generally undergo rapid enlargement during the proliferative phase, followed by gradual spontaneous involution but can rarely be complicated by high-output cardiac failure or Kasabach-Merritt syndrome.

Nonneoplastic Tumors

Ranulas

Ranulas are mucoceles that originate within the sublingual space from obstruction of the sublingual or minor salivary gland ducts.[24] When confined to the sublingual space, they are known as simple ranulas and when they herniate through a defect in the mylohyoid into the submandibular and sometimes even into the parapharyngeal spaces, they are known as diving or plunging

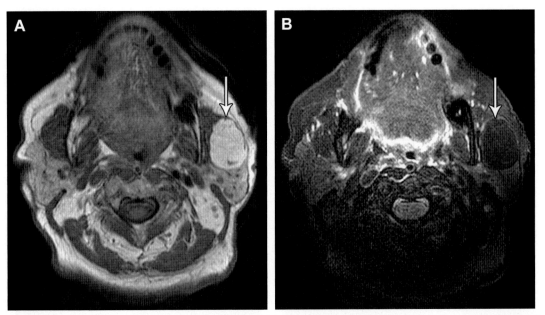

Fig. 13. Lipoma. Axial T1-weighted MR image (*A*) and fat-suppressed postcontrast T1-weighted MR image (*B*) show fat signal characteristics in the well-defined left parotid tumor (*arrows*).

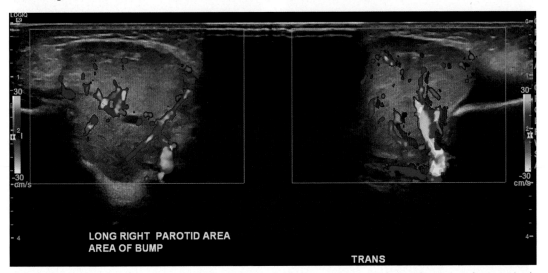

Fig. 14. Hemangioma or hemangioendothelioma. Doppler ultrasound images show a hypervascular mass in the right parotid gland.

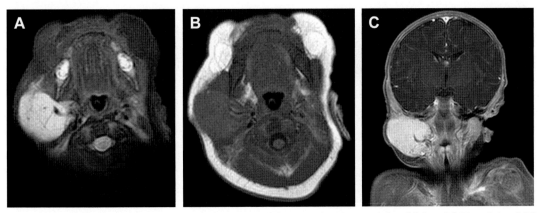

Fig. 15. Hemangioma or hemangioendothelioma. Axial fat-suppressed T2-weighted (*A*), axial T1-weighted (*B*), and coronal fat-suppressed postcontrast T1-weighted (*C*) MR images show a T2 hyperintense, avidly enhancing mass with prominent flow voids that encompasses the entire the right parotid gland.

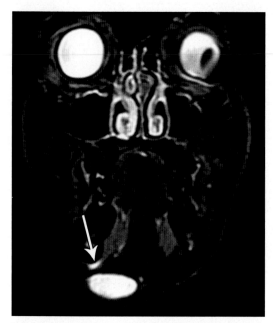

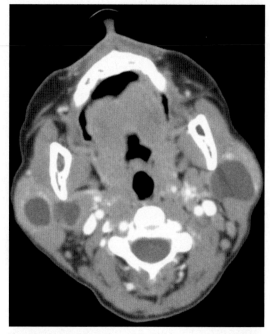

Fig. 16. Ranula. Coronal STIR MR image shows cystic lesion in the submandibular space with extension to the sublingual gland, or tail sign (*arrow*).

Fig. 17. Benign lymphoepithelial lesions. Axial CT image shows multiple bilateral cystic parotid gland lesions in the in a patient with HIV.

ranulas. Ranulas appear as well-defined, unilocular cystic masses on imaging.[24,25] A connection with the sublingual space is often apparent on imaging with plunging ranulas, which gives the appearance of the tail sign (**Fig. 16**).[25] Furthermore, the mass effect on adjacent muscles and vessels tends to be disproportionately minimal for the size of the lesion.[25]

Benign lymphoepithelial lesions
Benign lymphoepithelial lesions, or myoepithelial sialoadenitis, are the hallmark of human immunodeficiency virus (HIV)-associated salivary gland disease and represent lymphoid hyperplasia.

The lesions are often cystic, multiple, and involve the parotid glands bilaterally (**Fig. 17**) but can also be solid and involve the submandibular glands. In addition, there can be accompanying cervical lymphadenopathy. The histopathologic and imaging features of HIV-associated salivary gland disease are also analogous to lymphoepithelial sialadenitis related to Sjögren disease.[8] Sjögren syndrome can also be associated with reactive lymphadenopathy. Furthermore, the presence of lesions larger than 2 cm or rapidly growing lesions raises the possibility of superimposed lymphoma.[7]

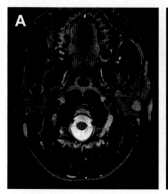

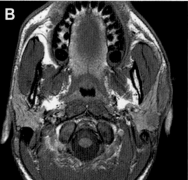

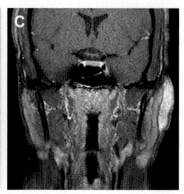

Fig. 18. Kimura disease. Axial STIR (*A*), axial T1-weighted (*B*), and coronal fat-suppressed postcontrast T1-weighted (*C*) MR images show enhancing left parotid space tumors in a young patient with eosinophilia.

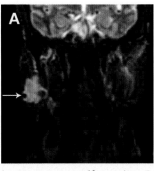
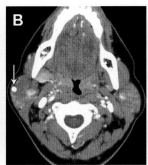
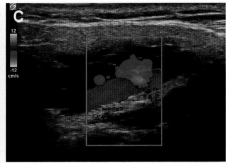

Fig. 19. Venous malformation. Coronal STIR MR image (*A*) shows a well-defined T2 hyperintense mass in the right parotid gland with a round low signal focus that corresponds to a phlebolith (*arrow*). The corresponding axial CT image (*B*) shows a low attenuation mass with a calcified phlebolith (*arrow*). Doppler ultrasound image (*C*) shows low-flow in the otherwise anechoic mass.

Kimura disease

Kimura disease is a chronic inflammatory disorder that consists of inflammatory masses with peripheral eosinophilia and elevated serum IgE, which predominantly affects young Asian male patients.[26] Most nonnodal lesions occur in the parotid and to a lesser extent in the submandibular regions, and are often bilateral and accompanied by cervical lymphadenopathy. On MR imaging, the lesions tend to be isointense to slightly hyperintense on T1-weighted images and hyperintense on T2-weighted sequences with respect to muscle and display moderate or marked enhancement (Fig. 18).[26] The lesions can infiltrate the salivary glands and subcutaneous extension, and the affected lymph nodes are enlarged. Kimura disease is difficult to diagnose based on the radiologic appearance alone.

Vascular malformations

Various types of vascular malformations can involve the salivary glands and can be broadly categorized as low-flow versus high-flow.[27,28] Low-flow lesions mainly include venous and lymphatic malformations, whereas high-flow lesions include arteriovenous malformations, although there may be combinations of these entities. Venous malformations typically display areas of high signal intensity on T2-weighted images and may contain phleboliths that appear as low signal foci, whereas on a CT scan, venous malformations appear as hypoattenuating or heterogeneous tumors that may contain rounded calcified phleboliths and tend to enhance gradually, with corresponding venous flow on Doppler ultrasound, although there may be thrombosed areas without flow or enhancement (Fig. 19).[29] Contrast-enhanced MR angiography can be useful for further classifying venous malformations.[30] Lymphatic malformations classically appear as transspatial multicystic masses with hemorrhage-fluid levels, which are best depicted on STIR or fat-suppressed T2-weighted MR imaging sequences (Fig. 20). Arteriovenous malformations are best characterized via CT angiography and/or catheter angiography and appear as serpiginous vessels that are often enlarged and clustered in a nidus (Fig. 21).[31] Alternatively, time-resolved imaging of contrast kinetics (TRICKS) MR angiography is a reliable, noninvasive modality for delineating feeding arteries, the nidus, and the draining veins of arteriovenous malformations within or near the salivary glands.[32]

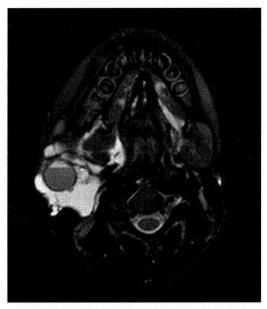

Fig. 20. Lymphatic malformation. Axial fat-suppressed T2-weight MR image shows a mass with multiple cystic components and a fluid-fluid level that engulfs the right submandibular gland.

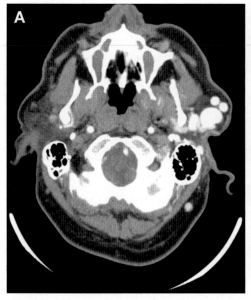
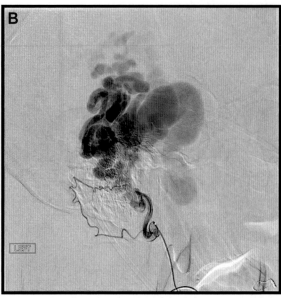

Fig. 21. Arteriovenous malformation. Axial CT angiography image (*A*) shows dilated vessels in the left parotid gland. The corresponding lateral digital subtraction angiogram (*B*) shows a large nidus of anomalous arteries and early draining veins.

SUMMARY

There is a wide variety benign salivary tumors, both neoplastic and nonneoplastic. Diagnostic imaging plays an important role in the diagnosis and treatment planning of these lesions. Familiarity with the characteristic imaging features of certain benign salivary tumors can help optimize radiological interpretation.

REFERENCES

1. Afzelius P, Nielsen MY, Ewertsen C, et al. Imaging of the major salivary glands. Clin Physiol Funct Imaging 2016;36:1–10.
2. Yousem DM, Kraut MA, Chalian AA. Major salivary gland imaging. Radiology 2000;216:19–29.
3. Christe A, Waldherr C, Hallett R, et al. MR imaging of parotid tumors: typical lesion characteristics in MR imaging improve discrimination between benign and malignant disease. AJNR Am J Neuroradiol 2011;32:1202–7.
4. Abdel Razek AA, Samir S, Ashmalla GA. Characterization of parotid tumors with dynamic susceptibility contrast perfusion-weighted magnetic resonance imaging and diffusion-weighted MR imaging. J Comput Assist Tomogr 2017;41(1):131–6.
5. Lechner Goyault J, Riehm S, Neuville A, et al. Interest of diffusion-weighted and gadolinium-enhanced dynamic MR sequences for the diagnosis of parotid gland tumors. J Neuroradiol 2011;38(2):77–89.
6. Tsushima Y, Matsumoto M, Endo K, et al. Characteristic bright signal of parotid pleomorphic adenomas on T2-weighted MR images with pathological correlation. Clin Radiol 1994;49:485–9.
7. Bialek EJ, Jakubowski W, Zajkowski P, et al. US of the major salivary glands: anatomy and spatial relationships, pathologic conditions, and pitfalls. Radiographics 2006;26:745–63.
8. Zaghi S, Hendizadeh L, Hung T, et al. MRI criteria for the diagnosis of pleomorphic adenoma: a validation study. Am J Otolaryngol 2014;35:713–8.
9. Ellis GL. Lymphoid lesions of salivary glands: malignant and benign. Med Oral Patol Oral Cir Bucal 2007;1(12):E479–85.
10. Pinkston JA, Cole P. Cigarette smoking and Warthin's tumor. Am J Epidemiol 1996;144:183–7.
11. Ikeda M, Motoori K, Hanazawa T, et al. Warthin tumor of the parotid gland: diagnostic value of MR imaging with histopathologic correlation. AJNR Am J Neuroradiol 2004;25:1256–62.
12. Jang M, Park D, Lee SR, et al. Basal cell adenoma in the parotid gland: CT and MR findings. AJNR Am J Neuroradiol 2004;25(4):631–5.
13. Ding J, Wang W, Peng W, et al. MRI and CT imaging characteristics of myoepithelioma of the parotid gland. Acta Radiol 2016;57(7):837–43.
14. Uchida Y, Minoshima S, Kawata T, et al. Diagnostic value of FDG PET and salivary gland scintigraphy for parotid tumors. Clin Nucl Med 2005;30:170–6.
15. Patel ND, van Zante A, Eisele DW, et al. Oncocytoma: the vanishing parotid mass. AJNR Am J Neuroradiol 2011;32:1703–6.

16. Sakai E, Yoda T, Shimamoto H, et al. Pathologic and imaging findings of an oncocytoma in the deep lobe of the left parotid gland. Int J Oral Maxillofac Surg 2003;32:563–5.

17. Caughey RJ, May M, Schaitkin BM. Intraparotid facial nerve schwannoma: diagnosis and management. Otolaryngol Head Neck Surg 2004;130:586–92.

18. McGuirt WF Sr, Johnson PE, McGuirt WT. Intraparotid facial nerve neurofibromas. Laryngoscope 2003; 113:82–4.

19. Shimizu K, Iwai H, Ikeda K, et al. Intraparotid facial nerve schwannoma: a report of five cases and an analysis of MR imaging results. AJNR Am J Neuroradiol 2005;26:1328–30.

20. Abreu E, Aubert S, Wavreille G, et al. Peripheral tumor and tumor-like neurogenic lesions. Eur J Radiol 2013;82:38–50.

21. Chikui T, Yonetsu K, Yoshiura K, et al. Imaging findings of lipomas in the orofacial region with CT, US, and MRI. Oral Surg Oral Med Oral Pathol Oral Radiol Endod 1997;84:88–95.

22. Nagao T, Sugano I, Ishida Y, et al. Sialolipoma: a report of seven cases of a new variant of salivary gland lipoma. Histopathology 2001;38:30–6.

23. Roebuck DJ, Ahuja AT. Hemangioendothelioma of the parotid gland in infants: sonography and correlative MR imaging. AJNR Am J Neuroradiol 2000;21:219–23.

24. Coit WE, Harnsberger HR, Osborn AG, et al. Ranulas and their mimics: CT evaluation. Radiology 1987;163:211–6.

25. Kurabayashi T, Ida M, Yasumoto M, et al. MRI of ranulas. Neuroradiology 2000;42:917–22.

26. Park SW, Kim HJ, Sung KJ, et al. Kimura disease: CT and MR imaging findings. AJNR Am J Neuroradiol 2012;33(4):784–8.

27. Mahady K, Thust S, Berkeley R, et al. Vascular anomalies of the head and neck in children. Quant Imaging Med Surg 2015;5:886–97.

28. Baker LL, Dillon WP, Hieshima GB, et al. Hemangiomas and vascular malformations of the head and neck: MR characterization. AJNR Am J Neuroradiol 1993;14:307–14.

29. Dubois J, Soulez G, Oliva VL, et al. Soft-tissue venous malformations in adult patients: imaging and therapeutic issues. Radiographics 2001;21: 1519–31.

30. Abdel Razek AA, Albair GA, Samir S. Clinical value of classification of venous malformations with contrast-enhanced MR angiography. Phlebology 2017;32(9):628–33.

31. Achache M, Fakhry N, Varoquaux A, et al. Management of vascular malformations of the parotid area. Eur Ann Otorhinolaryngol Head Neck Dis 2013; 130:55–60.

32. Razek AA, Gaballa G, Megahed AS, et al. Time resolved imaging of contrast kinetics (TRICKS) MR angiography of arteriovenous malformations of head and neck. Eur J Radiol 2013;82(11): 1885–91.

A Review of Salivary Gland Malignancies
Common Histologic Types, Anatomic Considerations, and Imaging Strategies

Remy Lobo, MD, Jeffrey Hawk, MD,
Ashok Srinivasan, MBBS, MD*

KEYWORDS

• Parotid • Submandibular • Sublingual • Minor salivary gland • Perineural tumor spread

KEY POINTS

- Most parotid neoplasms (approximately 4/5) are not malignant. Most sublingual neoplasms (approximately 4/5) are malignant. Approximately half of the minor salivary and submandibular neoplasms are malignant.
- The parotid gland has lymph nodes within its fascia, which makes it an important site in both primary and secondary malignancy evaluation.
- In addition to local aggressive features, important directions of spread for parotid malignancy include routes along the cranial nerves (CNs), most commonly trigeminal (CN V) and facial (CN VII), with their anastomotic connections. Knowledge of local tumor and nodal staging offers crucial prognostic and management information in tumor-node-metastasis staging of disease.

TUMOR EPIDEMIOLOGY AND PRESENTATION

Salivary gland malignancies are a rare group of heterogeneous neoplasms arising along the aerodigestive tract and its major secretory structures. They represent less than 8% of head and neck tumors and a total of less than 2500 new cases per year in the United States. Both viral and environmental factors have been implicated as potential causes of neoplasia.[1]

These tumors can present in various clinical scenarios. Major salivary gland malignancy typically manifests as a palpable abnormality to a clinician or patient. The major (parotid, submandibular, and sublingual) gland is often enlarged and may (or may not) be painful on examination. Pertinent features for the clinician involve the evaluation of the adjacent nervous structures. For example, cranial

nerve (CN) VII (facial) should be scrutinized in the setting of parotid enlargement because facial muscle weakness can alert a clinician to a parotid neoplasm affecting CN VII as it passes through the gland. Minor salivary gland malignancies present according to the surrounding tissue affected. For example, a hard palate tumor may be quite small, but if it affects a branch of CN V (trigeminal), the patient may present with numbness. Other scenarios can be imagined: a minor neoplasm along the optic canal could present with vision complaints and a nasal mass could present with obstruction. Nasopharyngeal masses often present late to the clinician and may already have invasion at the skull base.[2] If the primary site is more occult, a nodal mass may be the presenting sign, leading to imaging evaluation. Certain salivary malignancies (eg, mucoepidermoid carcinoma

Department of Neuroradiology, University of Michigan, B2-A209D, 1500 East Medical Center Drive, Ann Arbor, MI 48109, USA
* Corresponding author.
E-mail address: ashoks@med.umich.edu

Neuroimag Clin N Am 28 (2018) 171–182
https://doi.org/10.1016/j.nic.2018.01.011

[MEC]) have a tendency for nodal metastases. Close attention should be paid to the aerodigestive tract and associated salivary glands in all cases of pathologic nodal enlargement.

Most salivary gland neoplasms arise in the parotid gland, approximately 73% in 1 large study,[3] but they are not usually malignant; merely one-fourth (15%–32%) of parotid neoplasms are malignant on histology.[4] Less than 11% of salivary gland neoplasms arise in the submandibular gland, where they carry a 41% to 45% chance risk of being malignant. Less than 0.5% of salivary neoplasms arise in the sublingual gland, but they carry a 70% to 90% chance of being malignant. Minor salivary glands account for the remaining approximately 14% of salivary tumors.[1] Among the 450 to 750 minor salivary glands overall, approximately half of the tumors found are malignant. Risk of malignancy is stratified among the minor salivary glands; approximately half of the palatal neoplasms found are malignant; however, in the floor of mouth, the risk increases to 90%.[5] Although most large population studies are somewhat dated, recent studies have generally held these percentages stable over time.[6] The 1 addition is that more cancers are now diagnosed, yet causative factors remain elusive.

In summary, and as a rule, the risk of malignancy increases as the gland decreases in size. Although tumors are most commonly found in the parotid, they are least likely to be malignant in that location; the majority are adenomas. Although the sublingual gland is a small structure, tumors found within it are usually (almost 90% of the time) malignant. Still, given the overall disproportionate distribution of tumors to the parotid gland, the parotid is the most likely major salivary gland in which malignancy arises.

TUMOR HISTOLOGY

According to the World Health Organization (WHO), there are more than 25 types of distinct salivary gland tumors. New histologic and biochemical techniques allow for identification of different molecular and genetic subtypes (including hallmark translocations), which can help direct targeted therapy. The WHO updated their 2005[7] *Classification of Head and Neck Tumours* with a new list of salivary gland malignancies in 2017.[8] The most common salivary malignancies (**Box 1**) still include adenocarcinomas, carcinoma ex pleomorphic adenoma, acinic cell carcinoma, adenoid cystic carcinoma (ACCa), MEC, and lymphomas. Important additions include the mammary analog secretory carcinoma (an acinic cell variant based on gene fusion) and several differences in grouping (eg, low-grade

---

> **Box 1**
> **Common histologic types of salivary malignancies**
>
> *Primary*
>
> Adenocarcinomas
>
> Carcinoma ex pleomorphic adenoma
>
> Acinic cell carcinoma
>
> ACCa
>
> MEC
>
> Intraductal carcinoma
>
> Mammary analog secretory carcinoma
>
> Lymphomas
>
> *Secondary*
>
> Intraparotid lymph node metastases
>
> *Abbreviations:* ACCa, adenoid cystic carcinoma; MEC, mucoepidermoid carcinoma.

---

cribriform adenocarcinoma is now grouped in with intraductal carcinoma). The update grants pathologists increased flexibility to characterize the tumors according to which translocations and gene fusions are identified. Pathologists can also incorporate descriptions of high/intermediate/low-grade rates of mitoses into their analysis, and preference is now given to a new phrase, "high-grade transformation," which replaces dedifferentiation.[8] Genetic rearrangements are also described and help determine tissue of origin. Although much of the update revolved around primary neoplasms, it must be remembered that secondary malignant pathology can also occur in the salivary glands, specifically, malignant metastases to intraparotid lymph nodes.

IMAGING AND STAGING OF SALIVARY GLAND MALIGNANCIES

Major salivary gland malignancies have a separate, dedicated American Joint Committee on Cancer (AJCC) tumor-node-metastasis (TNM) staging system. Minor salivary gland malignancies are staged according to the local site of origin. AJCC TNM classifications for malignancies of the paranasal sinuses/nasal cavity, nasopharynx, oral cavity, oropharynx, hypopharynx, or larynx (with subsites) are used. Proper radiologic assessment of salivary gland malignancies requires having familiarity with the AJCC TNM staging schemes in the head and neck and apply these guidelines when mapping the extent of tumors.[9] Simply identifying the presence of a tumor or speculating as to the histologic type of tumor is not the primary role of the radiologist in these cases.

When imaging salivary gland malignancies, the goal is to determine the extent of tumor for treatment planning purposes. Four forms of extension should be considered (**Box 2**). These include direct extension (direct invasive growth of the primary tumor), perineural extension (extension along CNs and their branches) and metastatic extension (typically lymphatic extension to cervical lymph nodes); hematogenous metastasis to bone or brain as seen on head and neck imaging does occur but is far less common. Techniques for imaging salivary gland malignancies include ultrasound, Computed tomography (CT), MR imaging, and nuclear medicine (fluorodeoxyglucose [FDG] PET-CT).

Ultrasound

Superficial palpable masses are amenable to ultrasound evaluation. High-frequency linear transducers provide exquisite detail of the superficial anatomy and can be used as a convenient screening tool for lymphadenopathy. Ultrasound provides an inexpensive and portable means of early evaluation of superficial parotid and submandibular lesions. Ultrasound-guided procedures are also a useful adjunct for obtaining histologic samples that may help direct future imaging examiantions.[10] Ultrasound is of limited utility in the deep lobe of the parotid and of the minor salivary glands. Rare sublingual neoplasms, given inherent risk of malignancy, are usually evaluated with other cross-sectional modalities.

Computed Tomography

Salivary gland malignancies are often first imaged with (or incidentally detected) on routine CT imaging of the neck. Unless there is a contraindication,

contrast-enhanced imaging should always be used. Noncontrast imaging, either alone or in combination with contrast-enhanced imaging, is of limited value and is usually not indicated (discussed later).

CT imaging of the neck (**Table 1**) should begin at the midorbit and extend below the clavicular heads with the arms at a patient's side. A head holder may be helpful. The authors use a split bolus technique using a total of 125 mL of Isovue-300: an initial 50-mL bolus is followed 120 seconds later by a 75-mL bolus. The scan is initiated 60 seconds after the second bolus. Slice thickness is 1.25 mm with a 1.25-mm interval and a display field of view (DFOV) of 20 cm to 24 cm. Axial bone and soft tissue reformats are used in conjunction with the soft tissue sagittal and coronal reformats in all cases.

CT imaging is useful for identifying major and minor salivary gland tumors and determining the local direct extension of the tumor with attention to the nearby involved soft tissue and osseous structures. Bone algorithm CT nicely displays osseous cortical and trabecular destruction. Bone CT also demonstrates destruction of ossified cartilage from direct tumor extension. Perineural extension can be detected on CT by noting expansion of the respective skull base foramina or loss of fat on soft tissue images, but this occurs only after the nerves have been extensively involved by tumor. Direct and perineural extensions are critical components of the T component of TNM staging.

Lymphatic spread of tumor to cervical lymph nodes is well depicted with CT. Careful assessment of each cervical nodal level, including the retropharyngeal regions, should be performed after determining the local tumor extent. This determines the N component of the TNM staging. Presence or absence of extranodal extension was a new addition to the *AJCC Cancer Staging Manual, Eighth Edition*.[9] Extranodal extension (+) nodes have indistinct fat planes and may show strands of soft tissue directly invading the adjacent structures. Although many pathologic cervical nodes

---

Box 2
Imaging goals for assessing extent of salivary gland malignancies

Local extent (T staging, CT/MR imaging)

Direct extension

Perineural extension

Lymphatic spread (N staging, requires PET/dedicated chest, abdomen, pelvis imaging)

Nodal involvement

Hematogenous spread (M staging, requires PET/dedicated chest, abdomen, pelvis imaging, +/− MR imaging)

Anatomically remote structures (bone, brain, and so forth)

Table 1 Helical CT neck protocol	
Slice thickness	1.25 mm
Interval	1.25 mm
Pitch	0.97:1
Kilovolt (peak)	100
Auto milliamperes (minimum/maximum)	100/450
DFOV	20–24 cm

are clinically palpable, retropharyngeal nodes are not. Imagers can add value by drawing attention to the retropharyngeal nodes, possibly altering surgical approach. Assessment of the visualized intracranial structures and osseous structures on neck CTs remote from the primary tumor also assists with M component of TNM staging, although full staging requires PET and/or dedicated imaging of the chest, abdomen and pelvis (with or without MR imaging).

Dual-Energy Computed Tomography

Dual-energy CT (DECT) can be a useful technique to determine true tissue enhancement and identify differences in attenuation within glandular structures.[11] This technique, although not in common use, has potential for application in salivary imaging. DECT can generate a virtual noncontrast (VNC) image. VNC sequences are most useful for identifying calcifications seen in inflammatory sialolithiasis. Several higher-grade neoplasms (like salivary ductal carcinoma) can have calcifications,[12] and VNC sequences can increase the conspicuity of these foci. CT is limited in its detection of perineural tumor; DECT can (in part) overcome this with bone subtraction, which can increase the conspicuity of enhancement at the skull base foramina by removing the adjacent hyperattenuating osseous structures,[11] leaving the enhancing tumor floating in the foramen of interest. In an area of ongoing research, DECT may be useful in evaluating cervical lymphadenopathy.[13] DECT also has a benefit in assessing the primary malignant site. By creating virtual monochromatic sequences at a low kiloelectron voltage (eg, 50–70 keV), the conspicuity of tumors can be increased within the salivary glands. Salivary neoplasms can be occult on regular contrast-enhanced CT and obvious on MR imaging; virtual monochromatic sequences bridge this gap by creating a lower profile of photons; the native gland often becomes slightly hypoattenuated and the enhancing tumor becomes more conspicuous.[14] In cases of MR imaging not available, DECT may be a useful modality for analysis.

MR Imaging

MR imaging is useful for precise tumor mapping in certain circumstances and adds additional information for further soft tissue characterization of the primary tumor. The main uses for MR imaging are in the evaluation of salivary gland malignancies that arise near or extend to the skull base (more often minor salivary gland malignancies), evaluation of perineural tumor spread (important for parotid malignancies and minor salivary gland

malignancies near the skull base), and assessment for osseous marrow involvement, when applicable. MR imaging also provides better soft tissue resolution of head, neck, and intracranial structures.[15]

Dedicated MR imaging protocol (**Table 2**) for assessment of perineural spread, including protocols focused on the CN VII (for parotid malignancies) and CN V (for malignancies arising along the skull base or palate), should be performed in all applicable cases. This is particularly true when there is clinical evidence of CN deficits (eg, facial pain or numbness) or in the presence of a tumor with a high propensity (whether by location or histology) for perineural spread. MR imaging can detect perineural spread at a much earlier stage than CT and is the imaging standard in this assessment.[16]

Precontrast, non–fat-saturated T1 sequences are useful to detect intermediate to low T1-weighted image signal obliteration of high signal fat planes at the exocranial aspects of skull base foramina (stylomastoid foramen, foramen ovale, and so forth) or in the deep face (pterygopalatine fossa, inferior alveolar canal, orbital fissures, and so forth). Postcontrast, fat-saturated T1 sequences in the axial and coronal planes are useful for identifying abnormal enhancement in these same areas as well as asymmetric enhancement along the intraosseous and deeper courses of these nerves (intratemporal facial nerve, foramen rotundum,

Table 2 Skull base protocol	
Slice thickness, interval	3 mm, 1 mm
DFOV (cm), matrix	20, 512 × 512
Whole brain	Ax DWI, Ax FLAIR, Ax GRE, Sag T1, and Ax post-T1 (spin echo)
Precontrast skull base (third ventricle–hyoid)	Ax T1, Cor T1, Ax T2 FS, Cor STIR
Postcontrast skull base (third ventricle–hyoid)	Ax T1 FS, Cor T1 FS
Optional general (whole) neck	Precontrast Sag T1, Ax T2 FS or STIR, Ax T1, Cor T1, Cor STIR or T2 FS; and postcontrast Ax T1 FS, Cor T1 FS
Optional advanced imaging	T1 DCE, DWI (full-neck axial)

Abbreviations: Ax, axial; Cor, coronal; FLAIR, fluid-attenuated inversion recovery; FS, fat saturated; GRE, gradient recalled echo; Sag, sagittal.

vidian/pterygoid canal, palatine foramina, cavernous sinus, trigeminal/Meckel cave, and so forth). Caution should be used when evaluating the intratemporal facial nerve, because variable segments of the intratemporal perineural venous plexus enhance normally.[17] Enlargement and marked asymmetry are the hallmarks of pathology.

Precontrast non–fat-saturated and postcontrast fat-saturated T1 MR imaging are also useful for detecting involvement of marrow spaces of the mandible and skull base. In cases of minor salivary gland tumors of the larynx, they are helpful in detecting tracheal and cricoid cartilage infiltration.[18] These sequences, along with fat-saturated T2/short tau inversion recovery (STIR), are also useful for assessing invasion of soft tissues of the neck and skull base.

Advanced imaging is not ubiquitously used in the evaluation of salivary gland malignancies, although it may yet prove useful.[19] Techniques like diffusion-weighted imaging (DWI)/apparent diffusion coefficient (ADC) are well researched in the brain and many studies look at the hypointense signal on ADC as a marker of hypercellularity and as a surrogate marker of malignancy. The caveat is that multiple nonmalignant neoplasms (eg, Warthin tumors, also known as papillary cystadenoma lymphomatosum [PCL]) can also be hypointense on ADC. Because Warthin/PCL tumors are far more common than malignant neoplasms, this confounds data and overwhelms most studies. Dynamic contrast-enhanced imaging (DCE) uses contrast-enhanced curves to characterize tumoral angiogenesis, and tissue enhancement. DCE (Time to maximal contrast enhancement) has been shown helpful in distinguishing benign from malignant minor salivary gland neoplasms.[20] This was not replicated in major salivary glands, however.[21] Despite this, groups have tried a combination approach using DWI and DCE with varying degrees of success.[22] Continued research is ongoing in this area.[23]

PET-Computed Tomography

PET-CT is often an adjunct to other anatomic imaging in the evaluation of salivary gland malignancies. Primary lesions may be FDG avid, although several salivary carcinomas are not. More commonly incidental salivary lesions are found when imaging patients with PET-CT for a different cause. A reported 2% of cases have focal FDG-avid signal, although PET-CT is not reliable in distinguishing benign from malignant tissue (Warthin tumors can also be FDG avid). Tissue sampling is usually indicated in these cases because there is a reported one-third risk of malignancy.[24]

HISTOLOGIC TYPES OF SALIVARY GLAND MALIGNANCIES
Adenocarcinoma

Adenocarcinomas most commonly occur in the minor salivary glands of the palate and can be treated with surgical resection if caught early. Care must be taken to ensure clear margins because there is a risk of perineural extension and (less commonly) osseous invasion. Histologic progression[25] and transformation are also risks.[8] These adenocarcinomas were previously described as polymorphous low-grade adenocarcinoma. They stain positive for S100 on pathology,[26] have gene rearrangements of PRKD, and can have a targetoid appearance on histopathology.[8] **Fig. 1** shows a 49-year-old woman who initially presented with right facial numbness. She was worked up for stroke, but the cause of her numbness was actually a palatal adenocarcinoma affecting the maxillary division of CN V. Note the expansile lesion centered at the junction of the hard and soft palate, which, coincidentally, also has a targetoid appearance,

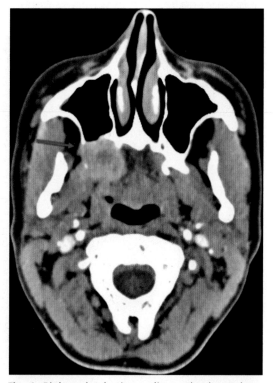

Fig. 1. Right palatal minor salivary gland neoplasm, adenocarcinoma, which initially presented with facial numbness in a 49-year-old woman. Axial image shows a right palate mass eroding the posterior right maxillary sinus and adjacent pterygoid plates (*arrow*). Incidental aerodigestive lesions can occasionally be identified on emergent stroke evaluation (CT angiogram, as shown, or MR imaging of the brain).

centrally hypoattenuating with increased peripheral attenuation/enhancement. Major salivary glands can also have adenocarcinomas, as shown in **Fig. 2**—a 51-year-old woman with left neck palpable lump. The parotid masses often present as painless abnormalities; key descriptions in **Fig. 2** involve the cystic change in the adenocarcinoma and irregular margins, suggesting a degree of infiltration. These have a nonspecific appearance on MR imaging and variable T2 signal (often hyperintense to the gland, although they can be hypointense) and usually enhance.

Carcinoma Ex Pleomorphic Adenoma

Carcinoma ex pleomorphic adenoma is a carcinoma that arises from a preexisting pleomorphic adenoma. This occurs in approximately 1.5% of pleomorphic adenoma cases at 5 years and almost 10% at 15 years.[27] The classic history is a painless mass for many years that has recently grown. That story was true in **Fig. 3**—a 52-year-old man with lump near the right submandibular gland that grew over the previous year. The peripherally calcified mass was excised en bloc,

with histologic features of carcinoma ex pleomorphic adenoma. Soft tissue invasion beyond the lesion capsule is common and should be quantified on pathology. Histologic hallmarks could include translocations of 8q12, 12q13-15, or 12q15.[8] Although most common in the parotid, they can occur in other secretory glands, even lacrimal. When positioned along bone, CT can show osseous erosions suggesting malignant degeneration.

Acinic Cell Carcinoma

Acinic cell carcinoma is a low-grade malignancy most commonly found in the parotid gland. The tumor is characterized by serous acinar differentiation and basophilic cytoplasmic granules on histology. Acinic cell carcinomas are not (typically) locally aggressive[28] and may be managed surgically. **Fig. 4** is an image of a 56-year-old woman with palpable left parotid mass. It is homogeneously intermediate/low in signal (see **Fig. 4A**) precontrast T1, distinguishing it from the remainder of the glandular architecture. It enhances uniformly (see **Fig. 4B**) and is intermediate

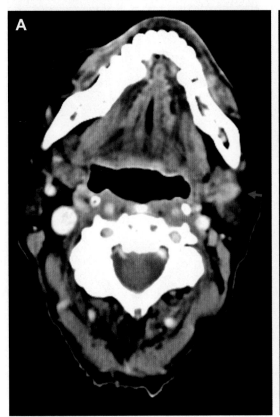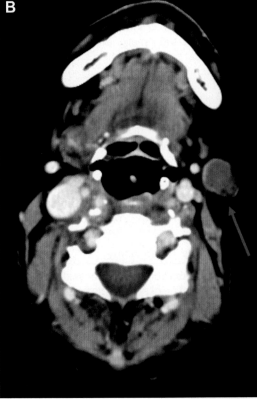

Fig. 2. Adenocarcinoma of the left submandibular gland in a 51-year-old woman with palpable nodule. Contrast-enhanced CT shows areas of hyperattenuation superiorly (*short arrow, A*) and cystic change more inferiorly (*long arrow, B*).

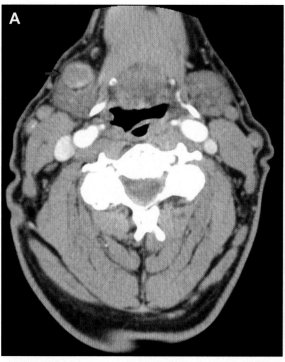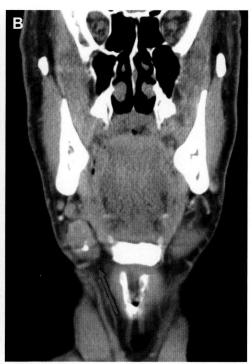

Fig. 3. Carcinoma ex pleomorphic adenoma in a 52-year-old man with "neck lump." Axial contrast-enhanced CT shows a peripherally hyperattenuating lesion (*small arrow, A*) in the right submandibular gland, with a punctate calcification on coronal contrast-enhanced CT (*long arrow, B*). Appearance is often nonspecific and requires histologic sampling.

on fluid-sensitive sequence (see **Fig. 4**C). Many malignancies previously believed acinic cell carcinomas are now characterized as mammary analog secretory carcinomas.[28]

Adenoid Cystic Carcinoma

ACCa occurs most commonly in middle-aged and elderly patients. ACCa occurs in both major and minor salivary gland tissue and has a strong propensity to spread by perineural growth. ACCa tumors are composed of ductal epithelial and myoepithelial cells. Architecturally, ACCa has 3 types, including solid, cribriform, and tubular, with cribriform the most common. ACCa can show distant metastasis as well as nodal metastasis.

On imaging, ACCa is intermediate to low signal on both T1 and T2. ACCa tumors enhance, and thickening and enhancement of CN V and/or CN VII raise concern for perineural tumor growth. **Fig. 5** shows a right parotid lesion in an 82-year-old woman who presented with facial weakness. The tumor is low/intermediate on T1 (see **Fig. 5**C) and enhancing (see **Fig. 5**B). Although T2 bright on fluid-sensitive sequences (see **Fig. 5**A), these tumors can have intermediate signal, as well. Subtle although true asymmetric enhancement of CN VII was positive at histology

for perineural tumor spread of ACCa. Lower-grade tumors often have better defined margins and high-grade tumors are generally more infiltrative on imaging. Histologically, they most commonly have 6q22-23 translocations, although they can also have 8q13 translocations.[8]

Mucoepidermoid Carcinoma

MEC is the most common salivary gland malignancy in both adults and children.[29] MEC originates from the epithelium of the salivary gland ducts and consist of a mixture of mucus-secreting cells, epidermoid cells, and intermediate cells. There can be cystic components and there is variability in the appearance of these tumors at pathology. MEC tumors are assigned a grade of low, intermediate, or high, based on features, such as necrosis, frequency of mitoses, and anaplasia. MEC metastasizes to lymph nodes and can show perineural tumor growth (although less frequently than ACCa).

On imaging, low-grade tumors may have a more circumscribed margin and higher-grade tumors may appear more infiltrative, ill-defined, and aggressive. MEC often demonstrates low to intermediate signal on both T1 and T2 imaging with cystic components appearing more T2

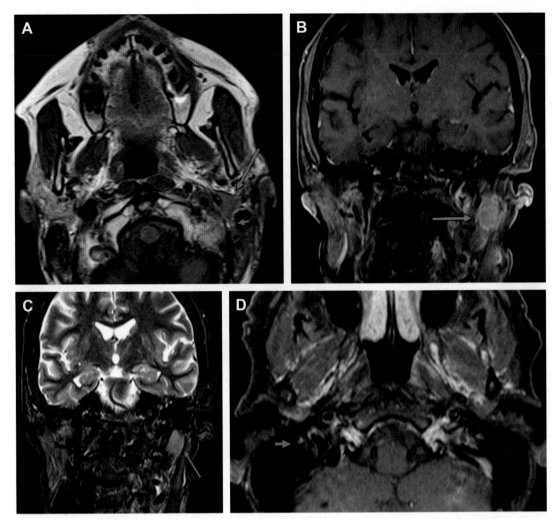

Fig. 4. Acinic cell carcinoma of the left parotid (*long arrows*) in a 56-year-old woman with facial swelling. Precontrast T1 axial shows a deep left parotid lobe lesion with intermediate to low T1 signal (*A*). Note the tail of tissue extending posteriorly toward the stylomastoid foramen (*short arrow, A*). Coronal postcontrast (*B*) shows uniform enhancement and slightly hyperintense T2/STIR (*C*) signal on coronal fluid-sensitive sequences. Note the asymmetric enhancement at the mastoid segment of the right facial nerve (*short arrow, D*).

hyperintense, as shown in **Fig. 6**—a 73-year-old man who presented with palpable right-sided neck mass. Low to intermediate on T1 (see **Fig. 6A**) and uniformly enhancing (see **Fig. 6B**),

The MEC showed relatively lower signal on coronal STIR (see **Fig. 6C**). The presence of ipsilateral enlarged nodes (see **Fig. 6C**) helped direct the differential to MEC over other neoplasms.

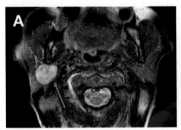
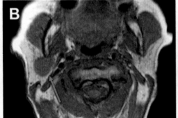
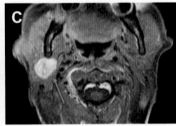

Fig. 5. ACCa of the right parotid in an 82-year-old woman. Axial T2 fat-saturated image (*A*) shows a slightly hyperintense lesion, precontrast T1 image (*B*) shows hypointense signal, and T1 with contrast fat-saturated image (*C*) shows homogenous enhancement (*long arrows*).

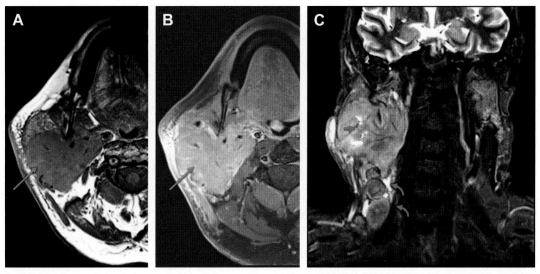

Fig. 6. Large MEC of the right parotid in a 73-year-old man who presented with slowly increasing neck masses. T1 hypointense on precontrast (*A*) and uniformly enhancing on T1 postcontrast (*B*) right parotid mass (*long arrows*) on initial scan. It had an almost stellate appearance on coronal STIR (*short arrow, C*) which raised concern for on-cocytoma. Ipsilateral enlarged and metastatic nodes (*curved arrows, C*) helped cement the diagnosis as a parotid malignancy, MEC, with ipsilateral lymphadenopathy.

Mammary Analog Secretory Carcinoma

Mammary analog secretory carcinoma is a new addition to the WHO classification and is characterized by a gene translocation, ETV6-NTRK3. These nonaggressive tumors may have previously been misdiagnosed as nonparotid acinic cell carcinomas.[28]

Lymphoma

Lymphoma can involve the salivary glands. This is true for all of the major salivary glands, including the parotid gland, which has intraglandular lymph nodes. Lymphoma in the salivary glands can be primary or secondary. Primary lymphomas of the salivary glands are often infiltrative and enlarge the glands diffusely, as shown in **Fig. 7**—CT in an 85-year-old woman who presented with constitutional symptoms and a left parotid mass. The bilateral nodal involvement helped narrow the differential in this case. Secondary lymphomas can have this appearance as well or present as enlarged lymph nodes in the parotid glands.

Metastasis to Intraparotid Lymph Nodes

The parotid gland is the only salivary gland that contains lymph nodes within the gland itself. These nodes are seen in normal patients, although they also serve as the primary drainage site for skin malignancies of the upper face, ear, and scalp. Common skin malignancies to metastasize to the parotid lymph nodes include squamous cell carcinomas and melanomas. These typically manifest with lymph node enlargement in a parotid gland on the side of the primary skin malignancy.

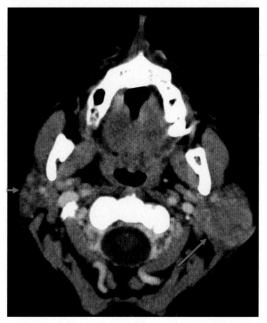

Fig. 7. Lymphoma, especially diffuse large B-cell variants, must be considered in the setting of enlarged parotid lymph nodes, especially with contralateral involvement (and systemic adenopathy, not shown). This 85-year-old woman presented with constitutional symptoms and a dominant left parotid mass (*long arrow*) with smaller contralateral intraparotid nodes (*short arrow*).

Parotid lymph nodes can also serve as the site of metastasis for systemic malignancies from other organs, such as kidney, breast, and lung. **Fig. 8** shows a case of osseous, parotid, and CN V (mandibular) lesions identified on a PET-CT for breast cancer staging. This 72-year-old woman had an FDG-avid palpable mass (a small left superficial lobe parotid nodule) and facial numbness under her chin due to tumor involvement on the mandibular division of CN V.

As with lymph node metastasis elsewhere, enlarged intraparotid lymph nodes or lymph nodes that are growing over time are a suspicious finding, particularly in patients with skin malignancies of the face, ear, and scalp. The nodes are often hypointense on T1 and intermediate to hyperintense on T2. They are most conspicuous on precontrast T1 sequences and on enhanced CT, where they contrast well with the fat in the parotid gland. Involved lymph nodes can become necrotic, demonstrating heterogeneity and areas of nonenhancement centrally, as can be seen elsewhere in the head and neck. PET-CT can be used to determine if nodes are involved, even those without suspicious morphologic features by CT assessment.[30,31]

Other Considerations

Hyperenhancement and/or enlargement in a salivary gland is not always a marker of malignancy. **Fig. 9** shows treatment-related changes from prior glossectomy and neck dissections for oral cavity squamous cell carcinoma. This 35-year-old man was treated with radiation; note the enlarged and hyperenhancing left sublingual gland, indicative of radiation-related inflammation. **Fig. 10** shows a complicated case of high-grade salivary ductal carcinoma in a 78-year-old man who had long-standing facial paralysis. The precontrast T1 image (see **Fig. 10**A) shows a T1 hypointense mass infiltrating the superficial and deep parotid lobes in the expected region of the auriculotemporal nerve. There was perineural spread of tumor from CN VII to CN V with spread intracranially through foramen ovale (mandibular CN V). There was also spread peripherally, with FDG-avid tissue along the pterygomaxillary fissure. Perineural spread of tumor can be central (toward the brain), peripheral (toward the end organ), or both, as in this unfortunate case.

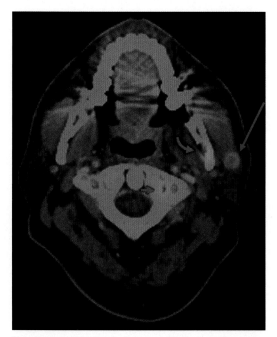

Fig. 8. Parotid glands have multiple lymph nodes; thus, metastatic disease can present with cheek swelling or facial numbness/pain as in this case. FDG-avid metastatic parotid nodule from breast cancer in a 72-year-old woman (*long arrow*). Note the adjacent involvement in the mandible, along the inferior alveolar nerve (*curved arrow*). Additional osseous lesions were also present (*short arrow*).

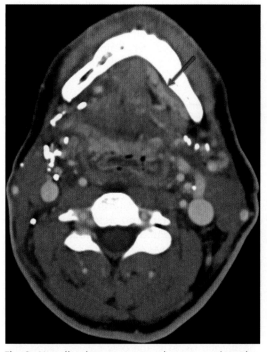

Fig. 9. Not all enlargement or enhancement is pathologic. Note the enlarged and hyperenhancing left sublingual gland (*arrow*) in a 35-year-old man with prior hemiglossectomy, bilateral neck dissections, chemotherapy, and radiation for oral cavity squamous cell carcinoma. Findings were related to treatment (radiation)-induced inflammation.

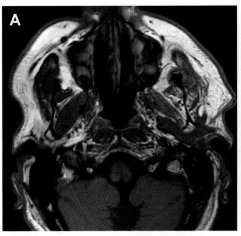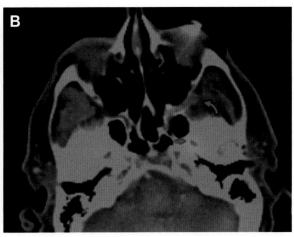

Fig. 10. Parotid malignancies often have an impact on facial nerve function (note the left eyelid gold weight). The trigeminal nerve can also be affected via anastomotic connections. This T1 hypointense mass (*long arrow, A*) insinuates along the expected path of the auriculotemporal nerve (connecting CN V and CN VII). FDG PET-CT showed avidity in the left foramen ovale (*short arrow, B*), pterygopalatine fossa, and pterygomaxillary fissure (*curved arrow, B*). This 78-year-old man also had direct brain parenchymal invasion (not shown) and was initially described as an "atypical schwannoma."

SUMMARY

Salivary gland malignancies represent a wide range of tumors from the indolent to the aggressive. The smaller the gland, the higher the malignant risk with (up to) 90% of sublingual gland tumors malignant. The most common location for a malignant tumor is the parotid gland because there are so many more parotid tumors overall. Patients may present with localized swelling, facial pain (suggesting trigeminal involvement), or facial paralysis (suggesting facial nerve involvement). CT and MR imaging both offer benefit in evaluating the extent of these tumors, although full staging (according to AJCC) may require additional imaging modalities.

REFERENCES

1. Guzzo M, Locati LD, Prott FJ, et al. Major and minor salivary gland tumors. Crit Rev Oncol Hematol 2010; 74(2):134–47.

2. Schramm VL Jr, Imola MJ. Management of nasopharyngeal salivary gland malignancy. Laryngoscope 2001;111(9):1533–44.

3. Eveson JW, Cawson RA. Salivary gland tumours. A review of 2410 cases with particular reference to histological types, site, age and sex distribution. J Pathol 1985;146(1):51–8.

4. Spiro RH. Salivary neoplasms: overview of a 35-year experience with 2,807 patients. Head Neck Surg 1986;8:177–84.

5. Batsakis JG, editor. Tumours of the head and neck. Clinical and pathological considerations. 2nd edition. London: Williams & Wilkins; 1982.

6. Boukheris H, Curtis RE, Land CE, et al. Incidence of carcinoma of the major salivary glands according to the WHO Classification, 1992 to 2006: a population-based study in the United States. Cancer Epidemiol Biomarkers Prev 2009;18(11):2899–906.

7. Barnes L, Eveson JW, Reichart P, et al, editors. Tumours of the salivary glands. Pathology and genetics of head and neck tumours. Lyon (France): World Health Organization; 2005.

8. Seethala RR, Stenman G. Update from the 4th edition of the World Health Organization classification of head and neck tumours: tumors of the salivary gland. Head Neck Pathol 2017;11(1):55–67.

9. Amin MB, Edge SB, Greene FL, et al, editors. AJCC cancer staging manual. 8th edition. New York: Springer; 2017.

10. Lee YY, Wong KT, King AD, et al. Imaging of salivary gland tumours. Eur J Radiol 2008;66(3):419–36.

11. Vogl TJ, Schulz B, Bauer RW, et al. Dual-energy CT applications in head and neck imaging. AJR Am J Roentgenol 2012;199:34–9.

12. Weon YC, Park SW, Kim HJ, et al. Salivary duct carcinomas: clinical and CT and MR imaging features in 20 patients. Neuroradiology 2012;54(6):631–40.

13. Tawfik AM, Michael Bucher A, Vogl TJ. Dual-energy computed tomography applications for the evaluation of cervical lymphadenopathy. Neuroimaging Clin N Am 2017;27(3):461–8.

14. Chawla A, Srinivasan S, Lim TC, et al. Dual-energy CT applications in salivary gland lesions. Br J Radiol 2017;90(1074):20160859.

15. Christe A, Waldherr C, Hallett R, et al. MR imaging of parotid tumors: typical lesion characteristics in MR imaging improve discrimination between benign

and malignant disease. AJNR Am J Neuroradiol 2011;32(7):1202–7.

16. Kato H, Kanematsu M, Makita H, et al. CT and MR imaging findings of palatal tumors. Eur J Radiol 2014;83(3):e137–46.

17. Gebarski SS, Telian SA, Niparko JK. Enhancement along the normal facial nerve in the facial canal: MR imaging and anatomic correlation. Radiology 1992;183(2):391–4.

18. Kuno H, Onaya H, Fujii S, et al. Primary staging of laryngeal and hypopharyngeal cancer: CT, MR imaging and dual energy CT. Eur J Radiol 2014;83(1):e23–35.

19. Yabuuchi H, Matsuo Y, Kamitani T, et al. Parotid gland tumors: can addition of diffusion-weighted MR imaging to dynamic contrast-enhanced MR imaging improve diagnostic accuracy in characterization? Radiology 2008;249:909–16.

20. Matsuzaki H, Yanagi Y, Hara M, et al. Minor salivary gland tumors in the oral cavity: diagnostic value of dynamic contrast-enhanced MRI. Eur J Radiol 2012;81:2684–91.

21. Aghaghazvini L, Salahshour F, Yazdani N, et al. Dynamic contrast-enhanced MRI for differentiation of major salivary glands neoplasms, a 3-T MRI study. Dentomaxillofac Radiol 2015;44(2). 20140166.

22. Eida S, Sumi M, Nakamura T. Multiparametric magnetic resonance imaging for the differentiation between benign and malignant salivary gland tumors. J Magn Reson Imaging 2010;31:673–9.

23. Hisatomi M, Asaumi J, Yanagi Y, et al. Diagnostic value of dynamic contrast-enhanced MRI in the salivary gland tumors. Oral Oncol 2007;43(9):940–7.

24. Seo YL, Yoon DY, Baek S, et al. Incidental focal FDG uptake in the parotid glands on PET/CT in patients with head and neck malignancy. Eur Radiol 2015; 25(1):171–7.

25. Seethala RR, Johnson JT, Barnes EL, et al. Polymorphous low-grade adenocarcinoma: the University of Pittsburgh experience. Arch Otolaryngol Head Neck Surg 2010;136(4):385–92.

26. Castle JT, Thompson LD, Frommelt RA, et al. Polymorphous low grade adenocarcinoma: a clinicopathologic study of 164 cases. Cancer 1999;86(2): 207–19.

27. Seifert G. Histopathology of malignant salivary gland tumours. Eur J Cancer B Oral Oncol 1992; 28:49–56.

28. Bishop JA, Yonescu R, Batista D, et al. Most nonparotid "acinic cell carcinomas" represent mammary analog secretory carcinomas. Am J Surg Pathol 2013;37(7):1053–7.

29. Jones AV, Craig GT, Speight PM, et al. The range and demographics of salivary gland tumours diagnosed in a UK population. Oral Oncol 2008;44(4): 407–17.

30. Razfar A, Heron DE, Branstetter BF, et al. Positron emission tomography-computed tomography adds to the management of salivary gland malignancies. Laryngoscope 2010;120:734–8.

31. Lee SK, Rho BH, Won KS. Parotid incidentaloma identified by combined 18F-fluorodeoxyglucose whole-body positron emission tomography and computed tomography: findings at grayscale and power Doppler ultrasonography and ultrasound-guided fine-needle aspiration biopsy or core-needle biopsy. Eur Radiol 2009;19(9): 2268–74.

Imaging of Sjögren Syndrome and Immunoglobulin G4-Related Disease of the Salivary Glands

Akifumi Fujita, MD, PhD

KEYWORDS

- Sjögren syndrome • Immunoglobulin G4-related disease • Salivary glands • Autoimmune disease
- CT • MR imaging

KEY POINTS

- MR imaging of chronic Sjögren syndrome shows a salt-and-pepper appearance of the parotid gland, and atrophy of the submandibular glands can be commonly detected incidentally with computed tomography and MR imaging in daily clinical practice.
- MR sialography can be replaced with conventional invasive sialography and is useful for grading Sjögren syndrome.
- Immunoglobulin G4-related disease (IgG4-RD) is a recently established disease that commonly shows involvement of the salivary glands. Mikulicz disease, Küttner tumor, and some inflammatory pseudotumors of the orbit are now considered to represent IgG4-RD.
- Bilateral symmetric diffuse swelling of the salivary glands (parotid, submandibular, and sublingual) and lacrimal glands is the classic finding of IgG4-RD.
- Isolated lesions of IgG4-RD are difficult to differentiate from tumors, especially malignant lymphoma, and usually require histopathological biopsy.

INTRODUCTION

Although salivary gland pathologic complications are relatively uncommon overall, the salivary glands are commonly affected in systemic autoimmune disease and diseases of unknown pathogenesis.[1,2] Bilateral symmetric involvement of multiple major salivary glands can easily result in suspicion of systemic disease; however, isolated salivary gland lesions often need to be differentiated from tumors, including malignancies. Imaging findings of salivary gland involvement in systemic disease is usually nonspecific; however, radiologists should be familiar with the clinical and imaging manifestations to avoid delays in diagnosis. Sjögren syndrome (SjS) is the most well-known autoimmune disease of the salivary glands, which can be affected both primarily and secondarily with other systemic diseases. Immunoglobulin (Ig)G4-related disease (IgG4-RD) is a recently introduced systemic inflammatory disease, now also considered an autoimmune disorder, that commonly affects salivary glands, as well as the pancreas, kidneys, lacrimal glands, and retroperitoneal periaortic lesions. This article discusses the details of SjS and IgG4-RD.

SJÖGREN SYNDROME
Background

SjS is a relatively common systemic autoimmune disease that is histologically characterized by

Disclosure Statement: The author has nothing to disclose.
Department of Radiology, Jichi Medical University School of Medicine, 3311-1, Yakushiji, Shimotsuke, Tochigi 329-0498, Japan
E-mail address: akifuji@jichi.ac.jp

Neuroimag Clin N Am 28 (2018) 183–197
https://doi.org/10.1016/j.nic.2018.01.003

lymphocytic infiltration and destruction of the salivary and lacrimal glands, leading to secretory dysfunction. Sicca syndrome is the term for the resulting dryness of the mouth and eyes. SjS is referred to as primary in patients who do not have any additional systemic disease, and secondary when sicca syndrome coexists in patients with other systemic diseases such as systemic lupus erythematosus, scleroderma, and rheumatoid arthritis, or other organ-specific autoimmune diseases such as Graves disease and Hashimoto thyroiditis. The diagnosis of SjS is often delayed for years after symptom onset owing to underestimation of the significance of sicca symptoms.[3–5]

Because cross-sectional imaging techniques such as ultrasonography (US), computed tomography (CT), and MR imaging now play an important role in daily clinical practice, radiologists may come across various imaging manifestations of SjS incidentally.[6–8] Although imaging results are not included in the diagnostic criteria and are not necessary for diagnosis, radiologists should be familiar with the imaging findings of SjS to avoid delaying the diagnosis. In particular, radiologists should be aware of associations with acute inflammation and secondary lymphoma in SjS patients.

Pathogenesis

The pathogenesis remains incompletely clarified; however, SjS is considered an autoimmune systemic disease. The characteristic lymphocytic infiltrates were initially observed to be proximal to salivary gland epithelial cells, which were subsequently shown to express numerous immunomodulatory molecules, such as cytokines, chemokines, adhesion molecules, and apoptosis-related molecules, as well as autoantigens and functional innate immunity receptors. Salivary gland epithelial cells seem to be able to function as professional antigen-presenting cells and to mediate the exposure of intracellular autoantigens to the immune system. Salivary glands are sites of autoantigen presentation and initiation of the autoimmune response in SjS.

Histopathology

SjS is characterized by lymphocytic infiltration of the exocrine glands, primarily the salivary and lacrimal glands. The principal pathologic lesion in SjS is focal lymphocytic sialadenitis, predominantly consisting of CD4-positive T cells and CD20-positive B cells, in the salivary glands. Analogous lesions may occur in the lacrimal glands. In the absence of SjS-associated serum autoantibodies, a positive labial salivary gland biopsy is a mandatory criterion for the classification of SjS.

Clinical Manifestations

Sicca syndrome and glandular enlargement represent the 2 major symptoms of SjS and are seen in more than 80% of patients at the time of diagnosis. Other systemic manifestations may also be seen, such as articular, cutaneous, Raynaud phenomenon, pulmonary, nervous system, renal, genitourinary, and hematologic findings.[3–5] The greatest concern for SjS patients is that SjS carries a substantially increased risk for the development of non-Hodgkin lymphoma.[4]

In the early phase, the parotid glands are diffusely enlarged with normal parenchyma (stage 0). In the intermediate phase, the salivary glands are diffusely enlarged with multiple, scattered cysts and solid masses. These cysts range in size from less than 1 mm (microcysts) to macrocysts and mixed solid-cystic masses of more than 2 cm (stage I–III). In the chronic phase, atrophy of the glands becomes evident (stage IV).[2]

Diagnostic Criteria

Several diagnostic classification criteria for SjS have been described by organizations in different countries[9,10]; however, none have been validated or universally accepted. **Box 1** shows the classification criteria recently described by the American College of Rheumatology.[11]

Imaging Modality for Diagnosis

Typically, histopathological examination of the labial gland is considered as the most promising method of diagnosis for SjS. Imaging is still not included in the diagnostic classification criteria; however, various imaging modalities have been recognized as useful for diagnosing and grading SjS. Because the subjective complaints of patients with xerostomia do not necessarily reflect salivary gland disease, more objective and reliable methods are necessary. Until the 1980s, conventional radiographic sialography and radionuclide scintigraphy were the typical imaging methods used for diagnosing SjS.[12] However, these examinations are invasive and require exposure to radiation. Recent noninvasive imaging modalities such as US and MR imaging, including MR sialography, might offer advantages for the diagnosis and management of SjS patients.

MR Imaging

In the early 1990s, Takashima and colleagues[13] compared MR imaging findings with the results of conventional sialography and histopathological examination. They reported heterogeneous signals on both T1-weighted and T2-weighted

---

Box 1
American College of Rheumatology 2012 classification criteria for Sjögren syndrome

The classification of SjS, which applies to individuals with signs or symptoms that may be suggestive of SjS, will be met in patients who have at least 2 of the following 3 objective features:

1. Positive serum anti-SSA/Ro antibody and/or anti-SSB/La antibody, or (positive rheumatoid factor and ANA ≥1:320)

2. Labial salivary gland biopsy exhibiting focal lymphocytic sialadenitis, with a focus score equal to or greater than 1 focus/4 mm^2, as assessed and defined in 2011 by Daniels and colleagues[60]

3. Keratoconjunctivitis sicca with ocular staining score equal to or greater than 3, as described in 2009 by Whitcher and colleagues[61], assuming that the individual is not currently using daily eye drops for glaucoma and has not had corneal surgery or cosmetic eyelid surgery in the last 5 years

Prior diagnosis of any of the following conditions would exclude participation in SjS studies of therapeutic trials because of overlapping clinical features of interference with criteria tests:

- History of head and neck radiations treatment
- Hepatitis C infection
- Acquired immunodeficiency syndrome
- Sarcoidosis
- Amyloidosis
- Graft-versus-host disease
- IgG4-related disease

Abbreviations: ANA; antinuclear antibodies; SS, Sjögren's syndrome.
Adapted from Rischmueller M, Tieu J, Lester S. Primary sjogren's syndrome. Best Pract Res Clin Rheumatol 2016;30(1):189–220; with permission.

---

images in SjS patients, which they termed a salt-and-pepper appearance (**Fig. 1**). Pathologically focal lymphocytic aggregates associated with increased interlobular fibrosis were considered responsible for the hypointense foci and decreased intensity ratio on T2-weighted images. Radiologists also often encounter severe atrophy of bilateral submandibular glands in SjS patients (**Fig. 2**). Whereas the salt-and-pepper appearance is seen in late-stage SjS patients, Izumi and colleagues[14] reported that quantitative analysis of conventional MR imaging can detect early-stage SjS among apparently normal subjects. They measured the standard deviation of signal intensity on T1-weighted images and found that SjS patients show reduced homogeneity of the parotid gland compared with normal subjects. They concluded that this quantitative method has potential for grading SjS. Another study by Izumi and colleagues[15] suggested that monitoring fat deposition might be useful for diagnosing SjS and assessing progression in patients with clinical and serologic findings suggestive of the disease.

MR hydrography is a method that uses a heavily T2-weighted sequence to enhance the fluid water content, providing a promising method for depicting the pancreaticobiliary system, urinary tract, inner ear, and cerebrospinal fluid system. This modality seems as useful for imaging the salivary duct system as MR sialography is. Although conventional radiographic sialography is considered the reference standard for imaging diagnosis of SjS, several studies have reported that MR sialography may replace the much more invasive conventional sialography.[16–19] Several studies have proposed MR sialographic staging of SjS according to the conventional sialographic criteria reported by Rubin and colleagues[12] (**Box 2; Figs. 3–5**).[18,19] The author prefers and recommends the double-echo steady state with water excitation sequence (DESS-WE) for salivary gland imaging because this method can clearly demonstrate both salivary ducts and nerves as areas of signal hyperintensity.[20,21]

Recent studies on the feasibility of diffusion-weighted imaging (DWI) in various diseases affecting the parotid glands have revealed promising results. The apparent diffusion coefficient (ADC) is used to quantify DWI and has been used to depict early cellular tissue damage. The ADC of the parotid glands in SjS correlates well with the salivary flow rate. The ADC of the salivary glands is increased in the early stages but becomes markedly decreased in the advanced stage.[22,23] Takagi and colleagues[24] reported

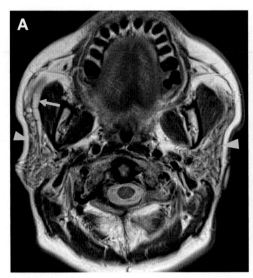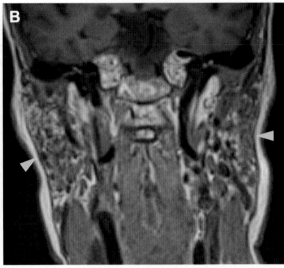

Fig. 1. Stage III SjS. (A) Axial T2WI. (B) Coronal T1WI. MRI demonstrates heterogeneous internal signal intensity of bilateral parotid glands on both T2WI and T1WI (arrowheads). Note the dilated parotid duct on the right on T2WI (arrow). This represents a case of Stage III SjS.

quantitative MR imaging using T1-weighted and fat-suppressed T2-weighted imaging using a microscopy coil to differentiate subjects with SjS from other subjects, and proposed criteria for imaging and staging SjS. Several studies have reported the usefulness of DWI for assessing SjS.[22,23,25] Kato and colleagues[26] reported that DWI may play an important role in detecting secondary lymphoma arising from SjS because of the restricted diffusion of water molecules in this pathologic state. Several other advanced imaging modalities are available, such as spin-lattice

relaxation time in the rotating frame (T1ρ) MR imaging and arterial spin-labeling perfusion imaging, and may have the potential to provide additional information for SjS.[27,28]

Ultrasound

Because US is noninvasive, inexpensive, and does not require exposure to radiation, recent studies have proposed US as a feasible alternative imaging modality to conventional sialography or scintigraphy for assessing SjS.[29,30] The characteristic

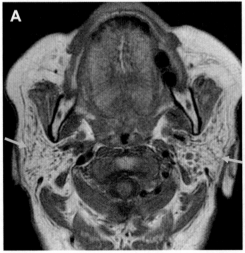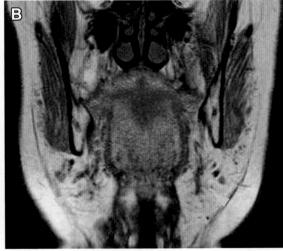

Fig. 2. Stage IV SjS. (A) Axial T1WI. (B) Coronal T1WI. MRI demonstrates diffuse fatty replacement of bilateral parotid glands with multiple nodular and linear areas of low intensity (arrows). Coronal T1WI shows severe atrophy of bilateral submandibular glands (arrowheads), as commonly seen in stage IV SjS.

Box 2
Staging with imaging findings of Sjögren syndrome

Conventional sialographic staging[12]

Stage 0: normal, no contrast material collection (no evidence of SjS)

Stage I: punctate, contrast material collection 1 mm in diameter or smaller

Stage II: globular, contrast material collection 1 to 2 mm in diameter

Stage III: cavitary, contrast material collection 2 mm in diameter or larger

Stage IV: destructive, complete destruction of the gland parenchyma

MR sialographic staging[18,19]

Stage 0: normal, homogeneous parenchymal signal intensity (no evidence of SjS)

Stage I: punctate, high-signal-intensity area 1 mm in diameter or smaller

Stage II: globular, high-signal-intensity area 1 to 2 mm in diameter

Stage III: cavitary, high-signal-intensity area 2 mm in diameter or larger

Stage IV: destructive, complete destruction of the gland parenchyma

for categorizing parotid lesions and predicting malignancy.[31]

Computed Tomography

Specific CT findings of SjS are heterogeneity, abnormal diffuse fat deposition, and diffuse punctate calcification (**Figs. 6 and 7**).[32] The author also often sees severe atrophy of bilateral submandibular glands in SjS patients. CT is not a primary imaging modality for diagnosing SjS; however, because this modality is heavily used in daily clinical practice for assessing diseases of the head and neck, radiologists should be familiar with the CT findings of SjS.

Radionuclide Scintigraphy

Salivary gland scintigraphy remains the gold standard for assessing salivary function. However, because bilateral decreased uptake and delayed excretion may be seen in patients with other systemic connective tissue disease, scintigraphic findings are not pathognomonic for SjS. 18F-Fluorodeoxyglucose (FDG) PET typically shows high tracer localization in the salivary glands in SjS.[33]

Secondary Lymphoma Associated with Sjögren Syndrome

SjS is considered as a risk factor for the development of malignant lymphoma. Salivary glands and ocular adnexa are the most common sites for secondary lymphoma with SjS. Various histologic subtypes of lymphoma have been described in patients with SjS; however, mucoid-associated lymphoid tissue (MALT) lymphoma is the most common.[34] Imaging findings for lymphoma of the salivary glands have been described as localized nodular or diffuse infiltrative lesions (see **Fig. 7**; **Fig. 8**). The nodular lesions are difficult to differentiate from intraparotid reactive lymphadenopathy.

US findings for gland involvement in SjS are hypoechoic spots and/or areas and hyperechoic streaks. Because US is easy to use in daily clinical practice, salivary gland US can be used as a primary imaging tool for the diagnosis and classification of SjS. The recently introduced parotid imaging reporting and data system (PIRADS) using US with power Doppler imaging offers a reliable noninvasive imaging modality that can be used

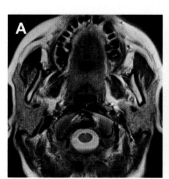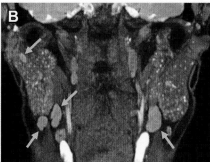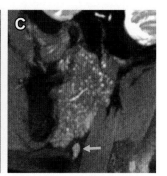

Fig. 3. Stage I SjS. (*A*) Axial T2WI. (*B*) Coronal DESS thin maximum intensity projection (MIP) image. (*C*) Sagittal DESS thin MIP image. Bilateral parotid glands look normal on T2WI. DESS images show multiple punctate areas of signal hyper-intensity (diameter, 1 mm), suggestive of stage I SjS. Lip biopsy confirmed the diagnosis. Note the multiple reactive swollen lymph nodes, including right intraparotid nodes (*arrows*).

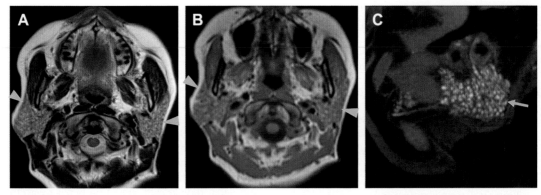

Fig. 4. Stage II SjS. (*A*) Axial T2WI. (*B*) Axial T1WI. (*C*) Sagittal DESS thin MIP image. MRI demonstrates heterogeneous signal intensity of bilateral parotid glands on both T2- and T1WI (*arrowheads*). DESS imaging shows globular areas of signal hyper-intensity (diameter, 1–2 mm), compatible with stage II SjS.

Nodular lesions are occasionally accompanied by multiple cystic foci that represent lymphoepithelial cysts within lymph nodes, salivary duct dilatation, or combinations of both (see **Fig. 8**; **Fig. 9**).[35] DWI or dynamic contrast-enhanced MR imaging has potential to detect secondary lymphoma in SjS patients.[35,36]

SUMMARY OF SJÖGREN SYNDROME

- Imaging findings of early-stage SjS are difficult to depict morphologically with routine CT or MR imaging. Analysis with advanced MR sequences has the potential to detect early-stage findings of SjS.
- MR imaging of chronic SjS shows a salt-and-pepper appearance of the parotid gland. Atrophy of the submandibular glands can be commonly detected incidentally with CT and MR imaging in daily clinical practice.

- MR sialography can be replaced with conventional invasive sialography and is useful for grading SjS.

IMMUNOGLOBULIN G4-RELATED DISEASE
Background

IgG4-RD is a chronic fibroinflammatory condition characterized by enlargement of the affected organs, elevated serum concentrations of IgG4, and infiltration of abundant IgG4-positive plasma cells into affected organs.[37–42] The concept of IgG4-RD has been developed and discussed based on the accumulation of evidence regarding autoimmune pancreatitis (AIP) with extrapancreatic lesions since 2002 when Hamano and colleagues[43,44] reported elevated serum concentrations of IgG4 in subjects with AIP in 2001 and the infiltration of IgG4-positive plasma cells into involved pancreatic and retroperitoneal tissues. Since then,

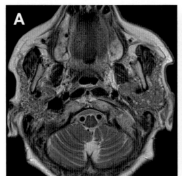
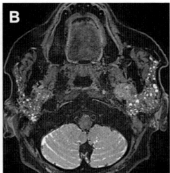
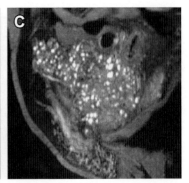

Fig. 5. Stage III SjS. (*A*) Axial T2WI. (*B*) Axial DESS image. (*C*) Sagittal DESS thin MIP image. T2WI demonstrates a heterogeneous signal with multiple small nodular regions of hyper-intensity in bilateral parotid glands. DESS images clearly show multiple globular to cavitary areas of signal hyper-intensity (diameter, >2 mm), compatible with stage III SjS.

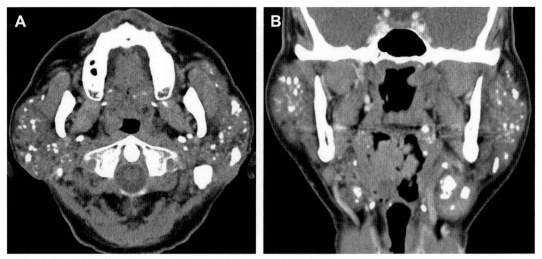

Fig. 6. Chronic SjS. (*A*) Axial contrast-enhanced CT. (*B*) Coronal contrast-enhanced CT. CT images demonstrate bilateral parotid gland swelling with multiple nodular and punctate calcifications. Calcifications are also noted within bilateral submandibular glands. This is a case of chronic SjS.

numerous reports on this novel entity have been published from Japan and, in 2011, 2 Japanese working groups made a joint proposal to unify the nomenclature as IgG4-RD, and suggested that IgG4-RD should include a wide variety of diseases, including Mikulicz disease, AIP, pituitary hypophysitis, Riedel thyroiditis, interstitial pneumonitis, interstitial nephritis, prostatitis, lymphadenopathy, retroperitoneal fibrosis, inflammatory aortic aneurysm, and inflammatory pseudotumor (**Box 3**).[45,46] This new disease entity and the nomenclature were accepted at an international symposium on IgG4-RD in the same year.[47] IgG4-RD is a multiorgan immune-mediated condition that mimics many malignant, infectious, and inflammatory disorders. The diagnosis links many conditions that were once regarded as isolated, single-organ diseases without any known underlying systemic conditions.[39,42]

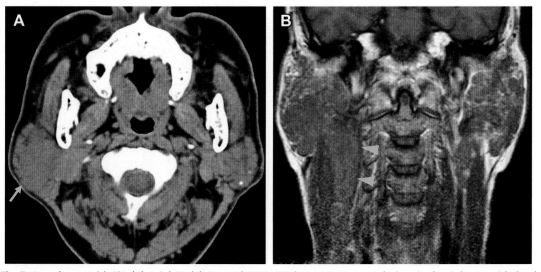

Fig. 7. Lymphoma with SjS. (*A*) Axial CT. (*B*) Coronal T1WI. CT demonstrates mass lesions in the right parotid gland (*arrows*), representing pathologically confirmed malignant lymphoma arising from SjS. Coronal T1WI shows associated lymph node swellings in the jugular chain (*arrowheads*). Note punctate calcification in the left parotid gland.

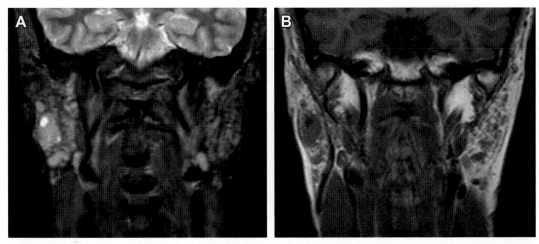

Fig. 8. Lymphoma with SjS. (*A*) Coronal short tau inversion recovery (STIR) imaging. (*B*) Coronal T1WI. MRI demonstrates multiple nodular lesions within bilateral parotid glands, suggesting lymphoepithelial lesions. A mass-like lesion with a cystic component is noted in the right parotid gland, compatible with lymphoepithelial cysts.

Pathogenesis

Although the pathophysiological mechanisms driving IgG4-RD remain unclear, an antigen-driven inflammatory condition or infection has been suggested, based on the features of this disease, including the chronic clinical course, effectiveness of steroid treatment, specific organ involvement, and common histopathological features shared by different unrelated organs. An elevated serum concentration of IgG4 is a distinctive feature of this disease. An immunologic response to an unknown antigen is postulated to drive mature plasma cell production of IgG4,

facilitated by cytokines secreted by activated type 2 helper T cells, which induce a prominent fibrotic reaction. Circulating B lymphocytes, particularly plasmablasts, may provide a biomarker of active disease and are increased in IgG4-RD.[48–50]

Histopathology

Tissue biopsy of the affected organ is the gold standard for diagnosing IgG4-RD, and the hallmarks of IgG4-RD include tissue infiltration by numerous IgG4-positive plasma cells. The 3 major pathologic features are lymphoplasmacytic

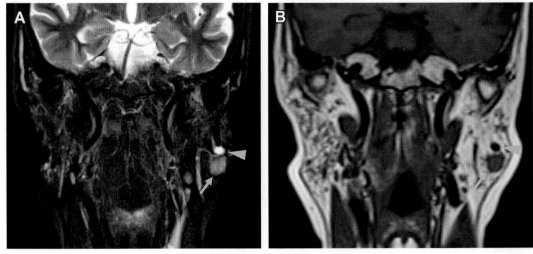

Fig. 9. Lymphoma with SjS. (*A*) Coronal STIR imaging. (*B*) Coronal T1WI. MRI demonstrates a nodular mass lesion in the left parotid tail (*arrows*), confirmed by biopsy as lymphoma. Note the lymphoepithelial cyst cranial to the mass lesion (*arrowheads*). Multiple punctate, nodular hyperintensities within the parotid glands suggest underlying SjS.

infiltration, fibrosis arranged at least focally in a storiform pattern, and obliterative phlebitis. In the head and neck region, submandibular gland or labial salivary gland biopsies are generally performed in cases with possible IgG4-RD to achieve accurate definitive and differential diagnoses.[37–39,42]

Clinical Manifestations

The head and neck region, particularly the salivary and lacrimal glands, is a common region for IgG4-RD involvement, along with the pancreas, kidneys, and retroperitoneum.[41,51] In the head and neck, IgG4-RD has been reported to involve not only the orbits but also the lacrimal glands, sinonasal cavity, temporal bone, perineurium of the V1 and V2 branches of the trigeminal nerve, larynx, thyroid glands, and cervical lymph nodes.[41,51–56]

Enlargement of both major and minor salivary glands is a common hallmark of IgG4-RD. A disorder known for Mikulicz disease, consisting of dacryoadenitis and enlargement of the lacrimal, parotid, and submandibular glands, is now recognized as a classic IgG4-RD.[40] The enlarged lacrimal and salivary glands in this condition have consistently been found to be elastic, painless, and persistent. Isolated enlargement of the submandibular glands is a common finding in IgG4-RD and was formerly known as Küttner tumor or chronic sclerosing sialadenitis. Although the submandibular glands are most frequently involved, the parotid, sublingual, and labial salivary glands may also be affected. In terms of gland function in patients with this disease, the flow of saliva is normal, or only slightly reduced, and improves with steroid treatment. Differentiation from lymphoma is important and usually requires histologic examination.

Diagnostic Criteria

The currently proposed diagnostic criteria include enlarged or hypertrophic organs, elevated serum levels of IgG4, and pathologic findings (**Box 4**). A definitive diagnosis requires all criteria to be met, whereas a probable diagnosis is considered when the clinical and histopathological criteria are met.[37,45] Serum concentrations of IgG4 are often elevated above 135 mg/dL, along with increased total IgG concentrations. Whether serum IgG4 levels offer an absolute marker of disease activity is not yet clear; however, these levels usually decrease after effective treatment and rise during relapses.

Imaging Modalities for Diagnosis

Because IgG4-RD frequently presents with organ enlargement and massive lesions, imaging can be helpful in diagnosing whether the component is malignant, and is usually used as the main modality for differential diagnosis. CT and MR imaging play an important role in depicting organ enlargement or tumor-like lesions.

Diffuse Multiglandular Disease

Diffuse enlargements of the parotid, submandibular, and sublingual glands are commonly seen manifestations of IgG4-RD of the salivary glands (**Fig. 10**). Bilateral lacrimal gland involvement is also associated with those patients (**Fig. 11**). Diffuse involvement is usually symmetric but some right-left differences can be seen.[48,49,55,56]

Localized Disease

Solitary mass-like lesions can be seen in the lacrimal and submandibular glands, which were formerly described as dacryoadenitis and chronic

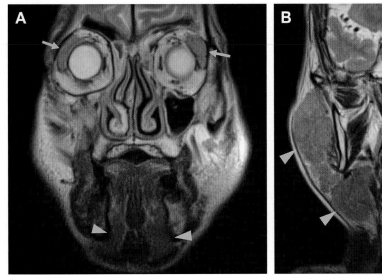

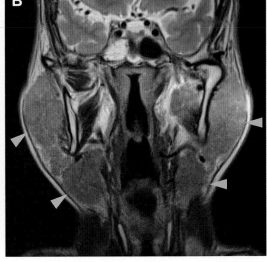

Fig. 10. Multiglandular IgG4-RD. (*A, B*) Coronal T2WI. Coronal T2WI demonstrates bilateral swelling of the lacrimal glands (*arrows*) associated with bilateral swelling of the parotid, submandibular, and sublingual glands (*arrowheads*). This represents a classic case of IgG4-RD.

sclerosing sialadenitis (Küttner tumor), respectively (**Fig. 12**).

MR Imaging

MR imaging can clearly demonstrate diffuse swelling of the salivary glands. Most lesions are well-defined and demonstrate relatively homogeneous signal intensity. T1-weighted and T2-weighted images demonstrate hypointense to isointense signals in the affected organs, and show homogeneous enhancement after injection of contrast medium; however, these findings are not specific for IgG4-RD (see **Figs. 10–12; Fig. 13**).[54–56] DWI usually shows mild ADC reduction, with the degree of this reduction depending on tissue cellularity and fibrosis, as well as signal intensity on T2-weighted images. Localized disease with these findings is distinguishable from malignancies, especially lymphoma.

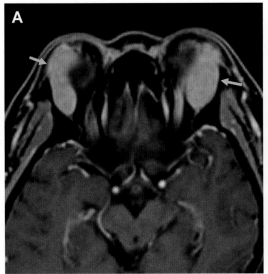

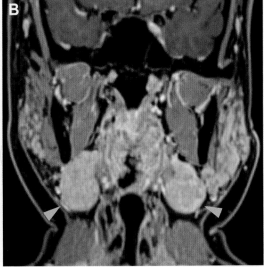

Fig. 11. Multiglandular IgG4-RD. (*A, B*) Coronal contrast-enhanced, fat-suppressed T1WI. Contrast-enhanced images demonstrate bilateral swelling of the lacrimal glands with marked enhancement (*arrows*) associated with bilateral swelling of the submandibular glands (*arrowheads*). Note the multiple nodular enhancement of bilateral parotid glands. This is another case of classic IgG4-RD.

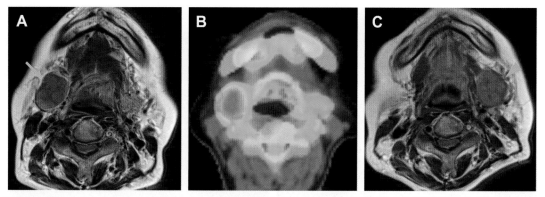

Fig. 12. Metachronal localized submandibular gland IgG4-RD. (*A*) Axial T2WI. (*B*) Axial T1WI. (*C*) Axial T2WI after 2 years. T2WI demonstrates swelling of the right submandibular gland (*arrow*), and PET-CT fusion images show marked uptake of FDG. Since cytology could not rule out the possibility of malignancy, surgical resection was performed and revealed IgG4-RD. Two years later, the patient returned with left submandibular gland swelling. T2WI shows the same findings as seen in the right submandibular gland lesion (*arrowhead*). Corticosteroid therapy was administered this time, and symptoms resolved.

Computed Tomography

CT can also be useful to demonstrate diffuse swelling of the salivary glands. CT is optimal for assessing osseous involvement; however, calcifications and associated stones are not noted in IgG4-RD of the salivary glands. Most lesions are well-defined and demonstrate relatively homogeneous attenuation. However, heterogeneous enhancement can be seen on CT (**Fig. 14**).[57]

Radionuclide Scintigraphy

Among patients with IgG4-RD with salivary gland involvement, associated extraglandular lesions are common, particularly in patients showing relapse. FDG PET-CT may be useful for evaluating systemic involvement of patients with IgG4-RD. This modality may also play an important role in evaluating response to corticosteroid treatment and targeting specific sites for biopsy (see **Figs. 12 and 13**).[52,58]

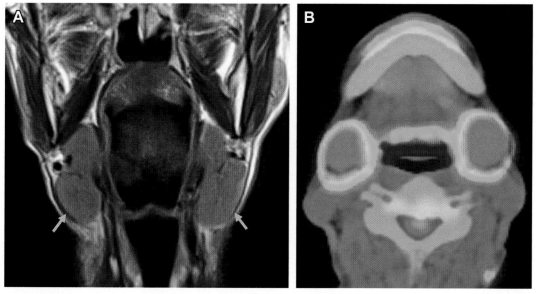

Fig. 13. Bilateral submandibular gland IgG4-RD. (*A*) Coronal T2WI. (*B*) Axial FDG PET-CT fusion image. Coronal T2WI demonstrates bilateral swelling of the submandibular glands (*arrows*). PET-CT fusion image shows marked uptake of FDG in the submandibular gland. This represents a case of pathologically confirmed IgG4-RD of bilateral submandibular glands.

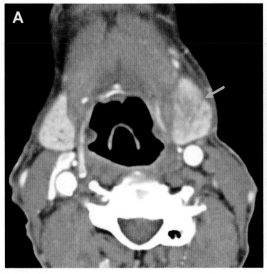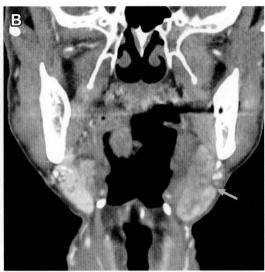

Fig. 14. Localized submandibular gland IgG4-RD. (*A, B*) Axial CT CT demonstrates swelling of the left submandibular gland (*arrows*), with internal signal heterogeneity. This is an isolated left submandibular lesion of IgG4-RD.

SUMMARY OF IMMUNOGLOBULIN G4-RELATED DISEASE

- IgG4-RD is a recently established disease that commonly shows involvement of the salivary glands.
- IgG4-RD typically shows both multiglandular and localized involvement, which is often difficult to differentiate from malignancies such as lymphoma or salivary gland carcinoma.
- Clinical findings, laboratory data, histopathological biopsy, and investigation of other commonly involved organs of IgG4-RD, may lead to early diagnosis.

DIFFERENTIAL DIAGNOSIS OF SALIVARY GLAND ENLARGEMENT

Salivary gland enlargement can be either bilateral multiglandular or localized. Both SjS and

IgG4-RD should be included in multiglandular disease. IgG4-RD is also an important differential diagnosis for localized disease (**Boxes 5** and **6**). Malignant diseases are considered among the differential diagnoses, particularly malignant lymphoma for multiglandular disease, and salivary gland carcinoma for localized disease.[48] Although the clinical distinction of SjS and IgG4-RD may be difficult, discriminating features also exist on histopathology and imaging. Involvement of sublingual glands or isolated involvement of the submandibular glands with sparing of the parotid glands is seen in IgG4-RD; however, this is uncommon in SjS. The glandular parenchyma in IgG4-RD usually appears homogeneous, in contrast to the heterogeneous appearance of SjS. MR sialography may help to differentiated IgG4-RD from SjS because IgG4-RD shows normal appearance on sialography, in contrast to SjS in which sialectasis is a typical feature.[59]

Box 5
Differential diagnosis of multiglandular salivary gland enlargement
SjS
IgG4-related disease (Mikulicz disease)
Malignant lymphoma
Sarcoidosis
HIV infection
Sialosis

Box 6
Differential diagnoses of localized salivary gland enlargement
Salivary gland benign tumor
Salivary gland carcinoma
Malignant lymphoma
IgG4-related disease (Küttner tumor)
Sialadenitis with sialolithiasis

REFERENCES

1. Hofauer B, Thuermel K, Gahleitner C, et al. Biomarkers in autoimmune salivary gland disorders: a review. ORL J Otorhinolaryngol Relat Spec 2017; 79(1–2):43–53.

2. Abdel Razek AA. Imaging of connective tissue diseases of the head and neck. Neuroradiol J 2016; 29(3):222–30.

3. Shiboski CH, Shiboski SC, Seror R, et al. 2016 American College of Rheumatology/European League Against Rheumatism classification criteria for primary Sjogren's syndrome: a consensus and data-driven methodology involving three international patient cohorts. Ann Rheum Dis 2017;76(1):9–16.

4. Rischmueller M, Tieu J, Lester S. Primary Sjogren's syndrome. Best Pract Res Clin Rheumatol 2016; 30(1):189–220.

5. Brito-Zeron P, Theander E, Baldini C, et al. Early diagnosis of primary Sjogren's syndrome: EULAR-SS task force clinical recommendations. Expert Rev Clin Immunol 2016;12(2):137–56.

6. Kojima I, Sakamoto M, Iikubo M, et al. Diagnostic performance of MR imaging of three major salivary glands for Sjogren's syndrome. Oral Dis 2017; 23(1):84–90.

7. Vogl TJ, Dresel SH, Grevers G, et al. Sjoegren's syndrome: MR imaging of the parotid gland. Eur Radiol 1996;6(1):46–51.

8. Spath M, Kruger K, Dresel S, et al. Magnetic resonance imaging of the parotid gland in patients with Sjogren's syndrome. J Rheumatol 1991;18(9): 1372–8.

9. Fujibayashi T, Sugai S, Miyasaka N, et al. Revised Japanese criteria for Sjogren's syndrome (1999): availability and validity. Mod Rheumatol 2004; 14(6):425–34.

10. Vitali C, Bombardieri S, Jonsson R, et al. Classification criteria for Sjogren's syndrome: a revised version of the European criteria proposed by the American-European Consensus Group. Ann Rheum Dis 2002;61(6):554–8.

11. Shiboski SC, Shiboski CH, Criswell L, et al. American College of Rheumatology classification criteria for Sjogren's syndrome: a data-driven, expert consensus approach in the Sjogren's International Collaborative Clinical Alliance cohort. Arthritis Care Res (Hoboken) 2012;64(4):475–87.

12. Rubin P, Holt JF. Secretory sialography in diseases of the major salivary glands. Am J Roentgenol Radium Ther Nucl Med 1957;77(4):575–98.

13. Takashima S, Takeuchi N, Morimoto S, et al. MR imaging of Sjogren syndrome: correlation with sialography and pathology. J Comput Assist Tomogr 1991;15(3):393–400.

14. Izumi M, Eguchi K, Ohki M, et al. MR imaging of the parotid gland in Sjogren's syndrome: a proposal for new diagnostic criteria. AJR Am J Roentgenol 1996; 166(6):1483–7.

15. Izumi M, Eguchi K, Nakamura H, et al. Premature fat deposition in the salivary glands associated with Sjogren syndrome: MR and CT evidence. AJNR Am J Neuroradiol 1997;18(5):951–8.

16. Tonami H, Higashi K, Matoba M, et al. A comparative study between MR sialography and salivary gland scintigraphy in the diagnosis of Sjogren syndrome. J Comput Assist Tomogr 2001;25(2):262–8.

17. Niemela RK, Paakko E, Suramo I, et al. Magnetic resonance imaging and magnetic resonance sialography of parotid glands in primary Sjogren's syndrome. Arthritis Rheum 2001;45(6):512–8.

18. Tonami H, Ogawa Y, Matoba M, et al. MR sialography in patients with Sjogren syndrome. AJNR Am J Neuroradiol 1998;19(7):1199–203.

19. Ohbayashi N, Yamada I, Yoshino N, et al. Sjogren syndrome: comparison of assessments with MR sialography and conventional sialography. Radiology 1998;209(3):683–8.

20. Fujii H, Fujita A, Yang A, et al. Visualization of the peripheral branches of the Mandibular division of the trigeminal nerve on 3D double-echo steady-state with water excitation sequence. AJNR Am J Neuroradiol 2015;36(7):1333–7.

21. Qin Y, Zhang J, Li P, et al. 3D double-echo steady-state with water excitation MR imaging of the intraparotid facial nerve at 1.5T: a pilot study. AJNR Am J Neuroradiol 2011;32(7):1167–72.

22. Regier M, Ries T, Arndt C, et al. Sjogren's syndrome of the parotid gland: value of diffusion-weighted echo-planar MRI for diagnosis at an early stage based on MR sialography grading in comparison with healthy volunteers. Rofo 2009; 181(3):242–8.

23. Sumi M, Takagi Y, Uetani M, et al. Diffusion-weighted echoplanar MR imaging of the salivary glands. AJR Am J Roentgenol 2002;178(4):959–65.

24. Takagi Y, Sumi M, Sumi T, et al. MR microscopy of the parotid glands in patients with Sjogren's syndrome: quantitative MR diagnostic criteria. AJNR Am J Neuroradiol 2005;26(5):1207–14.

25. Chu C, Zhou N, Zhang H, et al. Correlation between intravoxel incoherent motion MR parameters and MR nodular grade of parotid glands in patients with Sjogren's syndrome: a pilot study. Eur J Radiol 2017;86:241–7.

26. Kato H, Kanematsu M, Goto H, et al. Mucosa-associated lymphoid tissue lymphoma of the salivary glands: MR imaging findings including diffusion-weighted imaging. Eur J Radiol 2012;81(4):e612–7.

27. Kami YN, Sumi M, Takagi Y, et al. Arterial spin labeling imaging for the parotid glands of patients with Sjogren's syndrome. PLoS One 2016;11(3): e0150680.

28. Chu C, Zhou N, Zhang H, et al. Use of T1rhoMR imaging in Sjogren's syndrome with normal appearing parotid glands: initial findings. J Magn Reson Imaging 2017;45(4):1005–12.

29. Cornec D, Jousse-Joulin S, Marhadour T, et al. Salivary gland ultrasonography improves the diagnostic performance of the 2012 American College of Rheumatology classification criteria for Sjogren's syndrome. Rheumatology (Oxford) 2014;53(9): 1604–7.

30. Takagi Y, Kimura Y, Nakamura H, et al. Salivary gland ultrasonography: can it be an alternative to sialography as an imaging modality for Sjogren's syndrome? Ann Rheum Dis 2010;69(7):1321–4.

31. Abdel Razek AA, Ashmalla GA, Gaballa G, et al. Pilot study of ultrasound parotid imaging reporting and data system (PIRADS): Inter-observer agreement. Eur J Radiol 2015;84(12):2533–8.

32. Buch K, Nadgir RN, Fujita A, et al. Clinical associations of incidentally detected parotid gland calcification on CT. Laryngoscope 2015;125(6):1360–5.

33. Nishiyama Y, Yamamoto Y, Dobashi H, et al. Clinical value of 18F-fluorodeoxyglucose positron emission tomography in patients with connective tissue disease. Jpn J Radiol 2010;28(6):405–13.

34. Tonami H, Matoba M, Yokota H, et al. Mucosa-associated lymphoid tissue lymphoma in Sjogren's syndrome: initial and follow-up imaging features. AJR Am J Roentgenol 2002;179(2):485–9.

35. Kato H, Kanematsu M, Makita H, et al. CT and MR imaging findings of palatal tumors. Eur J Radiol 2014;83(3):e137–146.

36. Zhu L, Zhang C, Hua Y, et al. Dynamic contrast-enhanced MR in the diagnosis of lympho-associated benign and malignant lesions in the parotid gland. Dentomaxillofac Radiol 2016;45(4): 20150343.

37. Umehara H, Okazaki K, Nakamura T, et al. Current approach to the diagnosis of IgG4-related disease-combination of comprehensive diagnostic and organ-specific criteria. Mod Rheumatol 2017;27(3): 381–91.

38. Brito-Zeron P, Bosch X, Ramos-Casals M, et al. IgG4-related disease: advances in the diagnosis and treatment. Best Pract Res Clin Rheumatol 2016;30(2):261–78.

39. Kamisawa T, Zen Y, Pillai S, et al. IgG4-related disease. Lancet 2015;385(9976):1460–71.

40. Yamamoto M, Hashimoto M, Takahashi H, et al. IgG4 disease. J Neuroophthalmol 2014;34(4):393–9.

41. Bhatti RM, Stelow EB. IgG4-related disease of the head and neck. Adv Anat Pathol 2013;20(1):10–6.

42. Stone JH, Zen Y, Deshpande V. IgG4-related disease. N Engl J Med 2012;366(6):539–51.

43. Hamano H, Kawa S, Ochi Y, et al. Hydronephrosis associated with retroperitoneal fibrosis and sclerosing pancreatitis. Lancet 2002;359(9315):1403–4.

44. Hamano H, Kawa S, Horiuchi A, et al. High serum IgG4 concentrations in patients with sclerosing pancreatitis. N Engl J Med 2001;344(10):732–8.

45. Umehara H, Okazaki K, Masaki Y, et al. Comprehensive diagnostic criteria for IgG4-related disease (IgG4-RD), 2011. Mod Rheumatol 2012;22(1):21–30.

46. Umehara H, Okazaki K, Masaki Y, et al. A novel clinical entity, IgG4-related disease (IgG4RD): general concept and details. Mod Rheumatol 2012;22(1):1–14.

47. Stone JH, Khosroshahi A, Deshpande V, et al. Recommendations for the nomenclature of IgG4-related disease and its individual organ system manifestations. Arthritis Rheum 2012;64(10):3061–7.

48. Thompson A, Whyte A. Imaging of IgG4-related disease of the head and neck. Clin Radiol 2018;73(1): 106–20.

49. Takano K, Yamamoto M, Takahashi H, et al. Recent advances in knowledge regarding the head and neck manifestations of IgG4-related disease. Auris Nasus Larynx 2017;44(1):7–17.

50. Fragoulis GE, Zampeli E, Moutsopoulos HM. IgG4-related sialadenitis and Sjogren's syndrome. Oral Dis 2017;23(2):152–6.

51. Inoue D, Yoshida K, Yoneda N, et al. IgG4-related disease: dataset of 235 consecutive patients. Medicine (Baltimore) 2015;94(15):e680.

52. Tokue A, Higuchi T, Arisaka Y, et al. Role of F-18 FDG PET/CT in assessing IgG4-related disease with inflammation of head and neck glands. Ann Nucl Med 2015;29(6):499–505.

53. Tiegs-Heiden CA, Eckel LJ, Hunt CH, et al. Immunoglobulin G4-related disease of the orbit: imaging features in 27 patients. AJNR Am J Neuroradiol 2014;35(7):1393–7.

54. Toyoda K, Oba H, Kutomi K, et al. MR imaging of IgG4-related disease in the head and neck and brain. AJNR Am J Neuroradiol 2012;33(11):2136–9.

55. Katsura M, Mori H, Kunimatsu A, et al. Radiological features of IgG4-related disease in the head, neck, and brain. Neuroradiology 2012;54(8): 873–82.

56. Fujita A, Sakai O, Chapman MN, et al. IgG4-related disease of the head and neck: CT and MR imaging manifestations. Radiographics 2012; 32(7):1945–58.

57. Wang Z, Feng R, Chen Y, et al. CT features and pathologic characteristics of IgG4-related systemic disease of submandibular gland. Int J Clin Exp Pathol 2015;8(12):16111–6.

58. Nakatani K, Nakamoto Y, Togashi K. Utility of FDG PET/CT in IgG4-related systemic disease. Clin Radiol 2012;67(4):297–305.

59. Hong X, Li W, Xie XY, et al. Differential diagnosis of IgG4-related sialadenitis, primary Sjogren syndrome, and chronic obstructive submandibular sialadenitis. Br J Oral Maxillofac Surg 2017;55(2): 179–84.

60. Daniels TE, Cox D, Shiboski CH, et al. Associations between salivary gland histopathologic diagnoses and phenotypic features of Sjogren's syndrome among 1,726 registry participants. Arthritis Rheum 2011;63(7):2021–30.

61. Whitcher JP, Shiboski CH, Shiboski SC, et al. A simplified quantitative method for assessing keratoconjunctivitis sicca from the Sjogren's Syndrome International Registry. Am J Ophthalmol 2010; 149(3):405–15.

Imaging of Posttreatment Salivary Gland Tumors

Ahmed Abdel Khalek Abdel Razek, MD[a],*, Suresh K. Mukherji, MD, MBA[b]

KEYWORDS

• Postoperative • Postradiation • Parotid • Salivary • Recurrence • Malignancy

KEY POINTS

- Routine MR imaging is important for detecting the type of parotidectomy and reconstructive surgery for salivary gland tumors.
- Routine and advanced MR imaging, such as diffusion and perfusion MR imaging, is important for detection of locoregional recurrence of salivary glands cancer.
- 18F-Fluorodeoxyglucose–PET-computed tomography (CT) can detect distant metastasis and second cancer malignancy.
- Ultrasound and a routine CT scan are sufficient for the diagnosis of surgery-related complications of the salivary glands.
- Advanced MR imaging sequences can detect and quantify the radiation and radioactive iodine–induced sialadenitis.

INTRODUCTION

The treatment of choice of salivary tumors is surgery. Numerous surgical procedures are available to adequately treat tumors of salivary glands based on their biological aggressiveness. Radiotherapy is required in most patients with cancer of the salivary gland. Chemotherapy may be beneficial in certain tumor types.[1–8] MR imaging is the state-of-the-art imaging modality of choice in the evaluation of salivary glands after treatment.[6–8]

METHODS OF EXAMINATION
MR Imaging

MR imaging is superior to CT in detecting recurrent salivary tumors. Routine precontrast and postcontrast with diffusion-weighted MR imaging is the preferred modality for surveillance of salivary tumors after treatment. The T2 sequences provide the best signal discrimination. Enhanced fat-saturated T1 sequence is able to depict areas of enhancement.[6–8] Diffusion-weighted imaging is the most promising advanced magnetic resonance (MR) sequences that can be added to routine MR imaging.[9] Other advanced MR imaging methods, such as perfusion-weighted imaging, MR spectroscopy, and diffusion-tensor imaging, have a limited role and, proposed by some investigators, may be helpful in the assessment of recurrent head and neck cancer.[10–14]

Computed Tomography

A routine contrast CT scan may be used as a baseline study for detection of postoperative complications. Some recent studies have shown the diagnostic usefulness of 18F-fluorodeoxyglucose–PET (18-FDG-PET)/CT for posttreatment assessment of treated salivary gland tumors.[6–8] CT perfusion and dual-energy CT have a limited role in the assessment of patients with salivary gland tumors.[15,16]

[a] Department of Diagnostic Radiology, Mansoura University, Elgomheryia Street, Mansoura 35512, Egypt;
[b] Department of Radiology, Michigan State University, Michigan State University Health Team, 846 Service Road, East Lansing, MI 48824, USA
* Corresponding author.
E-mail address: arazek@mans.edu.eg

Neuroimag Clin N Am 28 (2018) 199–208
https://doi.org/10.1016/j.nic.2018.01.004
1052-5149/18/© 2018 Elsevier Inc. All rights reserved.

METHODS OF TREATMENT
Surgery

The treatment of choice for most salivary gland tumors is complete removal of the tumor with an adequate margin. Parotidectomy is considered a safer and more definitive procedure than parotid tumor enucleation, as the latter results in higher rates of recurrence and facial nerve dysfunction. Total parotidectomy is recommended for tumors with deep lobe involvement, suspected or confirmed high-grade tumors, or tumors with aggressive malignant potential, such as those with facial nerve involvement, multiple intraparotid masses, or cervical metastasis. Definitive surgery allows for very good local control, with rates approaching 97% in some series. Complete excision of the glands is recommended in submandibular tumors. Surgery followed by adjuvant radiotherapy is the treatment of choice for locally advanced malignant tumors of sublingual and minor salivary glands.[1,2,17]

Radiotherapy

Postoperative radiotherapy improves locoregional control for salivary cancers with high-risk features, such as nodal metastases, extracapsular spread, perineural invasion, advanced tumor (T) stage, high-grade malignancy, deep lobe and/or recurrent cancers, incomplete primary tumor resection, and secondary malignant tumors. High doses (>60 Gy) are necessary to achieve maximal local tumor control in the adjuvant setting. Options for radiation therapy include electron beam, photon beam, and particle beam (proton, neutron, carbon ion) therapies. Particle beam therapy has been shown to have the highest local control rates in adenoid cystic carcinoma.[1] Electron beam therapy may be used for superficial parotid lesions. Photon beam radiotherapy, such as intensity-modulated radiation therapy, allows precise dose escalation to the primary tumor site with significant reductions in dose exposure to normal tissues.[2-5]

Chemotherapy

Chemotherapy is reserved for patients with progressive local or metastatic disease that is not amenable to surgery or radiation therapy. The common chemotherapy used for salivary cancer is cisplatin, cyclophosphamide, doxorubicin, and 5-fluorouracil. Combination chemotherapy reveals response rates of 15% to 70%, with a median response duration of 6 to 7 months. Recent studies use platinum alone or as a combination chemotherapy, but further research is needed in this area.[1-3]

NORMAL POSTOPERATIVE
Parotidectomy

Parotidectomy is most commonly performed for parotid tumor resection. The different types of parotidectomy are (1) partial parotidectomy, excision of the tumor with a surrounding cuff of uninvolved parenchyma; (2) superficial parotidectomy, removal of all the parenchyma superficial to the facial nerve (Fig. 1); (3) total parotidectomy, removal of all parotid parenchyma (superficial and deep to the facial nerve) (Fig. 2); (4) radical parotidectomy, total parotidectomy with sacrifice of the facial nerve; and (5) extended radical parotidectomy, radical parotidectomy extended to at least one of the surrounding structures (skin, mastoid, mandible, masticatory muscles, and infratemporal fossa).[18-20]

Reconstructive Surgery

Reconstructive surgery restores the facial contour after parotidectomy with grafts and flaps that represent tissue transfer from one location to another. Grafts do not have their own blood supply, whereas flaps bring their own blood supply when transferred to a new location. Grafts survive on a blood supply acquired from the recipient bed, and the graft must lie within 1 to 2 mm of the recipient blood supply to survive. In contrast, flaps can be used to transfer much larger amounts of tissue. Various types of grafts consist of nonvascularized fat grafts, dermal-fat grafts, autologous flaps (platysma, temporoparietal fascia, sternocleidomastoid muscle, pectoralis major muscle flap), and microvascular flaps, such as the rectus abdominis myocutaneous flap and anterolateral thigh flap.[21] The imaging appearance varies according to tissue composition of flaps and the duration after surgery.

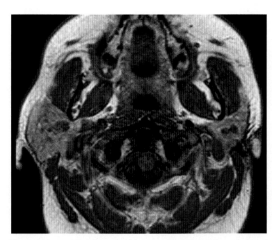

Fig. 1. Superficial parotidectomy: axial T1-weighted image shows partial resection of the superficial part of the left parotid gland.

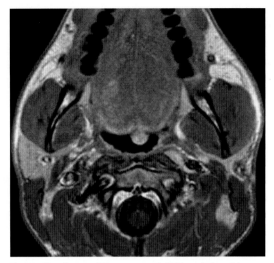

Fig. 2. Total parotidectomy: axial T1-weighted image shows a complete absence of superficial and deep lobes of the left parotid gland.

Myocutaneous flaps and grafts show muscle and fatty components. On MR, the muscle component demonstrates striations, a T1 signal similar to adjacent muscle, and a variable T2 signal; the fat component demonstrates signal intensity to the adjacent fat with suppression of the signal on fat-suppressed contrast T1-weighted images (**Fig. 3**). The muscle degenerates over time, as it is not innervated and the flaps gradually lose bulk with fatty infiltration. Viable flaps may demonstrate variable or no enhancement.[22,23]

POSTTREATMENT COMPLICATION

The complications after treatment of salivary tumors are the recurrence of pleomorphic adenomas; recurrence of salivary cancer; complications related

to surgery, such as facial nerve deficits (18%), sialocele (6%), infection with abscess (4%), hematoma (4%), and pseudoaneurysm; and radiation or radioactive-iodine (RAI)–induced sialadenitis.[1–5]

Recurrence of Pleomorphic Adenoma

The causes of recurrent pleomorphic adenoma are classified into pathology-related (capsule thickness or lack of capsule, high stromal chondroid/myxoid content, pseudopodia, satellite nodules, multicentricity) and surgery-related (rupture of the tumor, spillage of tumor contents, positive margin due to inadequate margin resection, inadequate excision related to the type of surgery) factors. The recurrence of pleomorphic adenoma occurs in 1% to 5% of patients after 5 to 15 years of parotidectomy and in relatively young patients. The recurrence is often multinodular (50%–100%) with an increased rate of postoperative complications, especially facial nerve paralysis (2%–20%), multiple recurrences (2.9%), and malignant degeneration (3.3%).[24,25]

MR accurately demonstrates a recurrent pattern as early clustered with bright T2 signal intensity. This feature results in a bunch-of-grapes appearance (**Fig. 4**). A lobular or multinodular appearance may represent tumor projections radiating from a central lesion. Recurrent pleomorphic adenomas are sometimes located in the subcutaneous tissues or adjacent neck spaces perhaps due to spillage during surgery. The enhancement pattern is variable, depending on the extent of cystic components, fibrosis, and necrosis.[24–27]

Recurrence of Salivary Gland Cancer

Seventy percent of the recurrences of salivary gland cancer occur within 3 years of treatment.

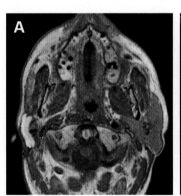
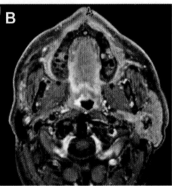
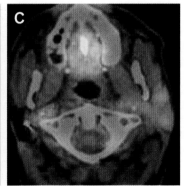

Fig. 3. Total parotidectomy: (*A*) Axial T1-weighted image shows a right total parotidectomy with small hyperintense fat in the postoperative right parotid bed. (*B*) Axial contrast fat-suppressed T1-weighted image shows absent right parotid gland with nonenhancing lesion denoting no recurrence. (*C*) PET-CT scan shows no recurrence could be detected.

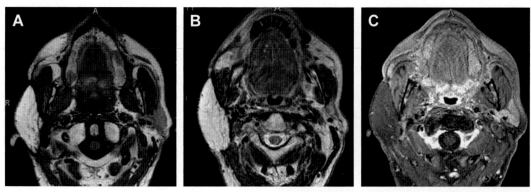

Fig. 4. Fat graft after total parotidectomy: (*A*) Axial T1-weighted image shows a right total parotidectomy with hyperintense fat graft overlies the parotid defect. (*B*) Axial T2-weighted image shows the fat graft shows less hyperintense signal intensity. (*C*) Axial contrast fat-suppressed T1-weighted image shows the suppressed signal intensity of fatty graft with no enhancing lesion denoting no recurrence.

The most common patterns of recurrence include local recurrence (13%), regional recurrence (22%), and distant metastases (33%) during a follow-up period of 10 years.[3] A baseline study (routine MR or CT) is recommended at 3 months after completion of therapy to facilitate early detection of recurrence during follow-up. However, there are no consensus recommendations for posttreatment surveillance imaging. Thus, the follow-up scans are guided by clinical factors, such as suspicion of tumor recurrence. Any enlarging posttreatment soft tissue mass or any new deep lesion or intracranial enhancement is concerning for recurrent disease. The rapid development of advanced MR imaging sequences (diffusion- and perfusion-weighted MR imaging) and the increasing availability of 18-FDG-PET/CT increased the applications of these techniques in the evaluation of the recurrence of salivary gland cancer. The selection of advanced MR and CT depends on availability and experience. At the authors' institution, patients with salivary cancer are scanned with routine contrast MR imaging and diffusion MR imaging every 6 months for 2 years after the baseline study. If there is clinical suspicion of recurrence, immediate scanning with MR is done.

Locoregional recurrence

Local and regional recurrence of salivary cancer is more likely to occur in patients with positive margins, regardless of the tumor grade. The 5-year overall survival of patients with salivary cancer is about 60%. Clinical findings suggestive of local recurrence of salivary cancer include a mass or diffuse fullness in the operative bed, pain in the operative bed, and recent facial paralysis in patients with a history of parotid malignancy.[3,28]

Contrast-enhanced MR imaging is the method of choice in the posttreatment setting. CT's sensitivity and specificity are low (**Fig. 5**), and PET-CT is not superior to MR for locoregional recurrence. MR imaging can differentiate mature scar tissue from recurrent tumor. Fibrotic scar tissue is characterized by a low T2 signal and no contrast enhancement. Recurrent tumor is typically expansile and has intermediate signal on a T2 signal with moderate T1 contrast enhancement (**Figs. 6** and **7**). However, there may be an overlap between a partially treated tumor and immature scar tissue. It is very important that postoperative studies be directly compared with the preoperative baseline study.[3–6] Surgical history is very helpful because a vascularized flap or graft could be mistaken for an enhancing recurrent tumor.[22,23]

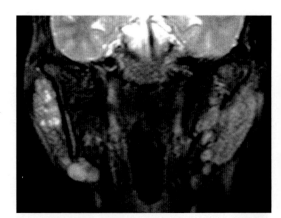

Fig. 5. Recurrent pleomorphic adenoma: coronal MR image shows multiple small well-defined clusters of bright T2 signal intensity with a bunch-of-grapes appearance in the superficial lobe of the right parotid gland that extends below the lower pole of the right parotid gland in a patient 10 years after surgery of pleomorphic adenoma.

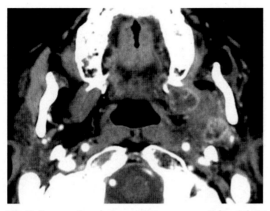

Fig. 6. Locoregional recurrent cancer parotid: axial CT scan shows an ill-defined mass of heterogeneous contrast enhancement seen in the left parapharyngeal space with involvement of the left pterygoid muscles and extension through the left stylomandibular tunnel.

Advanced MR sequences improve differentiation of recurrence from posttreatment changes. Diffusion-weighted MR imaging shows restricted diffusion with a low apparent diffusion coefficient (ADC) value of recurrence (**Fig. 8**) and unrestricted diffusion with a high ADC value of postoperative changes. Diffusion-weighted imaging is an excellent noninvasive imaging modality for monitoring patients after therapy.[28,29] Dynamic contrast MR imaging shows a significant difference in the wash-in and wash-out rates of recurrence and posttreatment changes with cutoff points of greater than 10.25 and greater than 6.25 for the wash-in and wash-out rates to predict recurrence, respectively.[30] Dynamic susceptibility contrast MR imaging shows a significant difference in the percentage of dynamic susceptibility contrast between recurrence and postradiation changes.[31] The percentage of changes

in choline levels at proton MR spectroscopy after chemoradiotherapy may serve as a marker of residual cancer in a posttreatment mass; however, the performance of MR spectroscopy of the head and neck is challenging.[12] Multi-parametric imaging with the combination of different MR sequences increased the accuracy for differentiation of recurrence from posttreatment changes.[3–5]

Advanced CT, such as CT perfusion, can help in this differentiation between post-therapeutic changes and tumor recurrence, which is characterized by significantly higher blood flow from post-therapeutic changes.[15] Although 18-FDG-PET/CT is accurate for initial staging, it does not demonstrate a significant contribution during surveillance. However, it is superior to detect distant metastases and/or second primary tumors.[3–6]

Perineural spread

Perineural spread is characteristic of adenoid cystic carcinoma but is also reported in other high-grade malignancies, such as adenocarcinoma and squamous cell carcinoma. The perineural spread may be antegrade or retrograde and contiguous or discontinuous resulting in skip lesions. MR imaging is the technique of choice to assess intracranial perineural spread of parotid malignancies along the facial (seventh) nerve (**Fig. 9**) to the geniculate ganglion or along the mandibular division of trigeminal (fifth) by way of the auriculotemporal nerve to the Meckel cave and cavernous sinus. Other cranial nerves may become involved with skull base invasion in advanced cancer. The skull base (**Fig. 10**) may be involved by direct spread of tumor as well as perineural spread of salivary gland malignancy.[32,33] Further data about perineural spread are discussed in Christopher Atkinson and colleagues' article,

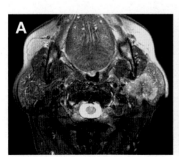
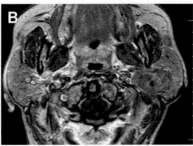
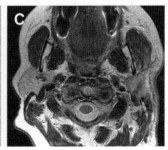

Fig. 7. Locoregional recurrent cancer parotid: (*A*) Axial T2-weighted image shows ill-defined lesion of mixed signal intensity seen in the left parotid gland after total parotidectomy. (*B*) Axial contrast T1-weighted image shows inhomogeneous enhancement of the mass denoting recurrence. (*C*) Axial T2-weighted image in another patient shows ill-defined hypointense lesion seen in the parotid bed after total parotidectomy surgery denoting recurrence.

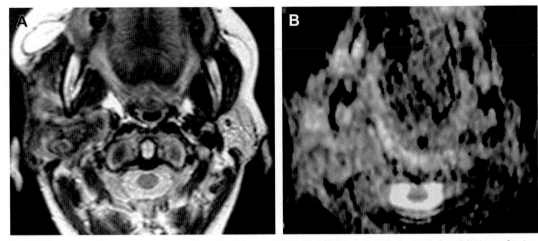

Fig. 8. Locoregional recurrent cancer parotid: (A) Axial T2-weighted image shows ill-defined lesion of mixed signal intensity seen in the postoperative bed. (B) ADC map shows low signal intensity with low ADC value cope with recurrent tumor. Axial T2-weighted image shows ill-defined hypointense lesion seen in the parotid bed after surgery denoting recurrence.

"Cross-Sectional Imaging Techniques and Normal Anatomy of the Salivary Glands," and Daniel Thomas Ginat's article, "Imaging of Benign Neoplastic and Non-neoplastic Salivary Gland Tumors," in this issue.

Nodal metastasis
Recurrence of high-grade salivary malignancy may be in the form of metastatic cervical lymph nodes. Diffusion-weighted MR imaging shows restricted diffusion of metastatic cervical lymph nodes. The iodine content at dual-energy CT is significantly lower for metastatic lymph nodes than reactive lymph nodes. The 18-FDG-PET/CT reveals an increase in FDG uptake in metastatic cervical lymph nodes.[34–37] Further data about nodal metastasis are discussed in Daniel Thomas Ginat's article, "Imaging of Benign Neoplastic and Non-neoplastic Salivary Gland Tumors," in this issue.

Distant metastasis
Distant metastasis is reported in more than 50% and is most commonly seen in high-grade adenoid

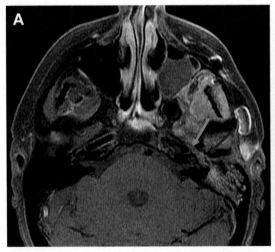
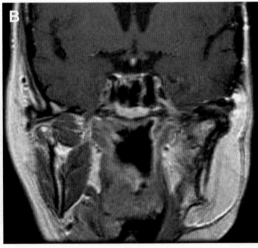

Fig. 9. Perineural spread of recurrent salivary cancer: (A) Axial contrast T1-weighted image shows recurrent adenoid cystic carcinoma with perineural spread along the facial nerve (red arrow) via the greater superficial petrosal nerve (blue arrow). (B) Coronal contrast T1-weighted image of the same patient shows thickening and enhancement of the mandibular nerve (red arrow) with extension through the foramen ovale into the cavernous sinus indicating perineural spread.

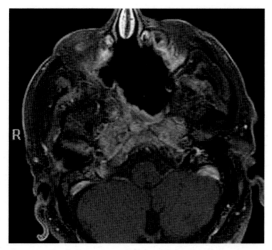

Fig. 10. Skull base invasion in recurrent salivary cancer: axial fat-suppressed T1-weighted image shows extensive enhancing recurrent malignancy with invasion of the skull base in patient with adenoid cystic carcinoma.

cystic carcinoma, adenocarcinoma not otherwise specified, and carcinoma ex-pleomorphic adenoma. Up to 90% of distant metastases are located within the lungs, 15% in the bones, and 5% in the liver and brain (**Fig. 11**). Whole-body diffusion-weighted MR imaging may be helpful in the detection of bony and pulmonary distant metastatic deposits in patients with salivary cancer.[3–6]

Postoperative Complications

The postoperative complications of salivary gland surgery include sialocele, hematoma, abscess, pseudoaneurysm, and graft stenosis. Other complications of salivary gland surgery, such as Frey syndrome, first bite syndrome,

and facial nerve dysfunction, do not require imaging.[1–5]

Sialocele
Sialocele arises from extravasation of the saliva into glandular and periglandular tissues secondary to disruption of the parotid duct/parenchyma after surgery. Imaging is required to determine the site of parenchymal/ductal injury. MR sialogram can detect the site of communication, information about the upstream ductal system, and the location of sialocele and its relationship with surrounding structures.[38–41]

Hematoma and abscess
Salivary gland tumors may show hematoma within tumor parenchyma that can occur after biopsy or surgery on salivary glands. Hematoma appears as a hyperdense area on CT (**Fig. 12**) and hyperintense on MR image with a hypointense rim. Abscess may develop after surgery and is characterized by a rim-enhancing fluid lesion on both CT and MR. The enhancing rim is more conspicuous on MR versus CT. Diffusion-weighted image shows restricted diffusion within the fluid compared with the uninfected fluid collection.[6,8,42]

Pseudoaneurysm and graft stenosis
Pseudoaneurysm arises from a disruption in arterial wall continuity during surgery with dissection of blood into the tissues around the damaged artery that communicates with the arterial lumen. This disruption results in direct weakening of the media or adventitia or creating of soft tissue fibrosis that surrounds the site of injury. Color Duplex ultrasound, CT angiography, and contrast MR angiography are noninvasive methods for diagnosis of pseudoaneurysm; but conventional

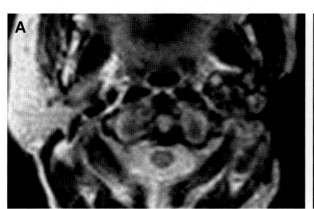
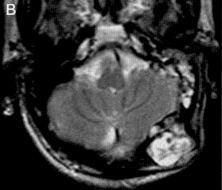

Fig. 11. Distant metastasis of recurrent salivary cancer: (*A*) Axial T2-weighted image shows an ill-defined lesion of mixed signal intensity seen in the bed of the left parotidectomy in patient with adenoid cystic carcinoma. (*B*) Axial T2-weighted image shows expansile bony lesion of the skull vault.

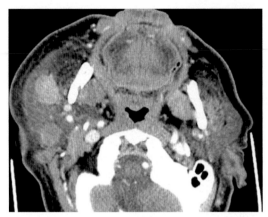

Fig. 12. Intraparotid hematoma: CT scan shows multiple hyperdense areas of hemorrhage after biopsy of Warthin tumor.

angiography is the gold standard for the final diagnosis.[43–45]

Radiation-Induced Sialadenitis

Radiation-induced sialadenitis occurs when external beam radiation involves the salivary glands and exceeds 15 to 20 Gy that occurs as part of a curative treatment of oral cavity or pharyngeal tumors. The involved gland is smaller, cellular, and fibrotic. The parotid gland is more severely affected by radiation than the submandibular and minor salivary glands. However, most intensity modulated radiotherapy regimens spare the parotid glands. Radiotherapy initially results in xerostomia, but salivary flow rates usually partially recover after 6 to 12 months because of hyperplasia of the surviving acini. Ultrasound shows features of acute or chronic sialadenitis depending on the time elapsed following treatment. On contrast CT the gland is small and avidly enhancing, and on MR imaging the affected gland is low to intermediate in signal intensity on all sequences (**Fig. 13**). The affected glands show a lower ADC value at diffusion-weighted MR imaging and a higher peak enhancement and time to peak on dynamic contrast MR imaging than unaffected glands.[46–50]

Radioactive Iodine–Induced Sialadenitis

RAI-induced sialadenitis occurs in 20% to 67% of patients with thyroid cancer who have received RAI therapy to ablate remnant thyroid tissues after thyroidectomy. RAI plays an effective role in the treatment of well-differentiated thyroid cancers. The RAI accumulates 30 to 40 times more in the salivary glands than in plasma through the sodium-iodide symporter. This accumulation damages the ductal epithelium and vascular endothelium of the salivary glands and results in obstructive sialadenitis characterized by pain and swelling over the affected area. Salivary gland scintigraphy can be used to evaluate salivary gland function after RAI. The salivary gland volume significantly decreased with an increase in the dysfunction grade on scintigraphy. The reduction in the volume of the salivary glands and the increase in attenuation of the parotid gland on nonenhanced CT can be indicators of the presence of RAI-induced sialadenitis. MR sialography may also be used to evaluate for sialectasis and duct stenosis.[51–53]

SUMMARY

MR imaging can diagnose recurrent pleomorphic adenomas and perineural spread of salivary cancer. Advanced MR imaging, such as diffusion

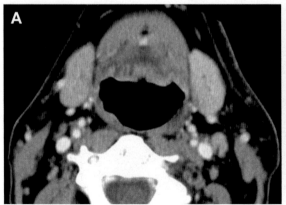
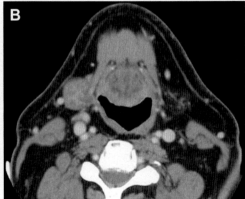

Fig. 13. Radiation sialadenitis: (*A*) Axial CT scan before radiations shows both normal submandibular glands. (*B*) After radiation therapy, there is reduction and small-sized left submandibular gland.

and perfusion MR imaging, can help in the detection of locoregional recurrence of malignancy and 18-PET-CT detect distant metastasis.

REFERENCES

1. Keller G, Steinmann D, Quaas A, et al. New concepts of personalized therapy in salivary gland carcinomas. Oral Oncol 2017;68:103–13.

2. Lewis AG, Tong T, Maghami E. Diagnosis and management of malignant salivary gland tumors of the parotid gland. Otolaryngol Clin North Am 2016;49:343–80.

3. Freling N, Crippa F, Maroldi R. Staging and follow-up of high-grade malignant salivary gland tumours: the role of traditional versus functional imaging approaches - a review. Oral Oncol 2016;60:157–66.

4. Friedman ER, Saindane AM. Pitfalls in the staging of cancer of the major salivary gland neoplasms. Neuroimaging Clin N Am 2013;23:107–22.

5. Abdel Razek AAK, Mukherji SK. State-of-the-art imaging of salivary gland tumors. Neuroimag Clin N Am 2018;28(2):303–17.

6. Lobert P, Srinivasan A, Shah GV, et al. Postoperative and postradiation changes on imaging. Otolaryngol Clin North Am 2012;45:1405–22.

7. Saito N, Nadgir RN, Nakahira M, et al. Posttreatment CT and MR imaging in head and neck cancer: what the radiologist needs to know. Radiographics 2012;32:1261–82.

8. Srinivasan A, Mohan S, Mukherji SK. Biologic imaging of head and neck cancer: the present and the future. AJNR Am J Neuroradiol 2012;33:586–94.

9. Razek AA. Diffusion-weighted magnetic resonance imaging of head and neck. J Comput Assist Tomogr 2010;34:808–15.

10. Gaddikeri S, Gaddikeri RS, Tailor T, et al. Dynamic contrast-enhanced MR imaging in head and neck cancer: techniques and clinical applications. AJNR Am J Neuroradiol 2016;37:588–95.

11. Abdel Razek AA, Samir S, Ashmalla GA. Characterization of parotid tumors with dynamic susceptibility contrast perfusion-weighted magnetic resonance imaging and diffusion-weighted MR imaging. J Comput Assist Tomogr 2017;41:131–6.

12. Abdel Razek AA, Poptani H. MR spectroscopy of head and neck cancer. Eur J Radiol 2013;82:982–9.

13. Koontz NA, Wiggins RH 3rd. Differentiation of benign and malignant head and neck lesions with diffusion tensor imaging and DWI. AJR Am J Roentgenol 2017;208:1110–5.

14. Abdel Razek AAK. Routine and advanced diffusion imaging modules of the salivary glands. Neuroimag Clin N Am 2018;28(2):245–54.

15. Razek AA, Tawfik AM, Elsorogy LG, et al. Perfusion CT of head and neck cancer. Eur J Radiol 2014;83:537–44.

16. Tawfik AM, Kerl JM, Razek AA, et al. Image quality and radiation dose of dual-energy CT of the head and neck compared with a standard 120-kVp acquisition. AJNR Am J Neuroradiol 2011;32:1994–9.

17. Abdel Razek AAK, Mukherji SK. Imaging of minor salivary glands. Neuroimag Clin N Am 2018;28(2):295–302.

18. Quer M, Guntinas-Lichius O, Marchal F, et al. Classification of parotidectomies: a proposal of the European Salivary Gland Society. Eur Arch Otorhinolaryngol 2016;273:3307–12.

19. Larian B. Parotidectomy for benign parotid tumors. Otolaryngol Clin North Am 2016;49:395–413.

20. Cracchiolo JR, Shaha AR. Parotidectomy for parotid cancer. Otolaryngol Clin North Am 2016;49:415–24.

21. Irvine LE, Larian B, Azizzadeh B. Locoregional parotid reconstruction. Otolaryngol Clin North Am 2016;49:435–46.

22. Syed F, Spector ME, Cornelius R, et al. Head and neck reconstructive surgery: what the radiologist needs to know. Eur Radiol 2016;26:3345–52.

23. Learned K, Malloy K, Loevner L. Myocutaneous flaps and other vascularized grafts in head and neck reconstruction for cancer treatment. Magn Reson Imaging Clin N Am 2012;20:495–513.

24. Dulguerov P, Todic J, Pusztaszeri M, et al. Why do parotid pleomorphic adenomas recur? A systematic review of pathological and surgical variables. Front Surg 2017;4:26.

25. Witt RL, Nicolai P. Recurrent benign salivary gland neoplasms. Adv Otorhinolaryngol 2016;78:63–70.

26. Moonis G, Patel P, Koshkareva Y, et al. Imaging characteristics of recurrent pleomorphic adenoma of the parotid gland. AJNR Am J Neuroradiol 2007;28:1532–6.

27. Merdad M, Richmon JD, Quon H. Management of recurrent malignant salivary neoplasms. Adv Otorhinolaryngol 2016;78:168–74.

28. Razek AA, Megahed AS, Denewer A, et al. Role of diffusion-weighted magnetic resonance imaging in differentiation between the viable and necrotic parts of head and neck tumors. Acta Radiol 2008;49:364–70.

29. Abdel Razek AA, Kandeel AY, Soliman N, et al. Role of diffusion-weighted echo-planar MR imaging in differentiation of residual or recurrent head and neck tumors and posttreatment changes. AJNR Am J Neuroradiol 2007;28:1146–52.

30. Samir S, El-Adalany MA, Hamed EE. Value of dynamic contrast enhanced magnetic resonance imaging in the differentiation between post-treatment changes and recurrent salivary gland tumors. Egypt J Rad Nuclear Med 2016;47:477–86.

31. Abdel Razek AA, Gaballa G, Ashamalla G, et al. Dynamic susceptibility contrast perfusion-weighted magnetic resonance imaging and diffusion-weighted magnetic resonance imaging in differentiating

recurrent head and neck cancer from post-radiation changes. J Comput Assist Tomogr 2015;39(6): 849–54.

32. Badger D, Aygun N. Imaging of perineural spread in head and neck cancer. Radiol Clin North Am 2017; 55:139–49.

33. Abdel Khalek Abdel Razek A, King A. MRI and CT of nasopharyngeal carcinoma. AJR Am J Roentgenol 2012;198:11–8.

34. Bradley PJ. Primary malignant parotid epithelial neoplasm: nodal metastases and management. Curr Opin Otolaryngol Head Neck Surg 2015;23:91–8.

35. Abdel Razek AA, Soliman NY, Elkhamary S, et al. Role of diffusion-weighted MR imaging in cervical lymphadenopathy. Eur Radiol 2006;16:1468–77.

36. Abdel Razek AA, Gaballa G. Role of perfusion magnetic resonance imaging in cervical lymphadenopathy. J Comput Assist Tomogr 2011;35:21–5.

37. Tawfik AM, Razek AA, Kerl JM, et al. Comparison of dual-energy CT-derived iodine content and iodine overlay of normal, inflammatory and metastatic squamous cell carcinoma cervical lymph nodes. Eur Radiol 2014;24:574–80.

38. Britt CJ, Stein AP, Gessert T, et al. Factors influencing sialocele or salivary fistula formation postparotidectomy. Head Neck 2017;39:387–91.

39. Meyer RA. Parotid sialocele or traumatic pseudocyst. J Oral Maxillofac Surg 2015;73:1240.

40. Abdel Razek AA, Ashmalla GA, Gaballa G, et al. Pilot study of ultrasound parotid imaging reporting and data system (PIRADS): inter-observer agreement. Eur J Radiol 2015;85:2533–8.

41. Gadodia A, Bhalla AS, Sharma R, et al. MR sialography of iatrogenic sialocele: comparison with conventional sialography. Dentomaxillofac Radiol 2011;40: 147–53.

42. Abdel Razek AA, Nada N. Role of diffusion-weighted MRI in differentiation of masticator space malignancy from infection. Dentomaxillofac Radiol 2013; 42(4):20120183.

43. Saad NE, Saad WE, Davies MG, et al. Pseudoaneurysms and the role of minimally invasive techniques in their management. Radiographics 2005;25(Suppl 1): S173–89.

44. Razek AA, Gaballa G, Megahed AS, et al. Time resolved imaging of contrast kinetics (TRICKS) MR angiography of arteriovenous malformations of head and neck. Eur J Radiol 2013; 82:1885–91.

45. Abdel Razek AA, Denewer AT, Hegazy MA, et al. Role of computed tomography angiography in the diagnosis of vascular stenosis in head and neck microvascular free flap reconstruction. Int J Oral Maxillofac Surg 2014;43:811–5.

46. Vissink A, van Luijk P, Langendijk JA, et al. Current ideas to reduce or salvage radiation damage to salivary glands. Oral Dis 2015;21:e1–10.

47. van Dijk LV, Brouwer CL, van der Schaaf A, et al. CT image biomarkers to improve patient-specific prediction of radiation-induced xerostomia and sticky saliva. Radiother Oncol 2017;122:185–91.

48. Abdel Razek AAK, Mukherji S. Imaging of sialadenitis. Neuroradiol J 2017;30:205–15.

49. Houweling AC, van den Berg CA, Roesink JM, et al. Magnetic resonance imaging at 3.0T for submandibular gland sparing radiotherapy. Radiother Oncol 2010;97:239–43.

50. Loimu V, Seppälä T, Kapanen M, et al. Diffusion-weighted magnetic resonance imaging for evaluation of salivary gland function in head and neck cancer patients treated with intensity-modulated radiotherapy. Radiother Oncol 2017; 122:178–84.

51. Hollingsworth B, Senter L, Zhang X, et al. Risk factors of (131)I-induced salivary gland damage in thyroid cancer patients. J Clin Endocrinol Metab 2016; 101:4085–93.

52. Choi JS, Lim HG, Kim YM, et al. Usefulness of magnetic resonance sialography for the evaluation of radioactive iodine-induced sialadenitis. Ann Surg Oncol 2015;22:S1007–13.

53. Nabaa B, Takahashi K, Sasaki T, et al. Assessment of salivary gland dysfunction after radioiodine therapy for thyroid carcinoma using non-contrast-enhanced CT: the significance of changes in volume and attenuation of the glands. AJNR Am J Neuroradiol 2012;33:1964–70.

Imaging of Pediatric Salivary Glands

Elliott Friedman, MD[a],*, Maria Olga Patiño, MD[a], Unni K. Udayasankar, MD[b]

KEYWORDS

- Pediatric salivary gland disease • Sialadenitis • Parotitis • Pediatric salivary gland tumor
- Hemangioma • Ranula • First branchial cleft cyst • Juvenile recurrent parotitis

KEY POINTS

- The incidence of salivary gland diseases in the pediatric age group differs greatly from the adult population. Infectious/inflammatory and vascular etiologies are the most common pathologies.
- The most common inflammatory salivary disorders worldwide are mumps and juvenile recurrent parotitis.
- Less than 5% of salivary gland neoplasms occur in children, with a roughly even split of epithelial tumors between benign and malignant tumors.
- Hemangioma and benign mixed tumor account for nearly 90% of benign salivary gland tumors in children. Mucoepidermoid carcinoma is the most frequent pediatric salivary malignancy.
- Congenital anomalies include first branchial cleft cysts and glandular aplasia or dysplasia, which may occur in isolation or as part of a syndrome.

INTRODUCTION

Salivary gland diseases in children are relatively uncommon compared with the adult population, with a different incidence of distribution of pathologies. In the pediatric population, diseases of the salivary gland are more frequently inflammatory or vascular in etiology. Some diagnoses, such as congenital anomalies of the salivary glands, including hypoplasia and aplasia, branchial cleft remnant lesions, and vascular malformations, are obviously more commonly seen in the pediatric population. Neoplastic masses are especially uncommon in children, with less than 5% of all benign and malignant tumors of the parotid glands estimated to occur in people younger than 16 years of age.[1,2]

NORMAL ANATOMY AND IMAGING TECHNIQUE

Normal anatomy of the salivary glands and imaging techniques have been described elsewhere in this issue. The imaging workup of salivary pathology depends on institutional preferences, resource availability, and technical expertise.

Ultrasound imaging is an excellent choice for the initial evaluation of suspected parotid or submandibular space lesions in pediatric patients, providing a readily available, noninvasive, and nonionizing means to evaluate superficial structures with good resolution. Higher frequency transducers are preferable, with 5 to 12 MHz wide-band linear transducers typically used.[3] Color Doppler imaging assesses the vascularity

Disclosure Statement: There is no funding source, commercial, or financial conflicts of interest for any of the authors with respect to this publication.
[a] Department of Diagnostic and Interventional Imaging, University of Texas Health Science Center at Houston, McGovern Medical School, 6431 Fannin Street, MSB 2.130B, Houston, TX 77030, USA; [b] Department of Medical Imaging, University of Arizona College of Medicine, 1501 North Campbell Avenue, Tucson, AZ 85724, USA
* Corresponding author.
E-mail address: Elliott.Friedman@uth.tmc.edu

neuroimaging.theclinics.com

of the gland and focal lesions. The normal salivary glands are homogenous in echotexture and hyperechogenic relative to adjacent muscles, with the degree of echogenicity of the parotid gland proportional to the amount of glandular fatty tissue, and not hypervascular on color Doppler imaging. Ultrasound imaging can assess gland size, distinguish cystic and solid masses, evaluate for ductal dilatation, and guide biopsy.

Cross-sectional imaging by computed tomography (CT) scanning and MR imaging provide excellent delineation of salivary gland masses. CT scanning is the most readily available imaging modality at most centers, and is not operator dependent. CT scanning and MR imaging are not limited in evaluation of deeper structures as with ultrasound examination, although CT scanning has the drawback of ionizing radiation exposure, and MR imaging may require sedation in younger children. CT scanning is an excellent modality to evaluate for the presence of air or calcifications. MR imaging provides superior soft tissue characterization and is the preferred imaging modality to evaluate a palpable mass. Echoplanar diffusion-weighted imaging can add additional information, with vascular and benign neoplastic lesions demonstrating higher apparent diffusion coefficient values than malignant tumors.[4] MR sialography uses heavily T2-weighted sequences (3-dimensional [3D] constructive interface in steady state, half Fourier acquisition single-shot turbo spin echo) to visualize the ductal system, and can be used in the evaluation of sialolithiasis and sialadenitis. MR sialography is noninvasive, and can evaluate up to the second-order ductal branches, but does not have as high of a spatial resolution as digital subtraction sialography.[5]

SALIVARY GLAND EMBRYOLOGY

The salivary glands develop as outgrowths of the oral epithelium that grow as solid cores of cells into the underlying mesenchyme. The parotid anlagen develop first at 4 weeks of gestation, followed by the submandibular and sublingual primordia at approximately 6 and 8 weeks of gestation, respectively. The cores undergo extensive branching, enlarge, and canalize to develop lumina. The enveloping mesenchyme divides the developing glands into lobules and forms a capsule. Minor salivary glands have a different embryogenesis, arising from mixed ectodermal and endodermal origins.[6,7]

The parotid glands are unique among the major salivary glands, because they contain intraglandular lymph nodes and lymphatic tissue, whereas the submandibular and sublingual glands do not. The parotid gland is the last of the salivary glands to encapsulate, occurring after development of the lymphatic system, resulting in entrapment of lymphatics within the glandular tissue.[6]

Accessory parotid tissue is most commonly located overlying the masseter muscle, and may also be found in the anterior and posterior triangles of the neck. Ectopic salivary gland tissue is commonly found in the parotid and periparotid lymph nodes, but is rarely reported in other locations, including the mandible, palatine and lingual tonsils, soft tissues of the neck, middle ear cavity, thyroid and parathyroid glands, cerebellopontine angle, and in a Rathke pouch remnant.[6]

CONGENITAL LESIONS
Aplasia and Hypoplasia

Absence of the major salivary glands is a rare anomaly that may affect single or multiple glands, unilaterally or bilaterally. The cause of salivary gland agenesis is unknown, but presumably related to a defect in early intrauterine development. Aplasias may occur as an isolated finding, or in association with other abnormalities, including ectodermal defects of the first branchial arch and malformations of the lacrimal apparatus and absence of the lacrimal puncta.[8]

Isolated major salivary gland aplasia can be asymptomatic, or may be associated with xerostomia and early dental caries, particularly with multiple gland aplasias. Radiographically, the contralateral salivary gland may be hypertrophied, and hypertrophy of the ipsilateral sublingual gland has also been reported, which can mimic a floor of the mouth mass[9] (**Fig. 1**).

Parotid and submandibular dysplasia and agenesis can be seen in association with Treacher–Collins syndrome (mandibulofacial dysostosis), an autosomal-dominant disorder characterized by mandibular/facial and zygomatic hypoplasias, ocular and otic abnormalities.[10] Lacrimoauriculodentodigital syndrome is characterized by hypoplasia or agenesis of the lacrimal system and salivary glands, deafness and ear abnormalities, and dental and digital anomalies[11] (**Fig. 2**).

First Branchial Cleft Cyst

First branchial cleft cysts (BCC) develop as a result of incomplete fusion of the cleft between the first and second branchial arches, and reflect duplication anomalies of the external auditory canal (EAC). These lesions are often asymptomatic until they present clinically as infections or repeated swelling in the periauricular soft tissues or parotid gland, or drainage into the EAC.[12] Radiographically, these cysts seem to be similar to other

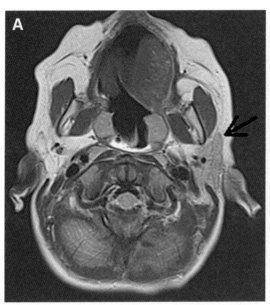
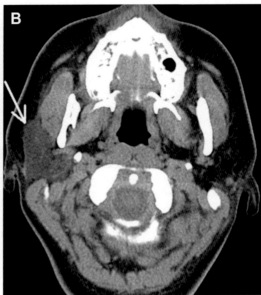

Fig. 1. Parotid aplasia. (*A*) Axial T2-weighted image in a 2-year-old boy showing absence of the right parotid gland with normal appearing parotid gland on the left (*arrow*). (*B*) Noncontrast axial computed tomography scan in a 13-year-old girl with an absent left parotid gland and normal gland on the right (*arrow*).

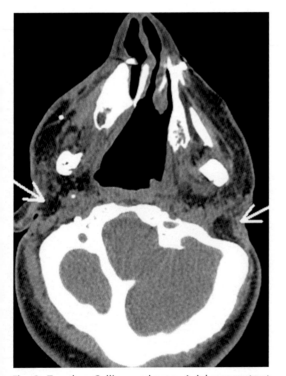

Fig. 2. Treacher–Collins syndrome. Axial noncontrast computed tomography image demonstrates bilateral parotid gland aplasia (*arrows*) in a patient with Treacher–Collins syndrome.

simple cysts, and may present with superimposed inflammatory changes or abscess formation.

Work described 2 types of first BCCs based on histology. Type I cysts, which are rare, are purely ectodermal, lined by squamous epithelium, and present as a cystic mass or fistula posterior to the pinna and concha. The cyst is characteristically located superior to the main trunk of the facial nerve, terminating in a cul-de-sac in the region of a bony plate at the level of the mesotympanum.[13]

Type II cysts reflect duplications of the membranous and cartilaginous portions of the EAC and contain skin (ectoderm) and adnexal structures as well as cartilage (mesoderm), and may be situated in the parotid gland. These lesions contain portions of the first and second branchial arches as well as the first cleft and are often associated with fistulous connections in the concha or EAC and fistulous openings in the neck[13] (**Fig. 3**).

Differential diagnosis of cystic parotid/periparotid lesion
- First BCC
- Sialocele
- Abscess/suppurative lymph node
- Lymphatic malformation
- Venous vascular malformation

Pearls
- Consider first BCC with a cystic lesion adjacent to the EAC, in the periauricular region, or extending between the EAC and angle of

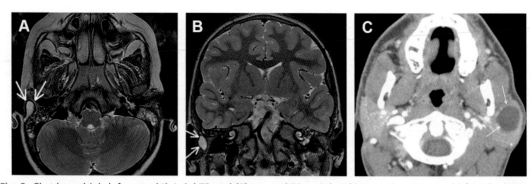

Fig. 3. First branchial cleft cysts. (*A*) Axial T2 and (*B*) coronal T2-weighted images in a 6-year-old female depict a T2 hyperintense periauricular lesion adjacent to the posterior superior margin of the right external auditory canal (*arrows*) compatible with a type I first branchial cleft cyst. Additional images (not shown) demonstrate no associated restricted diffusion or enhancement. (*C*) Axial post contrast CT demonstrating a circumscribed, nonenhancing low attenuation intraparotid lesion (*arrows*), reflecting a type II first branchial cleft cyst. ([*C*] *Courtesy of* Dr Kristen Baugnon, Emory University, Atlanta, GA.)

the mandible including any parotid or peripar-otid cyst.

- Recurrent parotid abscesses or unexplained otorrhea in a child should raise suspicion for a first BCC.

INFECTIOUS AND INFLAMMATORY SIALADENITIS

Infectious and inflammatory diseases are the most frequent causes of parotid gland swelling in children.[14] Infectious and inflammatory salivary diseases present with an overlapping and nonspe-cific radiographic picture of unilateral or bilateral diffuse salivary gland enlargement and enhance-ment in the acute or subacute phase. Concomitant cervical lymphadenopathy and adenotonsillar hypertrophy are commonly present. Chronic

inflammatory disorders may produce a heteroge-neous appearing atrophied gland, possibly with ductal dilatation and sialolithiasis. Acute inflamma-tion correlates with more T2 hyperintense signal and enhancement compared with chronically inflamed glands (**Fig. 4**).

Juvenile Recurrent Parotitis

Juvenile recurrent parotitis (JRP) is the most common inflammatory salivary gland disorder in children in the United States, and the second most common worldwide after the mumps virus.[15] JRP is a chronic condition of undetermined etiol-ogy manifested by repeat bouts of acute or subacute inflammation of the parotid glands, most commonly unilaterally, that are typically self-limited. Symptoms usually subside or

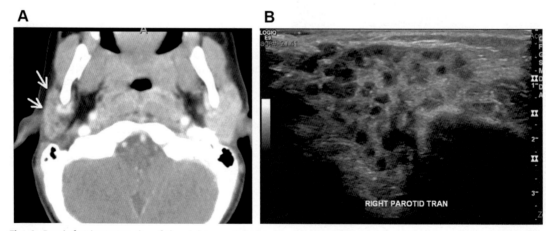

Fig. 4. Postinfectious atrophy of the right parotid gland in a 6-year-old girl. (*A*) Axial postcontrast computed to-mography scan through the parotid glands shows an atrophic right parotid gland with fatty infiltration (*arrows*). Normal appearance of the left parotid gland. (*B*) Grayscale ultrasound image of the right parotid gland obtained at the age of 4 years shows classic imaging appearance of acute parotitis.

completely resolve after puberty. The onset of symptoms is most commonly between 3 and 6 years of age, with repeated clinical exacerbations every 3 to 4 months, characterized by pain and swelling of the affected gland, and possibly a mildly elevated temperature.[15,16] Histologically, the affected glands demonstrate lymphocytic infiltration and chronic inflammatory changes with interlobular ductal dilatation.[16]

In the acute phase of JRP, nonspecific radiologic findings of inflammation are present: enlarged, enhancing gland with T2 hyperintensity on MR imaging. MR sialography demonstrates small intraglandular T2 hyperintense foci corresponding with cysts and tiny sialectasis, but normal caliber main parotid ducts. Ultrasound imaging demonstrates enlarged, heterogeneous glands with foci of hypoechogenicity corresponding with the sialectasis.[17]

Pearl
MR sialography clearly delineates intraglandular sialectasis with normal main parotid duct in JRP. Radiographic findings may be bilateral even though symptoms are usually unilateral.

Viral Sialadenitis

Viral sialadenitis most commonly affects the parotid gland, although the submandibular and sublingual glands may also be involved. Viral illnesses usually result from systemic infections, are self-limited, and imaging is not generally indicated unless a complication is suspected. The most common cause of viral parotitis is paramyxovirus (mumps). Mumps diagnosis can be made by serum immunoglobulin M or polymerase chain reaction.[18]

The parotid glands are usually affected bilaterally, although initial involvement may be unilateral.[19] Radiographic findings are nonspecific. Ultrasound imaging demonstrates an enlarged, heterogeneously hypoechoic gland with increased vascularity on power Doppler imaging.[20] On cross-sectional imaging, the gland is enlarged and enhancing, and T2 hyperintense on MR imaging (**Figs. 5 and 6**).

Pearl
Viral sialadenitis is most commonly bilateral, although initial involvement may be asynchronous or unilateral.

Bacterial Sialadenitis

Bacterial sialadenitis most commonly occurs in the parotid gland, but can also involve the submandibular gland, and is typically unilateral. The presence of purulence distinguishes bacterial etiologies

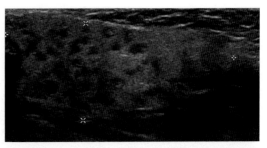

Fig. 5. Acute parotitis in a 9-year-old girl. Grayscale ultrasound image demonstrating multiple hypoechoic foci in the parotid gland.

from other causes of acute sialadenitis. Imaging is indicated to evaluate for complications such as abscess formation and locoregional spread with compromise of the airway or other adjacent structures. The most common involved organisms are *Staphylococcus aureus* and *Streptococcus* species.[19]

Imaging demonstrates an enlarged gland with edema in the gland and surrounding soft tissues. Ultrasound examination can assess for calculi and hypoechoic collections reflecting abscesses. The gland is generally enlarged, heterogeneously hypoechoic, and hypervascular. Radiographic sialography is contraindicated in cases of suspected acute suppurative sialadenitis.[20] CT scanning and MR imaging demonstrate glandular enhancement, except in areas of developing abscesses, which form peripherally enhancing collections, and the gland is usually diffusely T2 hyperintense with focal areas of high T2 signal that may reflect microabscesses or ductal dilatation (**Figs. 7–9**).

Granulomatous Disease

Mycobacterium
Mycobacterial infections may affect the intraparotid or other cervicofacial lymph nodes. Although the incidence of tuberculosis infection is decreasing in developed countries, infections with nontuberculous mycobacteria have increased. Nontuberculous mycobacteria infections most commonly present as slow-growing, unilateral, nontender nodes or nodal masses in immunocompetent children, less than 5 years old, who are otherwise healthy.[21,22] The nodal mass may eventually form a fistula to the skin surface.[22] Submandibular space lymph nodes are most commonly involved; however, parotid and preauricular area nodes may also be affected. Ultrasound examination reveals cystic nodes with nodal matting. CT scanning and MR imaging demonstrate centrally low attenuation, high T2 signal necrotic, peripherally enhancing nodes or

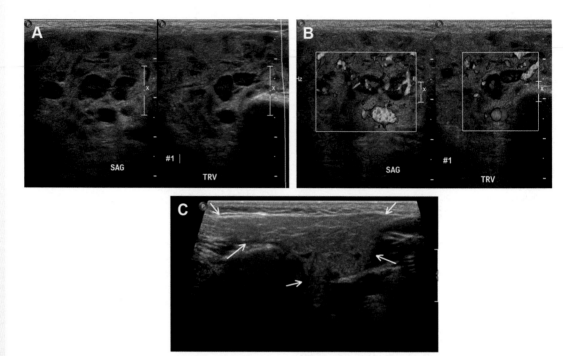

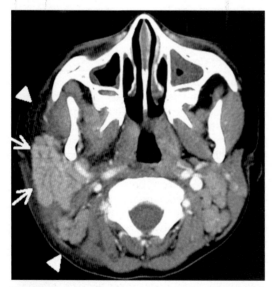

Fig. 6. Acute parotitis in a 5-year-old boy with mumps infection. (*A*) Grayscale ultrasound image shows an enlarged, hypoechoic right parotid gland with heterogeneous parenchymal echotexture. (*B*) Color Doppler imaging shows increased vascularity of the gland. (*C*) A normal left parotid gland (shown for comparison) demonstrates normal homogeneous echo pattern (outlined by *arrows*).

nodal masses with minimal surrounding inflammation (**Fig. 10**).[23]

Tuberculous lymphadenitis most commonly affects the posterior cervical, internal jugular, or

Fig. 7. Acute bacterial parotitis in a 6-year-old girl. Axial postcontrast computed tomography scan demonstrates asymmetric enhancement and enlargement of the right parotid gland (*arrows*), with diffuse subcutaneous edema in the soft tissues (*arrowheads*).

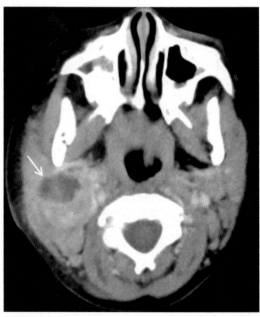

Fig. 8. Right parotid abscess in a 3-year-old girl with fever and right neck swelling. Axial postcontrast computed tomography scan shows an enlarged and hyperenhancing right parotid gland with a well-defined, low-density, peripherally enhancing collection (*arrow*). Note the extensive subcutaneous edema and inflammatory changes. The left parotid gland is normal.

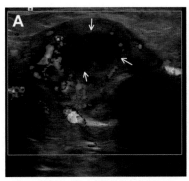
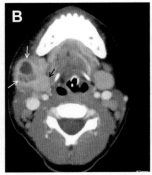
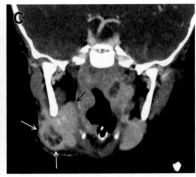

Fig. 9. Submandibular abscess in a 2-year-old girl. (*A*) Color Doppler ultrasound image of the right submandibular region shows a heterogeneous inflammatory mass with central anechoic areas (*arrows*) and increased vascularity peripherally. (*B*) Axial and (*C*) coronal postcontrast computed tomography images show a right submandibular region abscess with surrounding inflammatory changes (*arrows*). The abscess seems to arise from suppurative lymphadenopathy of the right submandibular lymph nodes with medially displaced submandibular gland (*black arrow*). The left submandibular gland is normal.

supraclavicular lymph nodes, often unilaterally, and frequently results from dissemination of pulmonary disease. Tuberculous nodes on CT scanning and MR imaging initially appear as homogenously enhancing enlarged nodes that later progress to central necrosis, and obliteration of surrounding fat planes with matted appearance. Chronically treated mycobacterial nodes may calcify. Tuberculosis of the parotid gland should be considered in cases of unilateral linearly arranged enhancing nodules in the superficial lobe of the parotid gland[24] (Fig. 10).

Differential diagnosis of nontuberculous mycobacteria lymphadenopathy
- Suppurative lymph nodes
- Tuberculous lymphadenopathy
- Second BCC
- Cat scratch disease
- Metastatic lymphadenopathy

Other granulomatous infections

Cat scratch disease is a typically self-limiting infection of children and young adults owing to the bacterium *Bartonella henselae*, classically acquired by a cat scratch or bite. Imaging demonstrates unilateral lymphadenopathy along the lymphatic drainage of the inoculation site, commonly in the mid cervical, parotid, and submandibular regions. Lymphadenopathy may be sharply delineated initially, but often becomes confluent with poorly defined borders.[24]

Sarcoidosis

Sarcoidosis is a systemic granulomatous disease of unknown cause that affects multiple organs in the body, primarily affecting the lungs and lymphatic systems.[25] Childhood sarcoidosis is rare. Infants and young children may present clinically with skin, joint, and eye involvement, lacking the typical lung disease, whereas older children

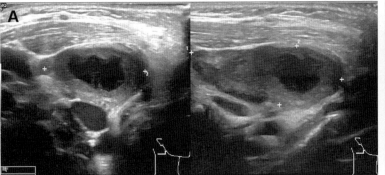
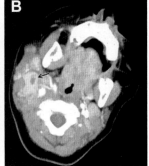

Fig. 10. Atypical mycobacterial infection of the right parotid gland lymph nodes in a 16-month-old girl. (*A*) Grayscale ultrasound images show enlarged lymph nodes with central suppuration. (*B*) Axial postcontrast computed tomography CT image also demonstrates multiple right parotid space lymph nodes with secondary inflammatory changes of the parotid gland. Note the central necrosis within an enlarged and inflamed node (*arrow*).

more often present with lung, lymph node, and eye involvement as seen in adults. Parotid gland enlargement is a relatively frequent finding in childhood sarcoidosis, particularly with the early onset type.[26] On MR imaging, the parotid glands are enlarged bilaterally, diffusely T2 hyperintense and enhancing, as well as possible lacrimal gland enlargement. Enlarged noncavitary intraparotid masses may be present, often in conjunction with cervical adenopathy.[27,28]

Human Immunodeficiency Virus Infection

Parotid gland enlargement is estimated to occur in up to 10% of human immunodeficiency virus (HIV)-infected individuals, and 3 forms of lymphocytic involvement have been described. Persistent generalized lymphadenopathy is the diffuse lymphadenopathy that occurs throughout the body and may involve the intraparotid nodes, histologically reflecting reactive follicular hyperplasia. Cervical lymphadenopathy and adenotonsillar hypertrophy are commonly present in HIV-infected individuals. Benign lymphoepithelial lesions are solid or mixed cystic and solid lesions that can also be seen in a number of other disease states, most commonly Sjögren syndrome (SS), thought to possibly represent expression of an autoimmune reaction. Benign lymphoepithelial lesions carry a long-term risk of transformation into malignant lymphoma. Benign lymphoepithelial cysts reflect cysts lined by hyperplastic and metaplastic squamous epithelium, and are unusual outside of the HIV-infected population.[29]

Imaging reveals multiple well-defined, cystic, solid, or mixed cystic and solid masses most commonly involving the parotid glands bilaterally, along with generalized lymphoidal hyperplasia in the neck.[27] Although the most common presentation of benign lymphoepithelial cysts is painless, multiple, bilateral, superficial lobe parotid cysts, unilateral disease, single cysts, intermittent pain, and deep lobe involvement may occur. Submandibular gland benign lymphoepithelial cysts have been reported rarely.[29]

Differential diagnosis of benign lymphoepithelial lesions
- HIV
- Sjögren syndrome
- Sarcoidosis
- Non-Hodgkin lymphoma
- Benign epithelial cysts

Pitfall

An uncommon presentation is as a unilateral single cystic or solid HIV-related parotid lesion that may mimic congenital cyst (first branchial cleft) or neoplasm, respectively.

Sialolithiasis

Pediatric sialolithiasis is rare compared with the adult population, and estimated to occur in less than 5% of all cases. As in adults, calculi are overwhelmingly most common in the submandibular duct, with at least 80% of stones estimated to occur there. The parotid duct is more commonly stenotic than the submandibular duct, predisposing to sialadenitis and sialolithiasis.[19] Recurrent periprandial pain and swelling is the characteristic clinical presentation. Pediatric patients tend to have smaller stones located more distally in the ducts, and on average present after a shorter duration of symptoms compared with adults.[30]

On ultrasound examination, the stones appear as focal hyperechoic foci that cast posterior acoustic shadows. Ultrasound examination is highly sensitive and specific for stones greater than 3 mm; however, sensitivity decreases for smaller stones.[31] Radiographs and cone beam CT sialography demonstrate calculi as radiopaque or radiolucent filling defects as well as clearly delineate ductal strictures in the main and intraglandular ducts. Cone beam CT sialography can visualize intraglandular ducts up to the sixth order branch while also allowing for visualization of the salivary gland parenchyma.[32] Routine CT scanning readily demonstrates calcified stones as well as their relation to glandular and ductal elements. MR sialography with heavily T2-weighted sequences provides a noninvasive technique to evaluate the salivary ducts, with complementary glandular evaluation by standard MR imaging sequences (Fig. 11).

Pitfall

On ultrasound examination, misinterpretations of ductal pathology may occur in cases of small noncalcified stones and focal strictures.

Juvenile Sjögren Syndrome

SS is an uncommon disease in children, and consequently underdiagnosed. SS is an autoimmune exocrinopathy, primarily affecting the lacrimal and salivary glands.[33] Patients may present with recurrent episodes of acute, tender glandular swelling, or chronic glandular enlargement with superimposed acute episodes of painless swelling. Ocular (keratoconjunctivitis sicca) and oral (xerostomia) symptoms are less frequent at presentation in children than adults with primary SS. Primary SS carries a risk of malignant transformation into non-Hodgkin lymphoma.[34]

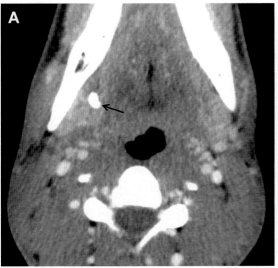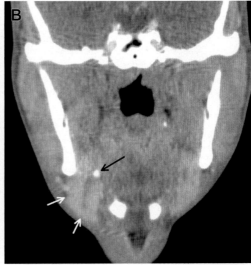

Fig. 11. Recurrent right submandibular sialadenitis secondary to sialolithiasis in a 16-year-old boy. (*A*) Axial and (*B*) coronal postcontrast computed tomography images show an enlarged and edematous right submandibular salivary gland (*white arrows*) with an obstructing radiodense calculus (*black arrows*) in the proximal submandibular duct. (*Courtesy of* Dr Ellen Park, Cleveland Clinic, Cleveland, OH.)

Ultrasound and MR imaging demonstrate small hypoechoic and T2 hyperintense glandular cystic foci in early stages of disease with increase in cyst size and glandular heterogeneity in later stages, including nodular foci corresponding to lymphocytic aggregates. Late stage SS may be associated with glandular calcifications, as well as atrophy and adipose deposition, with associated T1 hyperintensity.[35,36] CT scanning shows corresponding changes, and acute exacerbations demonstrate increased glandular density and may be unilaterally asymmetric. MR sialography is the most sensitive imaging modality to diagnose SS, clearly demonstrating glandular T2 hyperintense foci reflecting sialectasis, as well as abnormalities of the main duct.[37]

Pearl

Although SS is rare in children, it should be considered in cases of recurrent parotid gland swelling, even if the classic symptoms of xerostomia and xerophthalmia are not prominent at presentation.

Pitfall

Punctate sialectasis seen in early stage SS may seem similar to the changes of JRP.

RANULA

Ranulas are extravasation mucoceles of the sublingual gland or minor salivary glands in the floor of mouth that result from obstruction and consequent rupture of the main duct or acini, or disruption of submandibular ducts as a result of trauma or surgery. Extravasation of saliva results in formation of a floor of the mouth nonepithelialized pseudocyst that is lined by fibrous tissue and forms as the result of an inflammatory reaction to the extravasated mucus and subsequent granulation.[38]

Ranulas are defined as simple if they are confined to the sublingual space or diving/plunging if they extend around or through the mylohyoid muscle into the submandibular space or into the parapharyngeal space. On CT scanning and MR imaging, ranulas are thin-walled cystic lesions. Simple ranulas are confined to the sublingual space and are most closely mimicked by floor of the mouth epidermoids on CT scans, but are readily distinguishable by MR imaging because epidermoids have restricted diffusion. Plunging ranulas are often centered in the submandibular space, but a tail extending into the sublingual space is pathognomonic[39,40] (Fig. 12).

Differential diagnosis of cystic floor of the mouth lesion
- Ranula
- Lymphatic malformation
- Epidermoid/dermoid
- Oral cavity abscess/suppurative lymphadenopathy
- Submandibular duct sialocele
- Submandibular gland mucocele

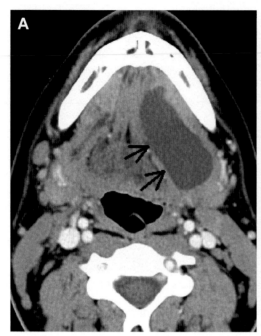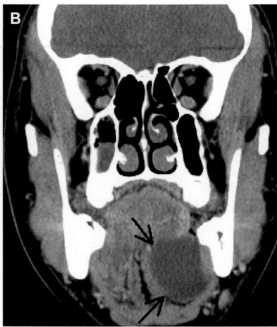

Fig. 12. Simple ranula in a 15-year-old girl. (*A*) Axial and (*B*) coronal postcontrast computed tomography images demonstrate a nonenhancing, low-attenuation lesion distending the left sublingual space (*arrows*).

Pearl

With a cystic submandibular space lesion, look for a collapsed tail of a cyst extending to sublingual space in plunging ranulas.

PNEUMOPAROTITIS

Pneumoparotid results from air blown retrograde through the excretory ducts of the parotid gland. The pathophysiology relates to increased intraoral pressure overcoming the valve system in the parotid duct, which may be contributed to by a patulous Stensen's duct, weak buccinator muscle, or masseter muscle hypertrophy. Activities that increase intraoral pressure or are associated with forced exhalation can be causative. In children, such activities may include wind instrument players, blowing up balloons, nose blowing, coughing fits, positive pressure ventilation during general anesthesia, or intentionally self-induced in adolescents. On ultrasound examination, tiny echogenic foci are present in the parotid gland. Air in the parotid duct and gland is clearly delineated on CT scans.[41]

HEMANGIOMAS AND VASCULAR MALFORMATIONS
Hemangiomas

Hemangiomas are benign vascular tumors of proliferating endothelial cells. Infantile hemangiomas appear in the first few months of life and characteristically undergo a proliferative phase in the first year of life followed by a protracted involuting phase that is typically completed by the end of the first decade.[42] Hemangiomas are the most common tumor of the parotid gland in children.[1,43] Of hemangiomas involving the major salivary glands, roughly 90% occur in the parotid gland, with the remaining minority occurring in the submandibular gland.[42]

Hemangiomas may present clinically as rapidly growing focal masses centered in the parotid space, or as a segmental lesion involving the parotid gland as well as adjacent soft tissues in the V3 trigeminal nerve distribution. Infantile hemangiomas of the head and neck, particularly the segmental type, may be accompanied by abnormalities of the PHACES association (posterior fossa malformation, carotid and cerebral arterial anomalies, cardiac defects, aortic coarctation, eye abnormalities, and sternal or other ventral developmental defects).[44,45] Segmental hemangiomas portend a greater likelihood of medical complications, including airway compromise, skin ulceration, and soft tissue and cartilage destruction.[43]

Most hemangiomas regress spontaneously; however, up to 10% may have complications of airway obstruction or vital structure compromise, or extensive facial disfigurement or skin ulceration, hemorrhage, or destruction. Hemangiomas can be effectively treated medically by propranolol, intra-lesional or systemic corticosteroids, or second-line interferon therapy.[41–43]

On MR imaging, proliferating infantile heman-giomas appear as intensely enhancing, well-defined masses, generally T1 isointense and T2 hyperintense relative to muscle, with increased vessels and associated flow voids within and adjacent to the mass. CT scanning demonstrates expected soft tissue mass, with diffuse enhancement. During the involuting phase, the mass is expected to contract in size and demonstrate signal and attenuation consistent with the ongoing fatty replacement. Doppler ultrasound imaging demonstrates diffuse hyper-vascularity in a noncalcified soft tissue mass[46] (**Figs. 13–15**).

Differential diagnosis of diffuse parotid enhancement
- Infantile hemangioma
- Arteriovenous malformation
- Venous vascular malformation
- Congenital hemangioma
- Sialoadenitis
- Primary epithelial neoplasm
- Other malignancy (lymphoma, sarcoma)

Pearl
If perilesional edema is present surrounding the enhancing mass, consider another type of mass instead of hemangioma.

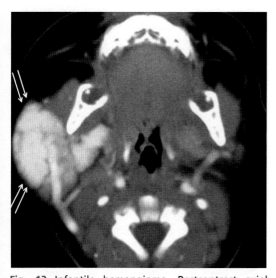

Fig. 13. Infantile hemangioma. Postcontrast axial computed tomography scan shows a diffusely enhancing mass (*arrows*) in the right parotid gland and parapharyngeal space. (*Courtesy of* Dr Patricia Hudgins, Emory University, Atlanta, GA.)

Vascular Malformations

As opposed to hemangiomas, vascular malforma-tions are slow growing congenital anomalies of vascular or lymphatic morphogenesis, with no endothelial cell hyperplasia, and no tendency toward spontaneous involution. Vascular malforma-tions are categorized as high-flow (arteriovenous malformations and fistulas) and low-flow (venous, lymphatic, capillary, mixed) malformations.[47]

Low-flow vascular malformations
Venous vascular malformations typically appear as compressible, heterogeneously hypoechoic le-sions with anechoic vascular spaces, and mono-phasic low-velocity venous flow. Lesions may be transspatial. The Valsalva maneuver and manual compression may accentuate intralesional flow signal. Echogenic phleboliths are evident in some lesions. MR imaging adequately delineates the extent of the lesion. Venous vascular malforma-tions are T2 hyperintense and hypointense or iso-intense on T1-weighted imaging, with areas of T1 hyperintensity reflecting hemorrhage or throm-bosis. Phleboliths, which are the hallmark of this entity, appear as focal signal voids on MR im-aging, and their presence is easily confirmed on CT scanning. Dynamic postcontrast imaging demonstrates heterogeneous and progressive enhancement.[46]

Pearl Phleboliths are pathognomonic of low flow vascular malformations with venous compo-nents. Phleboliths are not present in infantile hemangiomas.

Pitfalls
- Must distinguish phleboliths from sialoliths.
- Outdated terminology referred to venous vascular malformations as hemangiomas; however, this terminology should be avoided.

On ultrasound examination, macrocystic LMs are compressible, nonvascular, anechoic lesions that are most commonly multilocular with thin septae. Fluid–fluid levels or internal debris suggest prior hemorrhage. Lesions are often transspatial. Micro-cystic LMs are hyperechoic and more poorly defined. On MR imaging, LMs are low T1 and bright T2 signal lesions, usually multilocular cystic, without internal enhancement. Associated enhancement suggests a mixed venolymphatic malformation[46] (**Figs. 16–19**).

Pearl LMs may be complicated by hemorrhage or infection, and should be considered in the differen-tial diagnosis of suspected parotid abscess in an infant.

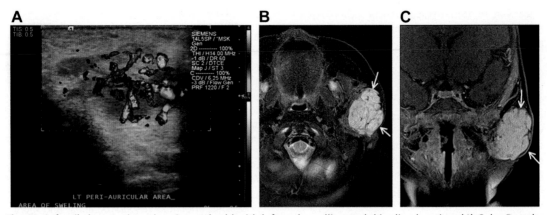

Fig. 14. Infantile hemangioma in a 6-month-old with left neck swelling and skin discoloration. (*A*) Color Doppler ultrasound image demonstrates a well-defined, hypervascular mass in the left preauricular region. (*B*) Axial fat-suppressed T2-weighted image shows a well-encapsulated, near homogeneously hyperintense left parotid mass (*arrows*) with internal septations and flow voids. (*C*) Coronal T1-weighted fat-suppressed postcontrast image demonstrates homogeneous enhancement of the mass (*arrows*), with internal vessels and septations evident.

High-flow vascular malformations

Imaging in arteriovenous malformations demonstrates dilated feeding arteries and draining veins with vascular nidus and little or no tissue matrix, in distinction to arteriovenous fistulas, which lack a nidus. Feeding arteries demonstrate an increased diastolic flow on Doppler ultrasound imaging and, in distinction to hemangiomas, arterialization of draining veins is the rule. Signal voids are present in enlarged and tortuous vessels. Angiographically, there is early venous filling, and intranidal or arterial aneurysms may be present.[46]

Traditionally, digital subtraction angiography has been considered the gold standard for high temporal and spatial evaluation of the arterial feeders, nidus, and venous drainage of arteriovenous malformations in the head and neck. However, digital subtraction angiography is an invasive technique with the risk of vascular injury or thromboembolism, ionizing radiation exposure, and is expensive and time consuming. Time resolved contrast-enhanced MR angiography, such as time-resolved imaging of contrast kinetics (TRICKS), has been demonstrated to be a reliable first-line noninvasive technique for delineating the feeding arteries, nidus, and draining veins of an arteriovenous malformation with high temporal and spatial resolution, that is comparable with digital subtraction angiography. Time resolved MR angiography techniques use a 3D spoiled gradient echo sequence to obtain sequential 3D volumes after contrast administration with oversampling of central k space.[48] Imaging with an isotropic high-resolution 3D T1 volumetric postcontrast sequence (magnetization prepared rapid acquisition gradient echo, fast spoiled gradient-recalled-echo) provides excellent spatial and contrast resolution.[46]

Pearl Vascular malformation or hemangioma should be considered when the lesion is transspatial.

EPITHELIAL SALIVARY NEOPLASMS

Neoplastic disease involving the salivary glands is much rarer in children than in adults. Less than 5% of all primary salivary gland neoplasms occur in patients younger than 16 year of age. Compared with adults, mesenchymal tumors are more common than epithelial tumors, of which hemangiomas are most frequent.[1] Nonepithelial tumors are the most common salivary neoplasms in neonates and infants in the first few years of life. Epithelial neoplasms are most common in the second decade of life.[1,49] In children, there is a higher relative incidence of malignant epithelial neoplasms than in adults, reflecting roughly one-half of epithelial tumors. Pediatric salivary tumors have a heavy parotid dominance, with the incidence of malignant lesions decreasing from the parotid to the submandibular to the sublingual glands, opposite the tendency in adults.[1,18]

The most common benign epithelial salivary neoplasm in children is benign mixed tumor (pleomorphic adenoma), and mucoepidermoid carcinoma is the most commonly encountered malignant epithelial neoplasm.[50] Mucoepidermoid carcinomas in children are most commonly of low histologic grade.[1]

The imaging characteristics are identical to those in the adult population, with benign mixed tumors typically appearing as circumscribed T2 hyperintense, enhancing masses, and low-grade mucoepidermoid carcinomas generally

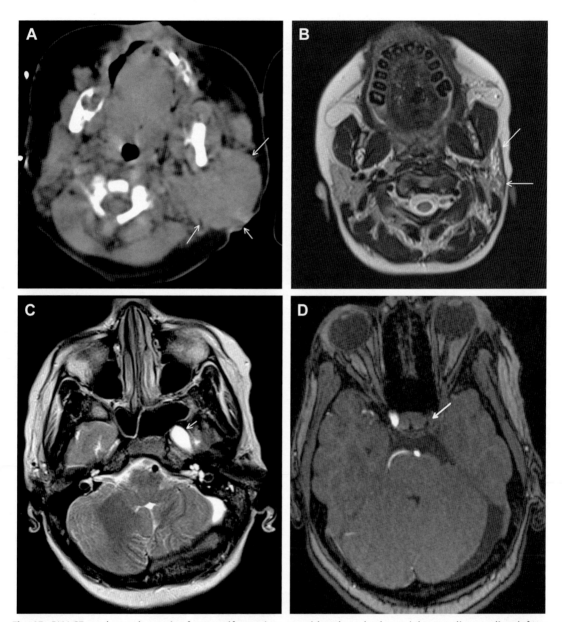

Fig. 15. PHACE syndrome (posterior fossa malformation, carotid and cerebral arterial anomalies, cardiac defects, aortic coarctation, eye abnormalities, and sternal or other ventral developmental defects) in an 11-year-old boy with left parotid gland infantile hemangioma first diagnosed at the age of 4 months. (*A*) Axial postcontrast computed tomography scan at age 4 months demonstrates a well-defined left parotid mass (*arrows*). Additional hemangiomas of the left neck and upper chest were also identified (not shown). (*B*) Axial T2-weighted MR image obtained at 10 years of age demonstrates changes secondary to spontaneous involution of the infantile hemangioma with atrophy and fatty infiltration within the left parotid gland (*arrows*). (*C*) Axial T2-weighted MR image through the posterior fossa shows dysplastic changes of the left cerebellar hemisphere with enlargement of the left Meckel's cave (*arrow*). (*D*) Axial time-of-flight image shows absence of flow-related signal in the left internal carotid artery (*arrow*).

well-defined masses demonstrating heterogeneous signal and attenuation and single to multiple variably sized cystic areas. Epithelial neoplasms of the minor salivary glands overwhelmingly are intraoral in location[1,47] (see **Fig. 19**; **Fig. 20**).

Differential diagnosis of focal salivary gland mass
- Primary epithelial neoplasm
- Reactive/metastatic lymph node
- Sialadenitis
- Lymphoma
- Sialocele

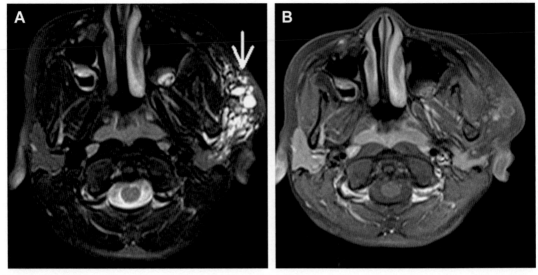

Fig. 16. Lymphatic malformation in a 4-year-old boy with left face swelling. (*A*) Axial fat-suppressed T2-weighted image demonstrates a transspatial, multicystic lesion involving the superficial lobe of the left parotid gland that extends anteriorly to the buccal fat pad (*arrow*). (*B*) Postcontrast axial T1-weighted image demonstrates no abnormal enhancement of the lesion.

Pearl

A benign parotid mass cannot be reliably distinguished from a low-grade malignancy by imaging appearance. However, a very high T2 signal (higher than cerebrospinal fluid) is suggestive of benign mixed tumor.

OTHER NEOPLASTIC DISEASES
Lymphoma and Nodal Metastatic Disease

Although uncommon, primary lymphoma, which is classified as a mucosa-associated lymphoid tissue, or secondary lymphoma may involve the lymph nodes of the parotid gland. Imaging may demonstrate focal nodal masses or an enlarged gland with diffuse infiltrative disease. Metastatic lymphadenopathy may also spread to the intraparotid nodes, although this finding is rare in the pediatric population[27] (**Fig. 21**).

Rhabdomyosarcoma

Rhabdomyosarcoma is the most common pediatric soft tissue sarcoma and, of these, 40% occur at sites in the head and neck. Most commonly, salivary gland involvement is from direct extension

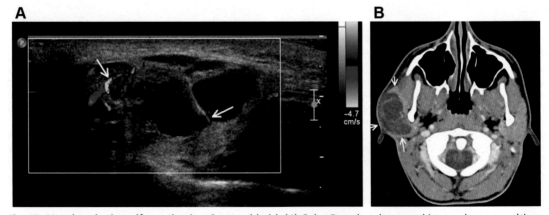

Fig. 17. Venolymphatic malformation in a 2-year-old girl. (*A*) Color Doppler ultrasound image shows a multiseptated complex cystic right parotid lesion with increased vascularity within the septations (*arrows*). (*B*) Axial postcontrast computed tomography image shows a predominantly cystic right parotid lesion with enhancing septae (*arrows*). Note the absence of surrounding inflammatory changes that help to differentiate this slow flow vascular malformation from an abscess.

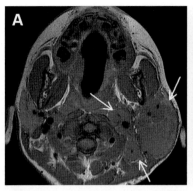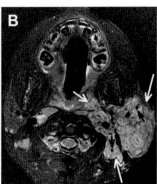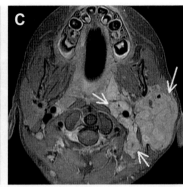

Fig. 18. Venolymphatic malformation in a 5-year-old boy. Axial (A) T1-weighted noncontrast, (B) T2-weighted with fat saturation, and (C) T1-weighted postcontrast with fat saturation images demonstrate a diffusely T2 hyperintense, enhancing transspatial mass centered in the left parotid space (arrows) and extending into the parapharyngeal, carotid, and posterior cervical spaces as well as smaller components in the posterior cervical and lateral retropharyngeal spaces on the right.

of disease. The mass typically demonstrates heterogeneous diffuse enhancement, with a T1 hypointense and a T2 hyperintense signal[27] (Fig. 22).

SYSTEMIC DISEASE

Sialosis (sialadenosis) refers to chronic bilateral, usually painless, swelling of the salivary glands, most commonly the parotid, without underlying inflammatory or neoplastic disease. Histologically, there is hypertrophy of the acinar cells, and chronically there may be fatty infiltration.[51] Among causes more common in the pediatric population are disorders of malnutrition, specifically bulimia and anorexia, which should be considered in unexplained bilateral parotid enlargement in adolescents.[52] The primary role of imaging is to exclude other etiologies of salivary gland enlargement.

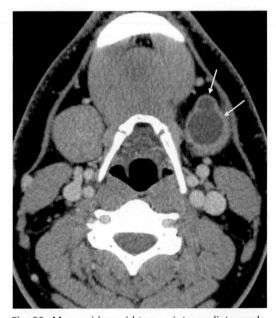

Fig. 19. Benign mixed tumor of the left parotid gland in an 18-year-old boy. Axial post–contrast-enhanced computed tomography scan demonstrates a well-defined enhancing mass within the superficial lobe of the left parotid gland (arrows). The absence of inflammatory changes of the overlaying subcutaneous tissue helps to differentiate this mass from acute inflammatory pathologies.

Fig. 20. Mucoepidermoid tumor, intermediate grade, in a 15-year-old patient. Axial postcontrast computed tomography scan shows a well-circumscribed lobular low-attenuation mass (arrows) in the left submandibular gland. (Courtesy of Lawrence Ginsberg, MD, Anderson Cancer Center, Houston, TX.)

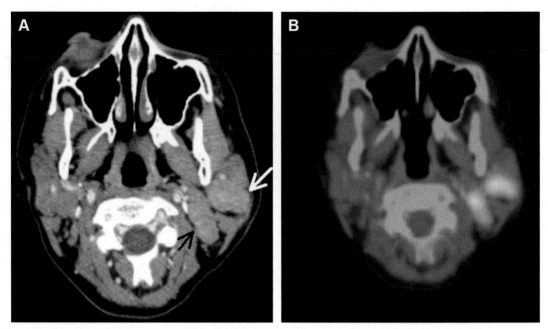

Fig. 21. A 13-year-old boy with Hodgkin lymphoma affecting the left parotid gland. (*A*) Axial postcontrast computed tomography scan demonstrates a lobulated enhancing mass in the posterior left parotid gland (*white arrow*) with additional level 2 lymph nodes (*black arrow*). (*B*) PET/CT fused image shows increased fluorodeoxy-glucose uptake within the parotid mass as well as the adjacent lymph nodes.

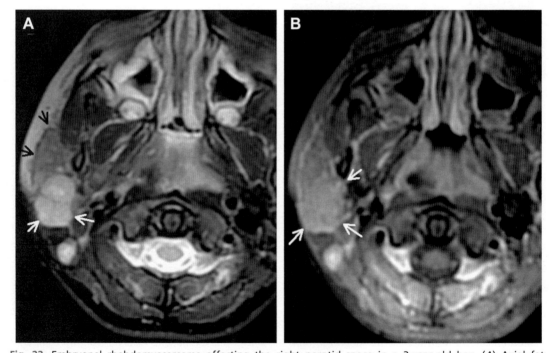

Fig. 22. Embryonal rhabdomyosarcoma affecting the right parotid space in a 3-year-old boy. (*A*) Axial fat-suppressed T2-weighted MR image shows a well-defined, lobulated, homogeneously hyperintense lesion in the right parotid space (*white arrows*) displacing the parotid gland anteriorly (*black arrows*). (*B*) Axial postcontrast T1-weighted fat-suppressed MR image demonstrates homogeneous enhancement of the lesion (*arrows*).

Progressive bilateral enlargement of the sub-mandibular glands may be seen in children with cystic fibrosis.[53]

SUMMARY

A wide variety of pathologies may affect the pediatric salivary glands. Uncomplicated viral and bacterial infections do not generally require imaging, except to evaluate for complications. In combination with the clinical history, salient imaging characteristics may either point to the specific diagnosis or narrow the differential diagnosis. Clinical and radiologic information will guide appropriate treatment.

REFERENCES

1. Luna MA, Batsakis JG, El-Naggar AK. Salivary gland tumors in children. Ann Otol Rhinol Laryngol 1991; 100:869–71.
2. Castro EB, Huvos AG, Strong EW, et al. Tumors of the major salivary glands in children. Cancer 1972; 29:312–7.
3. Bialek EJ, Jakubowski W, Zajkowski P, et al. US of the major salivary glands: anatomy and spatial relationships, pathologic conditions, and pitfalls. Radiographics 2006;26:745–63.
4. Abdel Razek AA, Gaballa G, Elhawarey G, et al. Characterization of pediatric head and neck masses with diffusion-weighted MR imaging. Eur Radiol 2009;19:201–8.
5. Kalinowski M, Heverhagen JT, Rehberg E, et al. Comparative study of MR sialography and digital subtraction sialography for benign salivary gland disorders. AJNR Am J Neuroradiol 2002;23: 1485–92.
6. Som PM, Miletich I. The embryology of the salivary glands: an update. Neurographics 2015; 5(4):167–77.
7. Johns ME. The salivary glands: anatomy and embryology. Otolaryngol Clin North Am 1977;10:261–71.
8. Dang NP, Picard M, Mondie JM, et al. Complete congenital agenesis of all major salivary glands: a case report and review of the literature. Oral Surg Oral Med Oral Pathol Oral Radiol Endod 2010;110: e23–7.
9. Srinivasan A, Moyer JS, Mukherji SK. Unilateral submandibular gland aplasia associated with ipsilateral sublingual gland hypertrophy. AJNR Am J Neuroradiol 2006;27:2214–6.
10. Osterhus IN, Skogedal N, Akre H, et al. Salivary gland pathology as a new finding in Treacher Collins syndrome. Am J Med Genet 2012;158A:1320–5.
11. Widemann HR, Drescher J. LADD syndrome: report of new cases and review of the clinical spectrum. Eur J Pediatr 1986;144:579–82.
12. Finn DG, Buchalter IH, Sarti E, et al. First branchial cleft cysts: clinical update. Laryngoscope 1987;97: 136–40.
13. Work WP. Newer concepts of first branchial cleft defects. Laryngoscope 1972;82:1581–93.
14. Orvidas LJ, Kasperbauer JL, Lewis JE, et al. Pediatric parotid masses. Arch Otolaryngol Head Neck Surg 2000;126:177–84.
15. Patel A, Karlis V. Diagnosis and management of pediatric salivary gland infections. Oral Maxillofacial Surg Clin N Am 2009;21:345–52.
16. Ericson S, Zetterlund B, Ohman J. Recurrent parotitis and sialectasis in childhood: clinical, radiologic, immunologic, bacteriologic, and histologic study. Ann Otol Rhinol Laryngol 1991;100:527–35.
17. Gadodia A, Seith A, Sharma R, et al. MRI and MR sialography of juvenile recurrent parotitis. Pediatr Radiol 2010;40:1405–10.
18. Iro H, Zenk J. Salivary gland diseases in children. GMS Curr Top Otorhinolaryngol Head Neck Surg 2014;13:Doc06.
19. Francis CL, Larsen CG. Pediatric sialadenitis. Otolaryngol Clin North Am 2014;47:763–78.
20. Orlandi MA, Pistorio V, Guerra PA, et al. Ultrasound in sialadenitis. J Ultrasound 2013;16:3–9.
21. Flint D, Mahadevan M, Barber C, et al. Cervical lymphadenitis due to non-tuberculous mycobacteria: surgical treatment and review. Int J Pediatr Otorhinolaryngol 2000;53:187–94.
22. Zimmermann P, Tebruegge M, Curtis N, et al. The management of non-tuberculous cervicofacial lymphadenitis in children: a systematic review and meta-analysis. J Infect 2015;71:9–18.
23. Lindeboom JA, Smets AM, Kuijper E, et al. The sonographic characteristics of nontuberculous mycobacterial cervicofacial lymphadenitis in children. Pediatr Radiol 2006;36:1063–7.
24. Razek A, Castillo M. Imaging appearance of granulomatous lesions of the head and neck. Eur J Radiol 2010;76:52–60.
25. Statement on sarcoidosis. Am J Respir Crit Care Med 1999;160:736–55.
26. Shetty AK, Gedalia A. Childhood sarcoidosis: a rare but fascinating disorder. Pediatr Rheumatol Online J 2008;6:16.
27. Lowe LH, Stokes LS, Johnson JE, et al. Swelling at the angle of the mandible: imaging of the pediatric parotid gland and periparotid region. Radiographics 2001;21:1211–27.
28. Koyama T, Ueda H, Togashi K. Radiologic manifestations of sarcoidosis in various organs. Radiographics 2004;24:87–104.
29. Dave SP, Pernas FG, Roy S. The benign lymphoepithelial cyst and a classification system for lymphocytic parotid gland enlargement in the pediatric HIV population. Laryngoscope 2007;117: 106–13.

30. Chung MK, Jeong H, Ko M, et al. Pediatric sialolithiasis: what is different from adult sialolithiasis? Int J Pediatr Otorhinolaryngol 2007;71:787–91.

31. Terraz S, Poletti P, Dulguerov P, et al. How reliable is sonography in the assessment of sialolithiasis? AJR Am J Roentgenol 2013;201:W104–9.

32. Kroll T, May A, Wittekindt C, et al. Cone beam computed tomography (CBCT) sialography—an adjunct to salivary gland ultrasonography in the evaluation of recurrent salivary gland swelling. Oral Surg Oral Med Oral Pathol Oral Radiol 2015;120: 771–5.

33. Nikitakis NG, Rivera H, Lariccia C, et al. Primary Sjögren syndrome in childhood: report of a case and review of the literature. Oral Surg Oral Med Oral Pathol Oral Radiol Endod 2003;96:42–7.

34. Cimaz R, Casadei A, Rose C, et al. Primary Sjogren syndrome in the paediatric age: a multicenter survey. Eur J Pediatr 2003;162:661–5.

35. Niemelä RK, Takalo R, Pääkkö E, et al. Ultrasonography of salivary glands in primary Sjogren's syndrome. A comparison with magnetic resonance imaging and magnetic resonance sialography of parotid glands. Rheumatology (Oxford) 2004;43: 875–9.

36. Izumi M, Eguchi K, Ohki M, et al. MR Imaging of the parotid gland in Sjogren's syndrome: a proposal for new diagnostic criteria. AJR Am J Roentgenol 1996; 166:1483–7.

37. Tonami H, Ogawa Y, Matoba M, et al. MR siaolgraphy in patients with Sjogren syndrome. AJNR Am J Neuroradiol 1998;19:1199–203.

38. Harrison JD. Modern management and pathophysiology of ranula: literature review. Head Neck 2010; 32:1310–20.

39. Coit WE, Harnsberger HR, Osborn AG, et al. Ranulas and their mimics: CT evaluation. Radiology 1987;163:211–6.

40. Kurabayashi T, Ida M, Yasumoto M, et al. MRI of ranulas. Neuroradiology 2000;42:917–22.

41. Ghanem M, Brown J, McGurk M. Pneumoparotitis: a diagnostic challenge. Int J Oral Maxillofac Surg 2012;41:774–6.

42. Sinno H, Thibaudeau S, Coughlin R, et al. Management of infantile parotid gland hemangiomas: a 40-year experience. Plast Reconstr Surg 2010;125: 265–73.

43. Greene AK, Rogers GF, Mulliken JB. Management of parotid gland hemangioma in 100 children. Plast Reconstr Surg 2004;113:53–60.

44. Weiss I, O TM, Lipari BA, et al. Current treatment of parotid hemangiomas. Laryngoscope 2011;121: 1642–50.

45. Oza VS, Wang E, Berenstein A, et al. PHACES association: a neuroradiologic review of 17 patients. AJNR Am J Neuroradiol 2008;29:807–13.

46. Dubois J, Alison M. Vascular anomalies: what a radiologist needs to know. Pediatr Radiol 2010;40: 895–905.

47. Mulliken JB, Glowacki J. Hemangiomas and vascular malformations in infants and children: a classification based on endothelial characteristics. Plast Reconstr Surg 1982;69:412–22.

48. Razek A, Gaball G, Megahed A, et al. Time resolved imaging of contrast kinetics (TRICKS) MR angiography of arteriovenous malformations of head and neck. Eur J Radiol 2013;82:1885–91.

49. Perez DE, Pires FR, Alves FA, et al. Salivary gland tumors in children and adolescents: a clinicopathologic and immunohistochemical study of fifty-three cases. Int J Pediatr Otorhinolaryngol 2004;68:895–902.

50. Ellies M, Laskawi R. Diseases of the salivary glands in infants and adolescents. Head Face Med 2010;6: 1–7.

51. Scully C, Bagan JV, Eveson JW, et al. Sialosis: 35 cases of persistent parotid swelling from two countries. Br J Oral Maxillofac Surg 2008;46:468–72.

52. Coleman H, Altini M, Nayler S, et al. Sialadenosis: a presenting sign in bulimia. Head Neck 1998;20: 758–62.

53. Barbero GJ, Sibinga MS. Enlargement of the submaxillary salivary glands in cystic fibrosis. Pediatrics 1962;29:788–93.

Imaging of Submandibular and Sublingual Salivary Glands

Amit K. Agarwal, MD[a],*, Sangam G. Kanekar, MD[b]

KEYWORDS

- Submandibular • Sublingual • Imaging • Salivary

KEY POINTS

- Submandibular and sublingual spaces have complex anatomies and are best evaluated on cross-sectional imaging.
- Magnetic resonance (MR) imaging provides the highest sensitivity for most of the neoplastic and vascular conditions involving these glands and spaces.
- Computed tomography still serves as the most commonly used modality worldwide and is well complemented by ultrasound on many occasions.
- MR has witnessed exponential growth for evaluation of deep neck space abnormality and for salivary gland evaluation.
- A wide spectrum of diseases can be seen in these regions, including inflammatory, infectious, vascular, and neoplastic conditions.

ANATOMY OF THE SUBLINGUAL AND SUBMANDIBULAR GLAND AND SPACES

The mylohyoid muscle divides the lower part of the oral cavity into 2 spaces: the sublingual (SL) space, which is located superior to the muscle, and the submandibular (SM) space, inferior to the muscle but superior to the hyoid bone. Most of the SM gland lies posterolateral to the mylohyoid muscle.[1,2]

Sublingual space contains the SL glands, the deep smaller portion of the SM gland, Wharton duct, the lingual artery and vein, the lingual nerve, and the hyoglossus muscle. The SM space contains the larger superficial portion of the SM gland, the facial artery and vein, the hypoglossal nerve, the anterior belly of the digastric muscle, and its lymph nodes (Fig. 1). The SL gland lies between the muscles of the oral cavity floor: the geniohyoid muscle, intrinsic muscles of the tongue, the hyoglossus muscle, and the mylohyoid muscle. Its lateral margins are adjacent to the mandibular body (Fig. 2).[2,3]

The SM gland is the second largest major salivary gland. The SM gland is divided into a superficial and a deep lobe. The superficial lobe lies in the digastric triangle and is bounded anteriorly by the anterior belly of the digastric muscle, posteriorly by the posterior belly of the digastric and stylohyoid muscles, and laterally by the lower border of the mandible and medial pterygoid muscle. Posteriorly, the stylomandibular ligament separates it from the parotid gland. The floor of the SM triangle is formed by the mylohyoid muscle anteriorly and the hyoglossus muscle posteriorly.[2–4] The superficial portion of the SM gland is covered by the platysma muscle and is traversed by the anterior facial vein and marginal mandibular

Disclosure Statement: The authors have nothing to disclose.
[a] Department of Radiology, UT Southwestern Medical Center, 5323 Harry Hines Boulevard, Dallas, TX 75390, USA; [b] Department of Radiology, Penn State University, 500 University Drive, Hershey, PA 17033, USA
* Corresponding author. 4102 Centenary Avenue, Dallas, TX 75225.
E-mail address: amitmamc@gmail.com

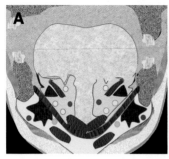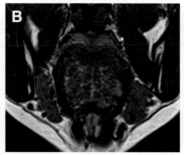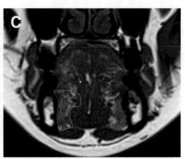

Fig. 1. Diagrammatic and MR imaging of the SM and SL space anatomy. (*A*) Diagram representing the SL and SM spaces with corresponding glanding. The SM space is seen as the green-shaded area (*B*) lying lateral to the mylohyoid sling (*brown arrow*) on coronal T1-weighted image. The SL space (*C*) is seen as the orange-shaded area lying lateral to the geniohyoid-genioglossus complex (*yellow arrow*) on T1-weighted coronal image.

nerve. The so-called deep portion of the SM gland lies deep to the posterior edge of the mylohyoid muscle (see **Fig. 2**). The lingual nerve lies above it and the hypoglossal nerve lies below. The middle layer of the deep cervical fascia encloses the SM gland. Wharton duct is around 5 cm long and exits anteriorly from the deep surface of the gland, coursing superiorly to the hypoglossal nerve while inferior to the lingual nerve and medial to the SL gland. It eventually lies between the mandible and the genioglossus muscle and empties lateral to the lingual frenulum through a papilla in the floor of the mouth behind the lower incisor tooth.[3,5]

Because there are no posterior fascial borders limiting the SL and SM spaces, communication is free between these spaces at the posterior margin of the mylohyoid (**Fig. 3**). In addition, no fascial border separates these spaces from the inferior parapharyngeal space. Thus, there is free communication among these 3 spaces, allowing lesions

occurring in the SL or SM space to extend into the parapharyngeal space. There is no true fascial capsule surrounding the SL gland, which is covered by oral mucosa on its superior aspect. Several ducts (of Rivinus) from the superior portion of the SL gland either secrete directly into the floor of mouth or empty into Bartholin duct that then continues into Wharton duct. The SL space has low attenuation similar to that of fat on computed tomography (CT), because of its primarily fatty content.[2–6]

A defect in the mylohyoid muscle is a common normal anatomic variant in the floor of the mouth that is seen in as many as 77% of CT examinations (**Fig. 4**).[7] Often in such cases, the SL salivary gland herniates through the defect into the adjacent SM space, sometimes producing a clinically palpable lump. Both the SM and the SL glands are supplied by the *submental* and *sublingual arteries*, branches of the lingual and facial arteries. The *facial artery*, the tortuous branch of the external carotid artery, is the main arterial blood supply of the SM gland.[3–8]

IMAGING TECHNIQUES FOR THE EVALUATION OF SUBMANDIBULAR AND THE SUBLINGUAL GLANDS

Plain films, sialography, ultrasound (US), nuclear medicine, CT, and magnetic resonance (MR) imaging are all commonly used in evaluation of salivary gland abnormality. CT is the most commonly used modality for salivary gland imaging with continuous improvement in the soft tissue differentiation, thinner sections, and excellent sagittal and coronal reconstructions along with the short examination time.[6,8,9] CT is very useful for evaluating infectious, inflammatory, and neoplastic processes and sialolithiasis. It is capable of depicting mandibular cortical bone erosion and destruction, cutaneous change, and

Fig. 2. Mylohyoid sling. Diagrammatic representation of the mylohyoid sling. The so-called deep portion of the SM gland lies deep to the posterior edge of the mylohyoid muscle and the lingual nerve lies above it.

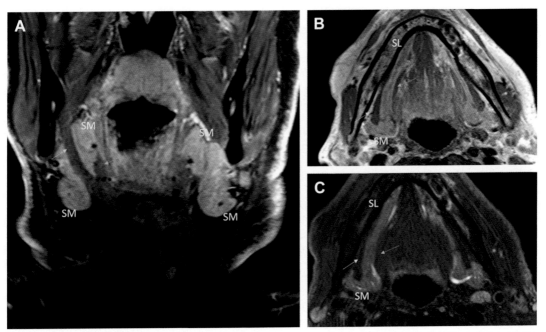

Fig. 3. Mylohyoid sling. The relationship of the superficial and deep lobe of the SM gland to the mylohyoid sling (*orange arrows*) is depicted on the (*A*) T1 coronal postcontrast (*B*) axial T1-weighted postcontrast and (*C*) axial T2-weighted images. The hyoglossus lies medially to the deep portion of SM gland (*green arrows*).

SM and SL gland and/or duct calculi. It is also very useful in evaluation of the associated neck lymphadenopathy. Streaky artifact from the dental hardware is one of the major limitations of CT in evaluation of the floor of the mouth and SL and SM glands. The SM and SL glands show a much higher attenuation on CT as compared with the parotid gland, because the latter has a higher content of fat in comparison to SM and SL glands. Direct postcontrast CT scan is preferred; however, in a suspected case of sialolithiasis, few unenhanced thin CT sections through the area of interest is performed to identify small calculi.[6,8–10]

MR imaging provides an excellent soft tissue resolution and therefore is predominately used staging oral cavity malignancies that involve the floor of the mouth and complex disease processes that extend through multiple anatomic spaces. Perineural spread of salivary gland tumors is better depicted by MR imaging than by CT. MR sialography uses specialized sequences that show the ductal anatomy in cases of suspected obstruction. Limitations of MR imaging of the salivary gland include artifacts produced by difficult breathing, especially in the patient treated for head and neck cancer with surgery and radiation, by swallowing-related movement, and by metallic dental amalgam. As compared with CT, it is less sensitive in diagnosis of calculus disease.[10–14] MR neurography is a new advanced technique with excellent depiction of the lingual and inferior alveolar nerve course and anatomy. This new

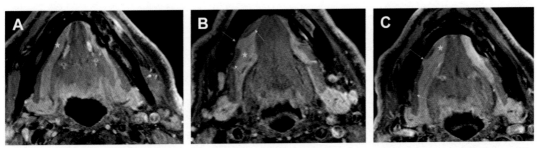

Fig. 4. Boutonniere. Multiple axial postcontrast T1 images of the oral cavity (*A-C*) show a small defect (*blue arrows*) in the mylohyoid muscle (*green arrows*). The right SL gland (*orange star*) protrudes through the defect into the SM space giving the impression of a boutonniere deformity. No defect is seen on the left side.

technique has the ability to differentiate intraneural from perineural masses and demonstrates nerve discontinuity in traumatic conditions (**Fig. 5**).

Plain radiographs, once more commonly used for detection of calculi, have a very limited role because of poor sensitivity and because of superimposition of bone on the areas of interest. Sialography is done less frequently nowadays but can still provide useful information in specific condition, such as duct dilatation (**Fig. 6**) and Sjogren syndrome (SS).[8–14]

US and Doppler are other commonly used imaging techniques for the evaluation of the salivary gland. The examination is usually performed with a high-resolution linear-array transducer, which provides excellent soft tissue resolution. Usually, 5- to 12-MHz, wide-band linear transducers (median frequency of 7–7.5 MHz) are used. The gland and the lesion present are usually evaluated in the 2 perpendicular planes for better definition. In addition, the whole neck can also be scanned to assess lymph nodes and search for concomitant or related disease. US is very useful in the evaluation of calculus disease, dilatation of the ducts, differentiating cystic masses from solid, and detection of associated neck lymphadenopathy.[8,9,15–18]

Advanced imaging techniques are increasingly being used for evaluation of head and neck tumors. These techniques include perfusion CT, perfusion MR imaging, and dedicated neck diffusion-weighted imaging (DWI). The basic principles for CT and MR perfusion studies are similar, with measurement of blood flow and blood volumes in the region of interest. Perfusion CT has more advantages, including having widespread availability, being less expensive, and having higher spatial resolution along with future prospects of integrating with PET-CT. Major clinical applications include differentiation of recurrent tumor versus posttreatment changes, which can be challenging on conventional studies. Perfusion scans can also better delineate the exact extent of tumor invasion, can serve as a guiding tool for biopsies, and can also help in characterizing neck lymphadenopathy. Diffusion imaging offers similar benefits and can be easily incorporated in MR imaging protocol given the short acquisition time and availability on most of the scanners. Diffusion imaging is also used to differentiate infective lesions, such as abscesses or suppurative lymphadenitis from their sterile counterparts.[19–22]

INFLAMMATORY DISEASES

Inflammatory diseases are the most common diseases affecting the major salivary glands. These inflammatory abnormalities may be either infectious or noninfectious, acute or chronic. Infectious abnormalities are most commonly viral or bacterial from the spread of a dental infection, usually from

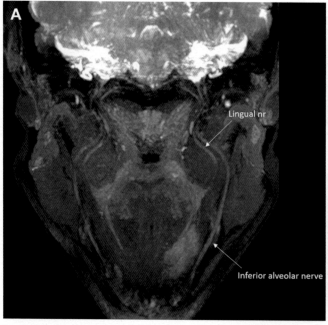
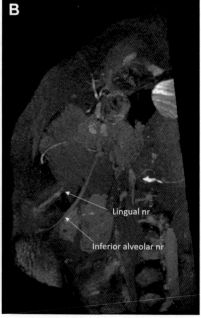

Fig. 5. MR neurography. Coronal (*A*) and sagittal (*B*) MR neurography images with depiction of the course and anatomy of the lingual and inferior alveolar nerves.

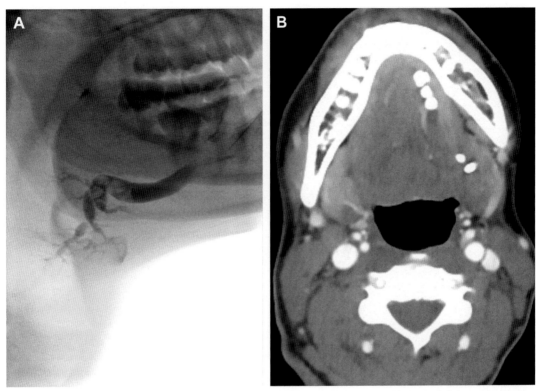

Fig. 6. Conventional sialogram with sialolith. Conventional sialogram (*A*) with dilatation of the main SM duct and numerous filling defects (calculus). Axial CT (*B*) in the same patient confirms the findings with better evaluation of gland morphology.

the premolar teeth or the first molar tooth or related to penetrating trauma, obstructing SM duct calculi, and intravenous drug use. Noninfectious inflammatory abnormalities include systemic disorders affecting the salivary glands, such as autoimmune diseases and sarcoidosis. From the clinical and imaging point of view, these abnormalities are classified into acute and chronic inflammatory abnormalities. Unilateral disease is usually secondary to ductal obstruction or bacterial infection. Bilateral involvement is commonly seen with viral infections (such as human immunodeficiency virus) and autoimmune inflammatory conditions, including immunoglobulin G4-related sialadenitis (IgG4 disease) and SS.

Acute Sialadenitis

Acute inflammation usually presents with painful swelling of the affected salivary gland. It may be unilateral or bilateral. Most commonly it is due to viral infections, which is most often bilateral and is most common in children. Viral infections are more common in parotid glands, whereas the acute bacterial infections are more common in SM and SL glands and are usually caused by *Staphylococcus aureus* or oral flora.[6,8,19]

Sonography can show an enlarged well-defined hypoechoic gland. They may be inhomogeneous, with multiple small, oval, hypoechoic areas, and may have increased blood flow at Doppler US. Concomitant painful enlarged cervical lymph nodes may be seen. Contrast-enhanced CT (CECT) shows diffuse enlargement of the affected gland, with or without inflammation of the surrounding soft tissue. The gland is diffusely hypodense due to edema and may show intraglandular ductal prominence. There may be associated extraglandular ductal dilatation, which may show wall enhancement on postcontrast CT. Bacterial infection may lead to an abscess formation within the salivary gland, which on CECT will show a central area of necrosis with surrounding capsular enhancement. MR imaging reveals diffuse edematous changes of the gland with increased T2 signal and hyperenhancement (**Fig. 7**). These changes are usually associated with enhancing enlarged lymph nodes.[15,18,23–25]

Chronic Sialadenitis

Chronic adult sialadenitis usually involves the parotid gland and presents with repeated episodes of acute inflammation of the salivary gland

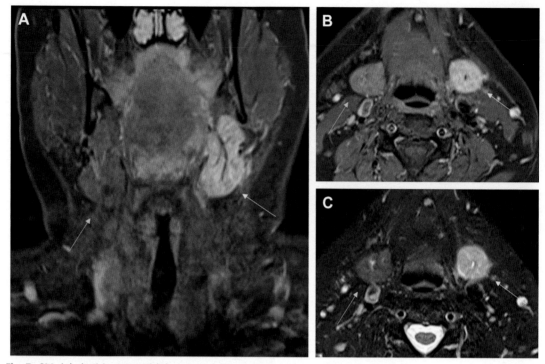

Fig. 7. SM sialadenitis. Coronal (*A*) and axial (*B*) contrast-enhanced T1-weighted images show avid enhancement of the left SM gland (*yellow arrows*) with normal enhancement pattern of the contralateral gland (*green arrows*). The left SM gland shows diffusely increased T2 signal (*C*) with normal signal of the right gland.

eventually resulting in acinar atrophy and ductal ectasia. Chronic sclerosing sialadenitis and granulomatous sialadenitis are 2 of the most common forms of chronic sialadenitis seen involving the SM and SL glands. It is clinically characterized by intermittent swelling of the gland, often painful. The imaging appearance is usually variable depending on the duration and severity of inflammation. The glands may be of normal size or smaller, may show normal density, or may appear hypodense. There may be associated intraglandular ductal dilatation and/or microcalcification. Chronic juvenile recurrent sialadenitis is much more common than adult sialadenitis, mainly seen in young male children and usually involving the parotid salivary gland.[15,24,25]

Ludwig Angina

Ludwig angina is a severe form of cellulitis, usually caused by streptococcal or staphylococcal bacteria. Ludwig angina is typically encountered in association with a 2- to 4-day history of prior mandibular dental extraction. Infections of the mandibular molars account for up to 90% of reported cases. Before the development of antibiotics, the infection would often spread inferiorly along fascial planes into the mediastinum, producing chest symptoms. The diagnosis of Ludwig angina requires 4 criteria to be met: (a) the process always involves both the SL and SM spaces and is usually bilateral; (b) there is gangrene or serosanguinous phlegmon but little or no frank pus; (c) it involves connective tissue, fascia, and muscle but spares glandular structures; and (d) it spreads by contiguity, not by lymphatics.[1,5,6,18,25]

On imaging studies, Ludwig angina appears as a diffuse cellulitis with increased attenuation on CT with associated enhancement involving the floor of the mouth. CECT typically shows diffuse aggressive inflammatory change and small fluid pockets representing serosanguinous accumulations in the floor of the mouth. Diffuse inflammation may involve the SL or SM glands and its surrounding soft tissue, which may extend deep into the SM and parapharyngeal spaces and the pharynx, leading to airway narrowing or obstruction. The role of imaging is to determine airway patency, document the presence of any gas-producing organisms, detect any underlying dental infection, detect osteomyelitis, and identify any drainable abscess. Early recognition and treatment are vital. Treatment is aimed at securing the airway and includes intravenous antibiotics and surgical decompression of the SM space. Ludwig angina is associated with a mortality rate of up to 10%.[1,6,26,27]

SIALOLITHIASIS

Sialolithiasis is most commonly seen in the SM gland (60%–90% of cases) followed by parotid glands (10%–20% of cases). The SM gland is more prone to calculous disease because of the high mucus content and viscous nature of its secretions. Between 80% and 90% of the calculi are opaque and therefore are visible on radiographs. US can reliably depict ductal obstruction and calculi as small as 3 mm, although there can be significant operator dependency. Sialolithiasis may cause partial or total mechanical obstruction of the salivary duct, resulting in recurrent swelling of a salivary gland during eating. It also predisposes the gland for bacterial infection.[2,5,6,28]

In a suspected case of calculus, unenhanced CT of the neck with thin sections is performed through the neck or region of interest. It is important to trace the entire Wharton duct in the floor of the mouth up to its opening. Axial images done parallel to the occlusal plane will project the entire SM duct below dental restorations and the potential artifact that they cause. CT has the highest sensitivity for the detection of SM gland calculi, particularly when they are small and multiple (see **Fig. 6**). CT may show intraglandular or extraglandular ductal calculus, with associated dilatation of the duct and ductules. If complicated, there may be associated inflammation of the gland and the surrounding soft tissues. Sialography may be used to demonstrate the location of the calculus and associated ductal stricture that is not evident at CT or US. Sialography is invasive and has a failure rate of around 14%. Today, MR sialography is more widely used because it is less invasive and used without ionizing radiation. MR sialography is performed by using T2-weighted 3-dimensional CISS (constructive interference in steady state) and HASTE (half-Fourier single-shot turbo spin-echo) sequences and is found to be comparable with that of conventional sialography for detecting the cause of ductal obstruction.[24,28,29]

GRANULOMATOUS LESIONS

Granulomatous disease is a unique form of chronic inflammatory condition characterized by the presence of epithelioid macrophages and can involve the SM and SL spaces. Infective granulomas are more common in the developing countries and can be secondary to bacterial (tuberculosis, nontuberculous mycobacterium, leprosy, syphilis) or a wide range of fungal infections (usually seen in immunocompromised patients). Noninfective granulomatous diseases are usually secondary to chronic autoimmune conditions, such as Wegener granulomatosis, sarcoidosis, and amyloidosis. These lesions are characterized by chronic soft tissue inflammatory changes, with or without suppuration. These lesions can be nodal or extranodal and can also involve the bone and the cranial nerves. Calcification and fibrosis can be seen in late stages of the disease, resulting in variable enhancement pattern on CT/MR. These lesions may also present as widespread nodular masses and mimic malignancy on imaging. Histopathology is usually required for diagnosis confirmation.[30,31]

VASCULAR LESIONS

The classification of and nomenclature based on the endothelial malformations have not been used in clinical practice. The most widely accepted classification system is by Mulliken and Glowacki,[32] which is based on the natural history, cellular turnover, and histology. It classifies the vascular malformation into 2 large groups: *hemangiomas* and *vascular malformations*.[1,6,32]

Hemangiomas tend to be small or absent at birth and often are not initially noticed by parents and caregivers. Shortly after birth, they undergo a proliferative phase, with rapid growth over several months followed by a stationary period, and then period of involution. Conversely, vascular malformations are always present at birth and enlarge in proportion to the growth of the child. They do not involute and remain present throughout the patient's life. Vascular malformations are subcategorized as lymphatic, capillary, venous, arteriovenous, and mixed malformations on the basis of their histologic makeup. Although MR imaging has been used to classify vascular malformations into one of these categories, contrast-enhanced or dynamic MR is more pertinent in classifying vascular malformations as either low-flow or high-flow lesions. Malformations with arterial components are considered high-flow lesions, and those without arterial components are considered low-flow lesions.[33–35]

Low-Flow Lesions

Infantile (capillary) hemangiomas are true vascular neoplasms that usually manifest by 3 months of age, proliferate in the first year, and involute by 9 years of age. The diagnosis is based on clinical history and examination, and imaging is required only to see the depth and extent of the lesion. This tumor shows a 3-phase evolution: rapid growth until the age of about 10 months, then stabilization, and finally, regression with sometimes an incomplete involution with residual calcifications. Imaging findings are a large solid mass that shows intermediate T1-weighted, high

T2-weighted signal intensities, and intense and fast enhancement with multiple enlarged vascular signal voids.[34–38]

Low-flow venous malformations in the head and neck occur most frequently in the buccal space or the floor of the mouth and may extend to involve SL or SM spaces. One of the commonly seen lesions is *cavernous hemangioma*. These lesions are compressible and have a hypoechoic, heterogeneous appearance with multiple anechoic sinusoidal spaces on US images. The slow flow in a lesion is often undetectable at power Doppler imaging and conventional angiography. MR imaging and CT are preferred because they allow a complete evaluation of the extent and transspatial dimensions of the lesions. Depending on the size of the venous channels, low-flow lesions range from predominantly cystic masses with high-signal-intensity venous lakes on T2-weighted image to more solid lesions that are isointense to the muscle. The lesions may contain calcified phleboliths, which are seen as dark hypointense foci on MR images and as calcific nodules on CT images.[1,18,34–38] These venous malformations can be classified into type I–IV, according to their venous drainage on angiography: type I is an isolated malformation without peripheral drainage; type II is a malformation that drains into normal veins; type III is a malformation that drains into dilated veins; and type IV is a malformation that represents dysplastic venous ectasia. This can be done on contrast-enhanced MR angiography (MRA) and can be very helpful in treatment planning.[39,40]

Lymphatic malformations (lymphangiomas/cystic hygromas) are the most common cystic masses within the first 2 years of life. They are most commonly located in the posterior triangle of the neck. Anteriorly, the SM space is much more frequently involved than the floor of the mouth. On imaging, a transspatial, multilocular mass with fluid-fluid levels, no central enhancement, and lack of phleboliths is suggestive of the diagnosis.[38,41]

High-Flow Lesions

Arteriovenous malformations (high-flow vascular malformations) of the head and neck are rare lesions with unclear pathogenesis. They usually present during childhood, growing proportionally to the child. The lesions are best depicted on MR images, where they appear as ill-defined masses with multiple flow voids, a large feeding artery or draining vein, and, occasionally, intraosseous extension. Dynamic contrast-enhanced MR is very helpful in evaluating the flow dynamics and

extent of arteriovenous shunting. Time-resolved imaging of contrast kinetics MRA is a newer technique for noninvasive assessment of arteriovenous malformations. This technique is based on multiple sequential 3-dimensional gradient acquisitions, which enable dynamic visualization of blood flow with high temporal resolution. This technique enables the capture of the early arterial phase without venous contamination with excellent characterization of arterial feeders and the nidus size. At present, digital subtraction angiogram (DSA) remains the gold standard to diagnose these lesions. These newer MR techniques, however, have the potential to replace DSA for vascular mapping before treatment (**Fig. 8**).[34,37–39,41,42]

CYSTIC LESIONS

SM and SL spaces both may be involved by the variety of cystic lesions. Most often, cysts in the floor of the mouth are benign and arise from salivary glands. Lesions such as ranula and dermoid or epidermoid cysts are more common in these spaces, whereas sialoceles, hydatid cysts, and thyroglossal duct cysts are rare. Cystic lesions in the SL/SM region are usually slow growing and often cause signs and symptoms only after they are large.

Ranula

A ranula is a mucous retention cyst or mucocele that arises from an SL gland or minor salivary gland. They have a peripheral epithelial layer, and depending on their capsule and extent, they are characterized as either simple or plunging (diving) ranula. They typically result from trauma or inflammation of the salivary glands, but rarely, can be congenital. There are 2 different concepts for the pathogenesis of ranula. One is a true cyst caused by ductal obstruction with an epithelial lining, and the other is a pseudocyst caused by injury of the duct and extravasation of mucus without an epithelial lining. Recently, typical ranulas have been considered an extravasation phenomenon of the SL gland. A simple ranula manifests clinically by swelling in the floor of the mouth.[43,44]

Imaging is useful for diagnosis and to determine the size, location, and extent of the lesion. On MR imaging, a ranula typically appears as a high-signal-intensity lesion in the SL space on T2-weighted images and may have abnormally high signal intensity on T1-weighted images because of its high protein content. A simple ranula occasionally involves the SM space by either herniating through a mylohyoid defect or arising from an ectopic SL gland. On CT, it is seen as a homogeneous, well-defined fluid density

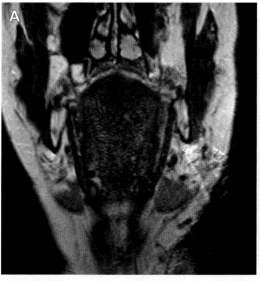 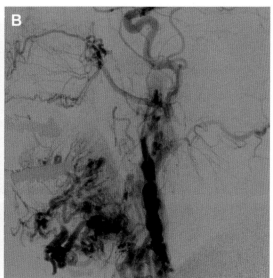

Fig. 8. High-flow vascular malformation. Coronal T1-weighted (*A*) images of the face reveal multiple prominent vessels in the SM region on the left (*red arrows*). Catheter angiogram (*B*) shows marked arteriovenous shunting with prominent arterial feeders from the external carotid artery branches suggesting a high-flow lesion.

mass on CT. On US images, a ranula typically appears as a simple cystic (anechoic) lesion deep to the mylohyoid muscle. It may contain fine internal echoes because of debris.[4,45]

A plunging or diving ranula develops after a rupture of simple ranula. The ruptured ranula usually extends posteriorly from the SL space into the SM space. Less commonly, it may extend anteriorly through a mylohyoid defect into the anterior SM space. The extension lacks epithelial lining, and therefore, a plunging ranula by definition is a pseudocyst. The lesion usually shows a narrow "tail" extending into the floor of the mouth. CT, MR imaging, and US all are capable of demonstrating the full extent of a plunging ranula.[43–45]

Dermoid/Epidermoid Cyst

Epidermoid and dermoid cysts in the floor of the mouth are mostly congenital. Epidermoid cysts are more frequently seen in the floor of mouth than in the SM space, whereas dermoid cysts are more often seen in the SM space than in the floor of mouth. Epidermoid cysts contain only epithelial elements, whereas dermoid cysts have both epithelial elements and a dermal substructure.

On MR, both types of lesions are well circumscribed and have high T2 signal with no enhancement or only thin rim enhancement. Dermoid can be differentiated by the presence of fatty and calcific components as well as fluid. This fat may coalesce into globules, creating a "sack of marbles" appearance, which is nearly pathognomonic

of dermoid (**Fig. 9**). On the other hand, epidermoid cysts are likely to be more homogeneous and, when occurring in the SL space, may be indistinguishable from simple ranulas, by presence of restricted diffusion on DWI (high diffusion and a low apparent diffusion coefficient), which is a characteristic feature for epidermoid.[1,6,10,45]

SYSTEMIC DISORDERS OF THE MAJOR SALIVARY GLANDS
Sialosis

Sialosis refers to a painless, noninflammatory enlargement of the salivary glands that may be caused by systemic disorders such as diabetes mellitus, alcoholism, hypothyroidism, and malnutrition. It may be also associated with medications such as antibiotics, diuretics, and psychotropic medications. Imaging appearance depends on the stage of the disease. In the early stages, MR imaging or CT will show uniformly homogenous, enlarged glands. On CT, in the early stages, glands show normal density (hyperdense), whereas in the later stages, there is diffuse enlargement with fatty infiltration (hypodense). Corresponding changes are also seen on MR of fat infiltration on T1-weighted image.[46]

Postirradiative Sialadenitis

Postirradiative sialadenitis is not uncommon especially following radiation therapy for head and neck cancer or for lymphoma. With improved radiation techniques, the acute painful form of postradiation

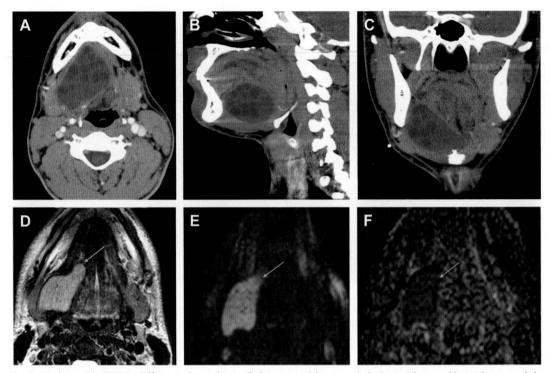

Fig. 9. SL dermoid. CECT in different planes (*A, B, C*) shows an oblong cystic lesion with round hypodense nodules in the right SL space, giving a "sack of marbles" appearance that is pathognomonic for dermoid cysts. Axial T2-weighted MR image (*D*) shows the lesion between the SL gland and the hyoglossus-geniohyoid muscles (*yellow arrow*). Lesion shows true restricted diffusion with bright signal (*green arrows*) on DWI (*E*) and appears dark on the ADC maps (*F*).

sialadenitis is exceedingly rare. In the subacute stages, CT shows hypodense edematous changes in SM and SL gland and spaces (**Fig. 10**). In the chronic stages, there is atrophy and fatty infiltration and intraglandular prominence of the duct possibly due to strictures or edematous blockage.[24,47]

Sjogen Syndrome

SS is an autoimmune exocrinopathy, which manifests with dysfunction of the salivary and lacrimal systems, typically presenting as complaints of oral and ocular dryness (xerostomia), respectively. SS may be *primary* (with no systemic autoimmune disorder) or *secondary* SS, which occurs in conjunction with another autoimmune connective tissue disease, such as rheumatoid arthritis, systemic lupus erythematosus, systemic sclerosis, or primary biliary cirrhosis. The disease may affect all salivary glands, parotid glands being the commonest followed by SM glands. On examination, the glands usually reveal bilateral, nontender, firm, and diffuse swelling.[10,48,49]

During the early phase of the disease, the glands are diffusely enlarged and both CT and MR have limited roles. As the disease progresses to intermediate phase, the imaging findings become more characteristic. The glands are diffusely enlarged in this phase with multiple microcysts (less than 1 mm) and macrocysts, along with solid masses. Atrophy of the gland is usually seen during the chronic phase. US features of advanced SS include inhomogeneous structure of the gland with scattered multiple small, oval, hypoechoic, or anechoic areas, usually well defined, and increased parenchymal blood flow. CT shows nonspecific honeycomb glandular appearance during the intermediate phase, which may progress to diffuse cystic appearance due to punctate, globular, cavitary, or destructive sialectasia. On MR imaging, a miliary pattern of small cysts are commonly seen in the subacute to chronic stages in a patient with SS. These characteristic changes are characteristically seen in the parotid gland and to a much lesser extent in the SM gland (**Fig. 11**). More commonly, the SM gland shows nonspecific enlargement.[18,48,49]

NEOPLASMS

Most of the salivary gland tumors are benign (70%–80%) and found most commonly in the

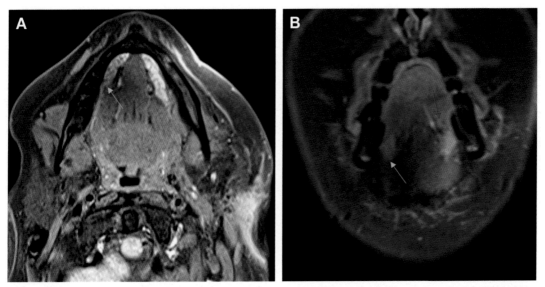

Fig. 10. Postradiation SL sialadenitis. Axial (A) and coronal (B) contrast-enhanced T1-weighted images show swelling and increased enhancement of the left SL gland (*red arrows*). Normal SL gland morphology is noted on the right (*green arrows*). Note the surgical absence of the left parotid gland for parotid tumor, which was followed by radiation.

parotid glands (80%–90%). About 10%–12% of all salivary gland neoplasms are located in the SM glands, of which approximately 50% are malignant. Pathologic rule of the salivary gland tumors is the smaller the salivary gland (eg, minor, SL), the higher are the chances of the tumor being a malignant lesion, and the larger the gland (parotid),

then the tumor is more likely benign. Approximately 25% of parotid, 50% of SM, and 80% of SL/minor salivary gland tumors are malignant. The most common salivary gland neoplasm is pleomorphic adenoma (benign), whereas mucoepidermoid carcinoma is the most common malignancy (overall). The commonest malignant

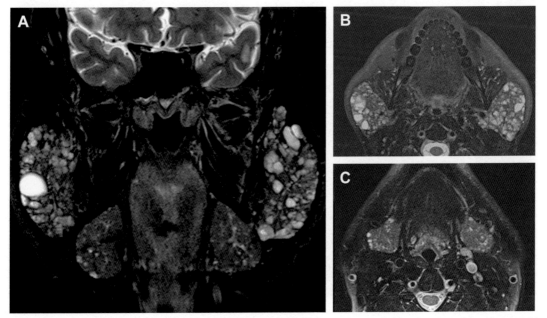

Fig. 11. SS. (A) Coronal T2 fat-suppressed images show diffuse enlargement of the parotid and SM glands with multiple tiny cysts within. Numerous tiny cysts are seen on the axial T2 images through the parotid (B) and the SM glands (C).

SM/SL/minor salivary gland tumor is however an adenoid cystic carcinoma.[50,51]

BENIGN NEOPLASMS
Pleomorphic Adenomas

The most commonly encountered benign tumor of the SM gland is pleomorphic adenoma, which comprises 53% to 64% of SM tumors. Pleomorphic adenomas rarely occur in the floor of the mouth. Only 1% of pleomorphic adenomas are found in the SL gland. Classical clinical presentation is that of a slowly growing, painless, discrete, hard mass. The histologic features and biologic behavior of pleomorphic adenoma of the SM gland are similar to those of the parotid gland.[50,51]

The imaging goal in a suspected case of an SM or SL mass is to determine the origin of the lesion, assess the extent, and identify the associated lymphadenopathy. On CT, pleomorphic adenomas typically appear as well-defined homogeneous lesions with attenuation slightly higher than that of muscle. Smaller lesions are usually quite homogeneous in appearance, whereas larger masses are heterogeneous, with areas of necrosis, hemorrhage, and cystic degeneration. The larger tumors tend to develop a lobulated

appearance. At MR imaging, the lesions have variable signal intensity depending on the presence and extent of necrosis, hemorrhage, or cystic change. These tumors have a nonhomogeneous appearance, with intermediate signal intensities on T1-weighted and proton density sequences. On T2-weighted images, there is usually a mixture of intermediate- and high-signal intensities. Associated hemorrhage may appear as high signal intensity on T1-weighted image. On US, pleomorphic adenomas are hypoechoic, well-defined, lobulated tumors with posterior acoustic enhancement and may contain calcifications (**Fig. 12**). The feature of lobulated shape is being emphasized in a differential diagnosis.[50–54]

The most common mass to be confused with an SM gland tumor, especially pleomorphic adenoma, is an enlarged lymph node. Distinction between these 2 becomes very important because treatment differs significantly. Cross-sectional imaging plays a vital role in defining the cleavage between the SM gland and the enlarged lymph nodes. However, in the case of a lymph node with perinodal spread, this distinction may be challenging. A neoplasm arising in the SM gland will not replace the entire gland. Some amount of normal gland almost always remains bordering the tumor. If this is not identified and the entire

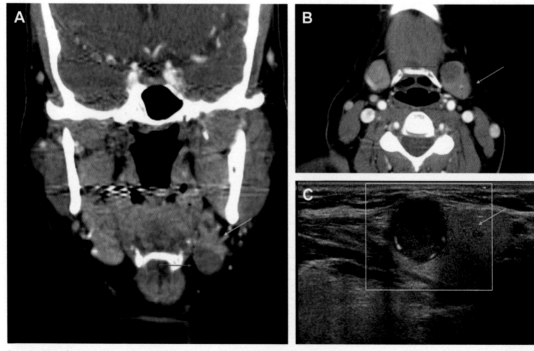

Fig. 12. SM pleomorphic adenoma. Coronal (*A*) and axial (*B*) CECT images show a round poorly enhancing lesion (*red arrows*) within the left SM gland (*green arrows*). US of the lesion (*C*) shows a hypoechoic mass (*red arrow*) with mild peripheral vascularity. The normal echotexture of the gland is shown with a green arrow. US-guided biopsy of the lesion was performed.

gland appears abnormal, then enlargement from obstruction is more likely and the course of the SM duct is carefully examined for calculus. In these cases, the floor of the mouth should be examined carefully on imaging to rule out early malignancy invading the duct.[6,50–54]

Other Benign Neoplasms

Lipomas are common mesenchymal tumors with the majority occurring in the posterior aspect of the neck. Rarely, they may be seen in the SL or SM spaces. Lipomas can be differentiated from normal fatty deposits by their internal architecture, their mass effect on adjacent structures, and their metabolic behavior. Most of the lipomas are well-defined encapsulated masses found just beneath the skin or between muscles and other connective-tissue structures. The imaging characteristics of classic lipomas include attenuation equivalent to that of subcutaneous fat on CT images and high signal intensity on both T1- and T2-weighted MR images. On fat-suppressed images, the signal within lipomas drops out completely. Thin septa occasionally can be seen within the tumors. There are numerous histopathologic variants of lipoma, such as fibrolipoma, angiolipoma, or intramuscular lipoma, which can present with atypical features on imaging, including thicker septa (more than 2 mm), nodularity, hemorrhage, and enhancement. Although uncommon, they are challenging to diagnose, and it may be impossible to distinguish them from their malignant counterparts. A vast majority of the lipomas are however simple with typical imaging appearance, and they rarely present a diagnostic challenge.[53–55]

Nerve sheath tumors (schwannomas and neurofibromas) are uncommon in this region. Neurofibromas are mostly associated with neurofibromatosis. Schwannomas (neurilemmomas) tend to occur in the fourth decade of life, arising from peripheral motor, sensory, and sympathetic nerves, most commonly in women (**Fig. 13**). Schwannomas arising from the lingual and hypoglossal nerves in the floor of the mouth have been reported. The lesions appear well defined and internally homogeneous, with attenuation of soft tissue on CT images and with signal isointense to that of muscle on T1-weighted MR images and hyperintense to that of muscle on T2-weighted images. Large lesions tend to become cystic and show contrast enhancement.[1,6,53,54]

MALIGNANT NEOPLASMS

Both SM and, rarely, SL gland spaces may be involved by a wide variety of malignant neoplasms.

These neoplasms may be primary, secondary, and local manifestations of systemic neoplastic diseases. Among primary malignant tumors, adenoid cystic carcinoma accounted for 42.2% of cases followed by mucoepidermoid carcinoma (22.2%), squamous cell carcinoma (17.3%), and adenocarcinoma (15.4%).[51–53]

Adenoid cystic carcinoma is very invasive and may develop over a short time. It usually presents as a painful mass that is fixed to the mandible (**Fig. 14**). Over one-third of these patients develop regional lymph node metastasis. Like in the parotid gland, this tumor has high propensity for nerve invasion. Because of the anatomic location of the SM gland, this poses a risk of perineural spread through the lingual and hypoglossal nerves toward the skull base and through the V3 division of the trigeminal but never extends into the Meckel cave. Perineural spread may also involve the mandibular or cervical branches of the facial nerve.[51–53]

Mucoepidermoid carcinoma is the second most common malignant neoplasm of the SM gland after adenoid cystic carcinoma. Metastatic cervical lymphadenopathy is more common in cases of mucoepidermoid carcinoma. Imaging features may be similar to any other malignant tumor but with less propensity for perineural invasion. *Squamous cell carcinoma* usually presents as a hard mass, often fixed, with a short history of 1 year or less and constitutes around 95% of oral cavity malignancies. In 20% of cases of squamous cell carcinoma of the floor of the mouth, metastases are identified in submental, SM, and upper deep cervical nodal groups. Tumors that involve the floor of the mouth may obstruct the SM duct, invade the adjacent mandible or tongue, and extend into the oropharynx. Invasion of the Wharton duct may cause dilatation of the duct, intraglandular ductal dilatation, and enlargement of the gland, making it more prone for infection. *Adenocarcinoma* arises infrequently in the SM gland. These very aggressive tumors invariably present with lymph node metastases and massive local extension to soft tissue and invasion of the mandible, resulting in poor local control, which adversely affects prognosis.

CECT and contrast-enhanced MR imaging are the modalities commonly used for initial evaluation and follow-up of the salivary gland malignancy. The main aim of the imaging is to establish whether the mass is intrinsic or extrinsic to the gland; to determine its relationship to the nerves; to evaluate the full extent of the lesion, with possible signs of invasion of surrounding structures; and to identify the enlarged/metastatic lymph nodes. MR imaging, with its superior soft tissue resolution, answers the above questions

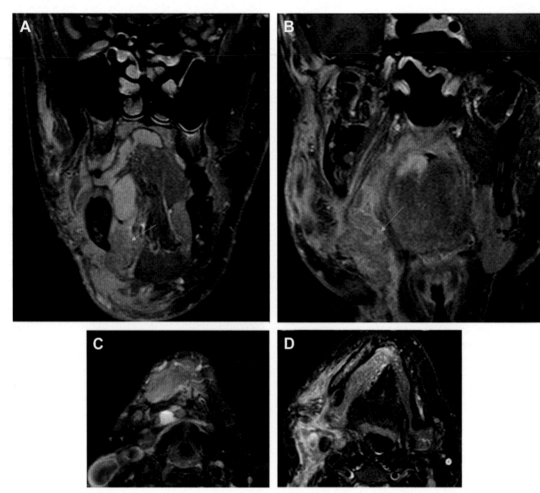

Fig. 13. Neurofibramotosis-1. Extensive multicompartment enhancing mass noted on the coronal contrast-enhanced MR images of the neck (*A, B*) involving the SM and SL spaces. The SM and SL salivary glands are enlarged (*yellow* and *green arrow*). Enlargement of the glands along with multiple neurofibromas with "target" appearance (*red arrows*) can be seen on the axial T2 images (*C, D*).

much better than CT. In addition, bone marrow involvement and perineural spread are better depicted by MR imaging. Perineural spread is best demonstrated on contrast-enhanced T1-weighted fat-saturated MR images presenting as thickened enhancing nerves.[1,12,50–54]

PSEUDOTUMORS

Nonneoplastic masses occasionally manifest in the floor of the mouth and should not be mistaken for tumors. Compensatory hypertrophy of the SL gland secondary to aplasia of the ipsilateral SM salivary gland is commonly mistaken for a palpable mass. An ectopic SM salivary gland also may appear as a mass in the floor of the mouth.[1] Rarely, ectopic thyroid tissue is observed in the floor of the mouth, where it appears as a well-defined, ovoid lesion with hyperattenuation

on unenhanced CT images and homogeneous enhancement on CECT images. It is sometimes associated with a coexistent cervical thyroid gland.[1,18]

Denervation muscle atrophy can result in hyperplasia of the contralateral side and mimic tumor. Cranial nerves provide motor supply to various muscles and muscle groups in the head and neck. When the innervation is interrupted by neural involvement with tumor or infection, there is a loss of motor function ipsilateral to the lesion.[56] This results in muscle wasting, fatty infiltration, and hemiatrophy of involved muscles. On imaging studies, the fatty atrophy is easily appreciated. However, the asymmetry can be mistaken for tumor because the normal side appears enlarged when compared with the atrophic side. The hypoglossal nerve provides motor innervation to the intrinsic and extrinsic muscles of the tongue. Lesions that affect

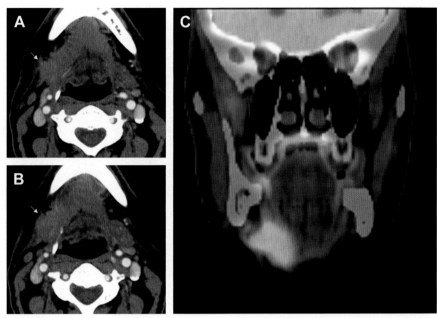

Fig. 14. Adenoid cystic carcinoma. Axial (*A, B*) CECT images of the neck show an infiltrative lesion of the right SM gland (*yellow arrows*) with signs of extracapsular spread, including thickening of the right platysma muscle. PET-CT coronal image (*C*) shows marked increased FDG activity in the right SM region.

the nerve can produce muscle atrophy and fatty replacement in 2 to 3 weeks. When present, a search for abnormality must be made along the entire course of the hypoglossal nerve, including the brainstem. The mandibular nerve (V3) provides motor innervation to not only the muscles of mastication, tensor tympani, and tensor palatini muscles but also the anterior belly of the digastric muscle and the mylohyoid muscle via the mylohyoid nerve. Injury to the mandibular nerve results in fatty atrophy of all the muscle bundles, whereas isolated injury to the mylohyoid nerve results in fatty infiltration and atrophy of only the anterior belly of the digastric and mylohyoid muscles. As with hypoglossal injury, a search for neural abnormality along the entire course of the nerve, back to the brainstem, is required when masticator muscle atrophy is identified.[57,58]

SUMMARY

Imaging remains the cornerstone for evaluation of SM and SL abnormality. Although CT remains the most widely accepted modality in use currently, there has been exponential growth in the usage of MR imaging for evaluation of SM and SL glands/spaces. US continues to provide strong complementary value to CT/MR imaging and serves as a vital tool for image-guided procedures. Good understanding of the complex anatomy of these spaces is vital for the radiologist to come

to an accurate diagnosis. Almost all the different categories of pathologic conditions (inflammatory, infectious, neoplastic, and vascular) can involve not only the SM and SL glands but also the surrounding structures in these spaces.

REFERENCES

1. La'porte SJ, Juttla JK, Lingam RK. Imaging the floor of the mouth and the sublingual space. Radiographics 2011;31(5):1215–30.
2. Laine FJ, Smoker WR. Oral cavity: anatomy and pathology. Semin Ultrasound CT MR 1995;16(6): 527–45.
3. Hermans R, Lenz M. Imaging of the oropharynx and oral cavity. Part I: normal anatomy. Eur Radiol 1996; 6(3):362–8.
4. Law CP, Chandra RV, Hoang JK, et al. Imaging the oral cavity: key concepts for the radiologist. Br J Radiol 2011;84(1006):944–57.
5. Sigal R. Oral cavity, oropharynx, and salivary glands. Neuroimaging Clin N Am 1996;6(2):379–400.
6. Yousem DM, Kraut MA, Chalian AA. Major salivary gland imaging. Radiology 2000;216(1):19–29.
7. White DK, Davidson HC, Harnsberger HR, et al. Accessory salivary tissue in the mylohyoid boutonnière: a clinical and radiologic pseudolesion of the oral cavity. AJNR Am J Neuroradiol 2001;22(2): 406–12.
8. Meesa IR, Srinivasan A. Imaging of the oral cavity. Radiol Clin North Am 2015;53(1):99–114.

9. Boyd ZT, Goud AR, Lowe LH, et al. Pediatric salivary gland imaging. Pediatr Radiol 2009;39(7):710–22.

10. Abdullah A, Rivas FF, Srinivasan A. Imaging of the salivary glands. Semin Roentgenol 2013; 48(1):65–7.

11. Otonari-Yamamoto M, Nakajima K, Tsuji Y, et al. Imaging of the mylohyoid muscle: separation of submandibular and sublingual spaces. AJR Am J Roentgenol 2010;194(5):W431–8.

12. Burke CJ, Thomas RH, Howlett D. Imaging the major salivary glands. Br J Oral Maxillofac Surg 2011; 49(4):261–9.

13. Silvers AR, Som PM. Salivary glands. Radiol Clin North Am 1998;36:941–66.

14. Thoeny HC. Imaging of salivary gland tumours. Cancer Imaging 2007;7:52–62.

15. Bialek EJ, Jakubowski W, Zajkowski P, et al. US of the major salivary glands: anatomy and spatial relationships, pathologic conditions, and pitfalls. Radiographics 2006;26(3):745–63.

16. Zengel P, Schrötzlmair F, Reichel C, et al. Sonography: the leading diagnostic tool for diseases of the salivary glands. Semin Ultrasound CT MR 2013; 34(3):196–203.

17. Ching AS, Ahuja AT. High-resolution sonography of the submandibular space: anatomy and abnormalities. AJR Am J Roentgenol 2002;179(3):703–8.

18. Agarwal AK, Kanekar SG. Submandibular and sublingual spaces: diagnostic imaging and evaluation. Otolaryngol Clin North Am 2012;45(6):1311–23.

19. Razek AA, Tawfik AM, Elsorogy LG, et al. Perfusion CT of head and neck cancer. Eur J Radiol 2014; 83(3):537–44.

20. Abdel Razek AA, Samir S, Ashmalla GA. Characterization of parotid tumors with dynamic susceptibility contrast perfusion-weighted magnetic resonance imaging and diffusion-weighted MR imaging. J Comput Assist Tomogr 2017;41(1):131–6.

21. Razek AA. Diffusion-weighted magnetic resonance imaging of head and neck. J Comput Assist Tomogr 2010;34:808–15.

22. Abdel Razek AAK, Mukherji S. Imaging of sialadenitis. Neuroradiol J 2017;30(3):205–15.

23. Francis CL, Larsen CG. Pediatric sialadenitis. Otolaryngol Clin North Am 2014;47(5):763–78.

24. Zenk J, Iro H, Klintworth N, et al. Diagnostic imaging in sialadenitis. Oral Maxillofac Surg Clin North Am 2009;21(3):275–92.

25. Madani G, Beale T. Inflammatory conditions of the salivary glands. Semin Ultrasound CT MR 2006; 27(6):440–51.

26. Barakate MS, Jensen MJ, Hemli JM, et al. Ludwig's angina: report of a case and review of management issues. Ann Otol Rhinol Laryngol 2001;110:453–6.

27. Smoker WRK. The oral cavity. In: Som PM, Curtin HD, editors. Head and neck imaging. 4th edition. St Louis (MO): Mosby; 2003. p. 1377–464.

28. Levy DM, Remine WH, Devine KD. Salivary gland calculi. Pain, swelling associated with eating. JAMA 1962;181:1115–9.

29. Williams MF. Sialolithiasis. Otolaryngol Clin North Am 1999;32:819–34.

30. Razek AA, Castillo M. Imaging appearance of granulomatous lesions of head and neck. Eur J Radiol 2010;76(1):52–60.

31. Robson C. Imaging of granulomatous lesions of the neck in the children. Radiol Clin North Am 2000; 38(5):969–77.

32. Mulliken JB, Glowacki J. Hemangiomas and vascular malformations in infants and children: a classification based on endothelial characteristics. Plast Reconstr Surg 1982;69(3):412.

33. Merrow AC, Gupta A, Patel MN, et al. 2014 revised classification of vascular lesions from the International Society for the Study of Vascular Anomalies: radiologic-pathologic update. Radiographics 2016; 36(5):1494–516.

34. Restrepo R, Palani R, Cervantes LF, et al. Hemangiomas revisited: the useful, the unusual and the new. Part 1. Overview and clinical and imaging characteristics. Pediatr Radiol 2011;41(7):895–904.

35. Liang MG, Frieden IJ. Infantile and congenital hemangiomas. Semin Pediatr Surg 2014;23(4):162–7.

36. Navarro OM, Laffan EE, Ngan BY. Pediatric soft-tissue tumors and pseudotumors: MR imaging features with pathologic correlation. Part 1. Imaging approach, pseudotumors, vascular lesions, and adipocytic tumors. Radiographics 2009;29(3):887–906.

37. Sadick M, Wohlgemuth WA, Huelse R, et al. Interdisciplinary management of head and neck vascular anomalies: clinical presentation, diagnostic findings and minimal invasive therapies. Eur J Radiol Open 2017;4:63–8.

38. Mahady K, Thust S, Berkeley R, et al. Vascular anomalies of the head and neck in children. Quant Imaging Med Surg 2015;5(6):886–97.

39. Abdel Razek AAK, Albair GA, Samir S. Clinical value of classification of venous malformations with contrast-enhanced MR angiography. Phlebology 2017;32(9):628–33.

40. Restrepo R. Multimodality imaging of vascular anomalies. Pediatr Radiol 2013;43(suppl 1): S141–54.

41. Flors L, Leiva-Salinas C, Maged IM, et al. MR imaging of soft-tissue vascular malformations: diagnosis, classification, and therapy follow-up. Radiographics 2011;31:1321–40.

42. Razek AA, Gaballa G, Megahed AS, et al. Time resolved imaging of contrast kinetics (TRICKS) MR angiography of arteriovenous malformations of head and neck. Eur J Radiol 2013;82(11):1885–91.

43. Lyly A, Castrén E, Aronniemi J, et al. Plunging ranula - patient characteristics, treatment, and comparison

between different populations. Acta Otolaryngol 2017;137(12):1271–4.

44. Li J, Li J. Correct diagnosis for plunging ranula by magnetic resonance imaging. Aust Dent J 2014; 59(2):264–7.

45. Edwards RM, Chapman T, Horn DL, et al. Imaging of pediatric floor of mouth lesions. Pediatr Radiol 2013; 43:523.

46. Scully C, Bagán JV, Eveson JW, et al. Sialosis: 35 cases of persistent parotid swelling from two countries. Br J Oral Maxillofac Surg 2008;46(6): 468–72.

47. Varoquaux A, Rager O, Dulguerov P, et al. Diffusion-weighted and PET/MR imaging after radiation therapy for malignant head and neck tumors. Radio-graphics 2015;35(5):1502–27.

48. Tonami H, Ogawa Y, Matoba M, et al. MR sialogra-phy in patients with Sjögren syndrome. AJNR Am J Neuroradiol 1998;19(7):1199–203.

49. Abdel Razek AA. Imaging of connective tissue dis-eases of the head and neck. Neuroradiol J 2016; 29(3):222–30.

50. Kato H, Kanematsu M, Mizuta K, et al. Carcinoma ex pleomorphic adenoma of the parotid gland: radiologic-pathologic correlation with MR imaging including diffusion-weighted imaging. AJNR Am J Neuroradiol 2008;29(5):865–7.

51. Spiro RH. Salivary neoplasms: overview of a 35-year experience with 2,807 patients. Head Neck Surg 1986;8:177–84.

52. Eveson JW, Cawson RA. Salivary gland tumors: a re-view of 2,410 cases with particular reference to his-tologic types, site, age and sex distribution. J Pathol 1985;146:51–8.

53. Furlong MA, Fanburg-Smith JC, Childers EL. Lipoma of the oral and maxillofacial region: site and subclas-sification of 125 cases. Oral Surg Oral Med Oral Pathol Oral Radiol Endod 2004;98:441–50.

54. Munir N, Bradley PJ. Diagnosis and management of neoplastic lesions of the submandibular triangle. Oral Oncol 2008;44:251–60.

55. Razek AA, Huang BY. Soft tissue tumors of the head and neck: imaging-based review of the WHO classi-fication. Radiographics 2011;31(7):1923–54.

56. Harnsberger HR, Dillon WP. Major motor atrophic patterns in the face and neck: CT evaluation. Radi-ology 1985;155:665–70.

57. Russo CP, Smoker WR, Weissman JL. MR appear-ance of trigeminal and hypoglossal motor denerva-tion. AJNR Am J Neuroradiol 1997;18(7):1375–83.

58. Kato K, Tomura N, Takahashi S, et al. Motor dener-vation of tumors of the head and neck: changes in MR appearance. Magn Reson Med Sci 2002;1(3): 157–64.

Routine and Advanced Diffusion Imaging Modules of the Salivary Glands

Ahmed Abdel Khalek Abdel Razek, MD

KEYWORDS

• Diffusion • MR imaging • Salivary • Parotid • Benign • Malignant • Recurrence • Radiotherapy

KEY POINTS

- Routine diffusion MR imaging can be incorporated into routine contrast MR imaging of salivary glands.
- Advanced diffusion imaging modules of salivary glands include diffusion tensor imaging, diffusion kurtosis imaging, and intravoxel incoherent motion MR imaging.
- Routine and advanced diffusion imaging modules help in differentiation of benign from malignant salivary gland tumors.
- Advanced diffusion imaging modules can detect radiation and radioiodine–induced sialadenitis.
- Routine and advanced diffusion imaging modules have a role in early diagnosis and staging of Sjögren syndrome.

INTRODUCTION

Over the past decade, there has been increasing interest in the use of diffusion-weighted imaging of the salivary glands. Routine diffusion-weighted MR imaging module can measure the mobility of water molecules diffusing in tissue, which is impacted by biophysical characteristics, such as cell density, membrane integrity, and microstructure.[1–4] Advanced diffusion imaging modules include additional sampling and analysis frameworks that represent other features, such as structural anisotropy (diffusion tensor imaging [DTI]), microvascularity (intravoxel incoherent motion [IVIM]), and microstructural complexity (diffusion kurtosis imaging [DKI]).[4–7] Routine and advanced diffusion imaging modules are noninvasive procedures without radiation exposure or administration of contrast medium. The examination has a short time and can be combined with routine MR imaging with multiparametric analysis of the salivary glands.[3–6]

TECHNIQUES

The routine diffusion imaging model of the salivary gland is a monoexponential form that may be either echo planar or non–echo planar imaging. The advanced diffusion imaging modules include DTI, DKI, and IVIM modules.

Monoexponential

A routine diffusion MR imaging module of the salivary glands is performed as a single-shot echo planar technique due to short acquisition time. Echo planar diffusion is commonly used in salivary glands imaging. Single-shot and multishot echo planar sequences differ in the number of repetition times used for filling the k-space, with the former using 1 repetition alone to fill the k-space and the latter using many repetitions.[2,8] The single-shot technique, although shorter in acquisition time, suffers from greater susceptibility effects, geometric distortion, and reduced spatial

Department of Diagnostic Radiology, Mansoura University, Elgomheryia Street, Mansoura 35512, Egypt
E-mail address: arazek@mans.edu.eg

Neuroimag Clin N Am 28 (2018) 245–254
https://doi.org/10.1016/j.nic.2018.01.010

resolution, which all are improved with the multi-shot technique. Non–echo planar diffusion can provide further improvement in image quality with lesser susceptibility artifacts and higher spatial resolution but take longer time and have lower signal-to-noise ratio, which necessitates multiple averages.[2,9]

Biexponential Intravoxel Incoherent Motion (Microvascularity)

The IVIM imaging is a technique with the potential for simultaneously assessing both tissue perfusion and diffusion by using a single diffusion-weighted imaging with a different number of b values. The signal decay at low b values is primarily attributed to perfusion, whereas data obtained at high b values are mainly dominated by diffusion. The IVIM parameters are perfusion fraction (f), pure diffusion coefficient (D), pseudo-diffusion coefficient (D*), and apparent diffusion coefficient (ADC). The D value represents true diffusion and D* value represents pseudodiffusion in microcirculation.[6,10]

Diffusion Kurtosis Imaging (Intravoxel Heterogeneity)

DKI quantifies nongaussianity (kurtosis) of the water displacement distribution, which is measurable in a quadratic order expansion of the signal b-value dependence. Metrics from DKI reflect excess kurtosis of tissues, representing its deviation from gaussian diffusion behavior. The water diffusion probability distribution function can be referred to as nongaussian because of the presence of barriers (eg, cell membrane) and compartments (eg, intracellular and extracellular spaces) in many biological tissues. So the nongaussian distribution may be a true condition in tissue, and a diffusion kurtosis model is established to provide a complete characterization of water diffusion. The mean diffusional (MD) kurtosis is significantly higher in malignant tumors compared with benign lesions.[6,11]

Diffusion Tensor Imaging (Anisotropy)

DTI extends routine diffusion imaging module to characterize the orientational variability of the diffusion process, allowing assessment of diffusion directionality or anisotropy.[12,13] DTI requires the acquisition of a greater number of diffusion gradient directions, 6 or more, and expresses the diffusion coefficient as a function of direction in the form of a tensor. The calculated DTI tensor parameters include the MD or ADC and associated anisotropy indices expressing variability between the eigenvalues, such as the normalized index of fractional anisotropy (FA).[6,12]

Diffusion Tensor Tractography

Diffusion tensor tractography is the postprocessing imaging analysis after reconstructing the nerve fibers, allowing displaying the nerve or white matter fascicle. At DTI, there is a decrease in FA of the facial nerve that contacts or infiltrated with the salivary gland tumors. Diffusion tensor tractography can localize the position of the main trunk of the facial nerve and its major branches in relation to salivary gland tumors. The results best at higher 3T scanner. These data are important to avoid facial nerve injury during surgery.[1,14]

IMAGE ANALYSIS

Image analysis of diffusion imaging modules can be performed by visual assessment and region of interest analysis. Advanced image analysis, including histogram analysis, texture analysis, and machine learning, has recently been introduced and still is in research.

Visual Assessment

Qualitative evaluation is performed by means of visual assessment of the signal intensity on images acquired at high b values and their corresponding ADC maps. Malignancy shows high signal intensity on a high b-value image and low signal intensity on the corresponding ADC map, whereas most benign tumors commonly appear as areas of low signal intensity on high b-value images with high signal intensity on corresponding ADC maps.[2]

Region of Interest Analysis

The region of interest analysis is the most common method for quantification of ADC. Simple methods of acquiring a mean ADC include the drawing of multiple small regions of interest on 1 or several sections or a single large region of interest on 1 section or calculation of ADC from the entire lesion. Regions that are frankly necrotic should be excluded from the ADC calculation. The standard region of interest summary statistics is mean or median.[2–4]

Histogram Analysis

Histogram analysis is reflect the intensity distribution of a volume of interest but not the spatial distribution of the intensities on pixel distribution. It is commonly referred to as first-order statistics. ADC histogram features, including ADC, mean

ADC percentiles (5th, 10th, 25th, 50th, 75th, and 90th percentiles), skewness, kurtosis, and entropy. ADC histogram analysis ADC histogram analysis has been successfully used for differential diagnosis, histologic differentiation, and assessing therapeutic response in various tumors.[5]

Texture Analysis

Texture analysis based on ADC maps is an emerging modality to extract texture features describing local and regional relationships between pixels within the regions of interest, which can better reflect intratumoral heterogeneity. The ADC texture features include correlation, autocorrelation, entropy, and homogeneity. It has shown promise in the field of oncology in diagnostics, quantifying tumor heterogeneity, separating tumor tissue from surrounding tissue, tumor grading and classification, and predictions of treatment response and survival.[15]

Machine Learning Analysis

Machine learning is the subfield of artificial intelligence in which algorithms are trained to perform tasks by learning patterns from data rather than by explicit programming that has been recently applied for analysis of diffusion MR imaging.[16]

Diffusion Imaging of Normal Salivary Glands and Gustatory Stimulation

One study reported that the ADC of the parotid glands is lower than that of the submandibular glands in volunteers because the parotid glands had significantly greater fat content compared with the submandibular glands.[17,18] At IVIM, both D and f values correlated inversely with the age in healthy parotid glands, whereas D* value did not. The parotid glands of men showed higher IVIM MR imaging parameters than those of women.[19] The IVIM method allows for simultaneous quantification of changes in perfusion and diffusion effects after gustatory stimulation of the parotid gland.[20]

CLINICAL APPLICATIONS
Differentiation Malignant from Benign Tumors

A routine diffusion module is used for assessment of parotid, submandibular, and minor salivary glands tumors.[21–23] At diffusion MR imaging, the mean ADC value of benign lesions is significantly higher than that of malignant lesions. The mean ADC value of pleomorphic adenoma (**Fig. 1**) is significantly higher than those of both Warthin tumor and malignant tumors, and there is insignificant difference between the mean ADC values of the Warthin tumor and malignant tumors.[24,25] Few studies discuss the value of combined diffusion-weighted imaging with dynamic contrast MR imaging.[26–29] A recent study reported, however, that parotid lesions with ill-defined margin, adjacent tissue infiltration, presence of cervical lymphadenopathy, an ADC of 1.3×10^{-5} mm^2/s, and plateau time intensity curve pattern are more likely malignant. The diagnostic value of routine MR imaging is increased when diffusion-weighted MR imaging is applied in combination, whereas additional dynamic contrast study did not improve differential ability of conventional MR imaging.[28]

Few studies discuss the role of DTI in the differentiation of malignant from benign salivary gland tumors (**Fig. 2**). One study reported that there is a significant difference in the ADC and FA ($P = .032$ and $P = .011$, respectively) between benign and malignant parotid tumors. The cutoff points between benign and malignant parotid tumors for ADC and FA are 1.02×10^{-3} mm^2/s and 0.24, respectively.[30] Another study added that the FA values of malignant salivary gland

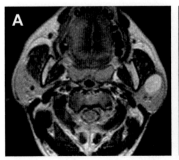
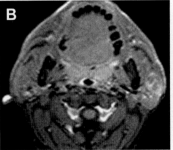
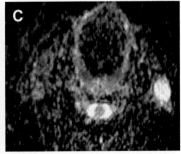

Fig. 1. Routine diffusion-weighted image of pleomorphic adenoma. (*A*) T2-weighted image shows a well-defined hyperintense mass in the right parotid gland. (*B*) Contrast T1-weighted image shows intense contrast enhancement of the mass. (*C*) ADC map shows unrestricted diffusion of the tumor with high ADC value.

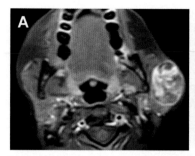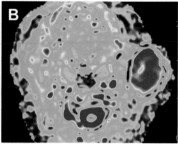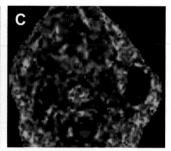

Fig. 2. DTI of pleomorphic adenoma. (*A*) Contrast T1-weighted image shows well-defined mass of inhomogeneous pattern of contrast enhancement. (*B*) ADC map shows unrestricted diffusion with high MD of the mass. (*C*) FA map shows the tumor with low FA value.

tumors are significantly higher than those of benign tumors (0.26 ± 0.06 vs. 0.17 ± 0.05, respectively), with an insignificant difference in ADC value.[31] Combined values FA and MD can differentiate malignant from benign salivary gland tumors.[32]

At DKI, benign salivary gland tumors show lower mean kurtosis and FA value and higher MD value than that of malignancy. The cutoff point between benign and malignant parotid tumors for mean kurtosis is 1.053.[33] The IVIM module may help distinguish benign from malignant salivary gland tumors by using high D* to reflect higher pseudodiffusion in microcirculation of Warthin tumors and high D value to reflect less restricted pure diffusion of pleomorphic adenomas (**Fig. 3**). The D values of malignant tumors (0.96 ± 0.22 × 10^{-3} mm²/s) are significantly different from those of benign tumors (pleomorphic adenomas, 1.38 ± 0.30 × 10^{-3} mm²/s; P = .002, and Warthin tumors, 0.61 ± 0.11 × 10^{-3} mm²/s; P = .005). The D* values of malignant tumors (21.99 ± 19.01 × 10^{-3} mm²/s) were significantly smaller than those of Warthin tumors (42.64 ± 20.17 × 10^{-3} mm²/s; P = .022). The combination of D and D* criteria provided the best diagnostic accuracy (100%) for differentiation among the 3 tumor types.[34]

Benign Salivary Gland Tumors

Characterization of benign salivary gland tumors is important because management of pleomorphic adenoma is different from warthin tumor. Routine diffusion imaging associated with dynamic contrast and conventional MR imaging can predict the subtype of benign salivary gland tumors; however, there is overlap in the imaging features and ADC value of some salivary gland tumors.

Pleomorphic adenomas
Pleomorphic adenomas are the most common benign tumor of the salivary gland. They exhibit unrestricted diffusion and high ADC value because these tumors show a heterogeneous component of epithelial, myoepithelial, and stromal cells with areas of fluid within the epithelial glandular areas. The range of ADC value of pleomorphic adenoma varies among different studies (1.5–2.2 mm²/s × 10^{-3} mm²/s).[24,35]

Warthin tumor
Warthin tumor is the second most common benign tumor of the salivary glands. This tumor reveals a low ADC value, ranging from 0.72 mm²/s to 0.96 mm²/s × 10^{-3} mm²/s, due

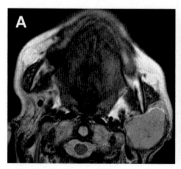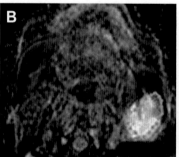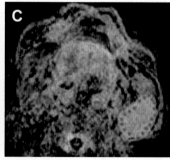

Fig. 3. IVIM of pleomorphic adenoma. (*A*) T2-weighted image shows a well-defined mass involving almost of the right parotid gland. (*B*) Pseudodiffusion map shows the mass with low D* value. (*C*) True diffusion map shows the tumor with high D value of the tumor. (*Courtesy of* Ann King, MD, Hong Kong.)

to the presence of epithelial and lymphoid stroma with microscopic slitlike cysts filled with proteinous fluid. The low ADC value of Warthin tumor is simulating malignancy (**Fig. 4**). Advanced diffusion imaging modules help in this differentiation.[36] At DTI, the FA of Warthin tumor is significantly lower than that of malignant tumors.[32] At IVIM, the D* values of Warthin tumors are significantly higher than those of malignant tumors because Warthin tumors are highly vascular compared with malignant salivary gland tumors. The f values of Warthin tumors are significantly larger than those of pleomorphic adenomas.[34]

Other benign salivary gland tumors

Few studies have reported the ADC value of other benign tumors of the salivary glands. One study reported that the mean ADC value of basal cell adenoma (1.24 mm^2/s $\pm$ 0.18 mm^2/s $\times$ 10^{-3} mm^2/s) is significantly lower than that of pleomorphic adenoma.[37] Another study reported that the myoepithelial adenomas have high ADC value (1.86 mm^2/s $\pm$ 0.18 mm^2/s $\times$ 10^{-3} mm^2/s) that simulates pleomorphic adenoma due to the presence of myepithelial components.[24] Oncocytomas reveal low ADC value (1.06 mm^2/s $\pm$ 0.06 mm^2/s $\times$ 10^{-3} mm^2/s) that simulates the Warthin tumors. The ADC value of oncocytomas is higher than that of Warthin tumors.[38] Hemangiomas show intense homogenous contrast enhancement with high ADC value (1.69 mm^2/s $\pm$ 0.16 mm^2/s $\times$ 10^{-3} mm^2/s) at diffusion MR imaging[39] (**Fig. 5**).

Malignant Salivary Gland Tumors

Malignant salivary gland tumors show restricted diffusion with low ADC value (**Fig. 6**). There is an insignificant difference in the ADC of histopathologic subtypes of malignant salivary gland tumors. The high ADC value of mucoepidermoid carcinoma may be attributed to the presence of excess mucus content of this tumor.[22] Lymphomas revealed restricted diffusion with lower ADC values due to the presence of high cellularity of lymphoid tissue.[40] The ADC value of high-risk malignancy is lower than that of low-risk malignancy but does not reach a significant level ($P = .13$).[22] Diffusion-weighted MR imaging helps selection of biopsy from the viable solid part of the malignancy[41] and has a role in nodal and distant staging of the salivary cancer.[42,43] More details about the role of diffusion MR imaging in staging of salivary cancer are in another article in this issue.[3]

Post-Treatment of Salivary Glands

Recurrent salivary cancer

Recurrent or residual salivary gland cancer shows restricted diffusion with low ADC value (**Fig. 7**). The mean ADC value of residual or recurrent salivary gland cancer after surgery is significantly less than ($P = .001$) that of post-therapeutic changes. This is attributed to high cellularity with the restricted diffusion of recurrence tumor and edema of postoperative changes.[44,45]

Radiation-induced sialadenitis

Radiation-induced salivary gland damage and consequential xerostomia are among the most common and distressing adverse effects of radiotherapy for head and neck cancer. Diffusion-weighted imaging combined with salivary stimulation may be a potential tool for noninvasively assessing salivary gland function and diagnosis

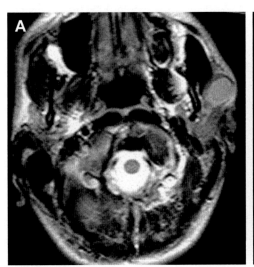
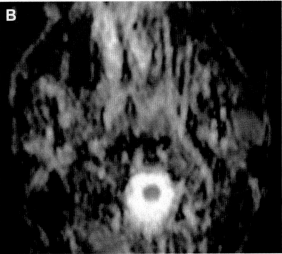

Fig. 4. Warthin tumor. (*A*) T2-weighted image shows small mass is seen in the tail of the left parotid gland with intermediate signal intensity. (*B*) ADC map shows unrestricted diffusion of the mass with low ADC value.

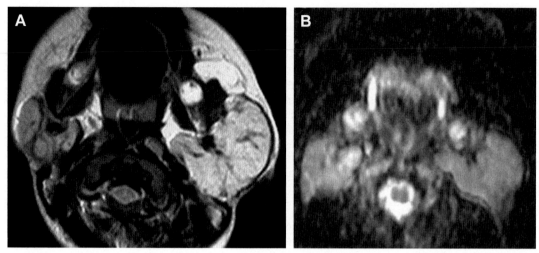

Fig. 5. Hemangioma of parotid gland. (*A*) T2-weighted image shows hyperintense mass of the left parotid gland in a child with multiple signal void regions. (*B*) ADC map shows unrestricted diffusion of the mass with high ADC value.

of radiation-induced xerostomia.[46] As a result of gustatory stimulation of salivary gland, the ADC shows a biphasic response with an initial increase and subsequent decrease. This pattern was seen both before and after radiotherapy.[47] The reduction of parotid volume and an increase of parotid ADC are dominated by the effect of acinar loss rather than edema at early to intermediate phases and the following recovery of parotid volume, and ADC toward the baseline values might reflect the acinar regeneration of parotid glands.[48] The ADC histogram analysis has been successfully introduced into the evaluation of radiation-induced parotid damage in nasopharyngeal cancer patients undergoing radiotherapy. The author found that parotid volume, skewness, and kurtosis decreased, whereas all the other ADC histogram

parameters, including ADC mean; minimum ADC; kurtosis; and 25th, 50th, 75th, and 90th percentiles increased after radiotherapy.[49]

At IVIM, there are significant changes in all diffusion parameters, including ADC, D*, and F values during the course of radiotherapy. The pretreatment f and D* values are the best independent predictors of the percentage shrinkage of salivary glands. Therefore, perfusion-related coefficients of IVIM can predict the diagnosis of radiation-induced sialadenitis and guide treatment strategy in radiotherapy.[50] Another study added that postradiotherapy, all of the IVIM parameters increased significantly and the change rates of ADC, f, and maximum relative enhancement are negatively correlated with the atrophy rate of the salivary glands.[51] Radiation-induced sialadenitis in

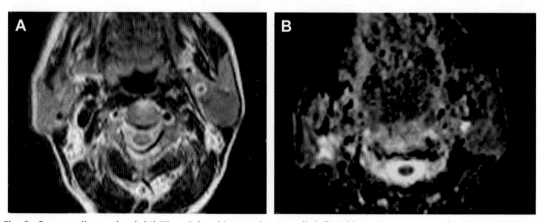

Fig. 6. Cancer salivary gland. (*A*) T2-weighted image shows well-defined hypointense mass of left parotid gland. (*B*) ADC map shows restricted diffusion of the mass with low ADC value.

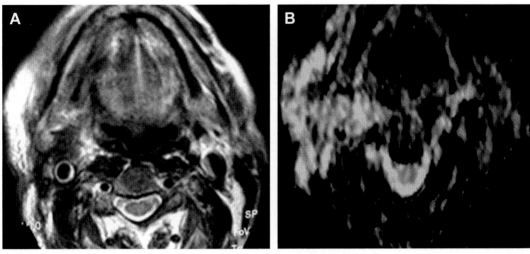

Fig. 7. Recurrent cancer parotid. (*A*) T2-weighted image shows ill-defined lesion is seen at operative bed after right parotidectomy. (*B*) ADC map shows unrestricted diffusion lesion is seen in the postoperative region with low ADC value.

patients with nasopharyngeal carcinoma undergoing radiotherapy can be effectively evaluated by DKI in the early stage. The parotid ADC and D parameters are increased and parotid volume and K values are decreased significantly during the course of radiotherapy, and the change rate of D values is positively correlated with radiation dose postradiotherapy.[52]

Radioiodine therapy–induced sialadenitis
The IVIM can detect changes of parotid glands after radioiodine therapy for differentiated thyroid cancer. The f and D values differ significantly between patients at less than and more than 3 months of therapy. The f and D values of patients less than 3 months therapy are significantly higher than those of volunteers. There is a significant positive correlation between f value and symptom score of the patients.[53]

Immunologic Disorders

Sjögren syndrome
Sjögren syndrome is an autoimmune disorder of the salivary and lacrimal glands.[54,55] In the early stages to mid-stages (stages 1–3), the ADC is gradually increased (**Fig. 8**), whereas in the advanced stage (stage 4), the ADC is markedly decreased.[56,57] At IVIM, all IVIM parameters of parotid glands in Sjögren syndrome at grade 0 are significantly higher than those in volunteers, and there are significant differences in the D and f values of parotid glands in Sjögren syndrome among different grades (*P* = .003 and *P* =.001, respectively). The D and f values of parotid glands at early stages and advanced stages in patients with Sjögren syndrome are significantly higher

and lower, respectively, than those in volunteers.[58] All IVIM parameters of the Sjögren syndrome group are significantly higher than those of the volunteers. The f value is the best diagnostic performance for detection of early Sjögren syndrome.[59] All parotid DKI parameters have great potential for diagnosis of early stage of Sjögren syndrome. The parotid ADC, D, and K values in Sjögren syndrome are significantly higher than those of volunteers. The parotid ADC and D values correlated negatively, whereas the K values correlated positively with the magnetic resonance nodular grade of Sjögren disease.[60]

Immunoglobulin G4–related sialadenitis
Immunoglobulin G4–related sialadenitis shows restricted diffusion and low ADC value of the submandibular gland. These may be attributed to the presence of abundant infiltration of immunoglobulin G4–positive plasma cells and lymphocytes with excess fibrosis.[22]

Inflammatory Disorders

The mean ADC value of salivary malignancy is significantly lower than that of inflammatory process of the salivary glands, and the ADC value is increased in sialoadenitis and decreased with abscess formation.[61] Diffusion-weighted MR imaging seems to display the physiologic changes of the parotid gland after gustatory stimulation in patients suffering from acute or chronic inflammation and is useful for discriminating healthy from affected glands.[62] Chronic granulomatous lesions, such as tuberculous infection, may involve the salivary glands that show restricted diffusion with low

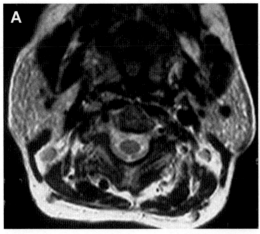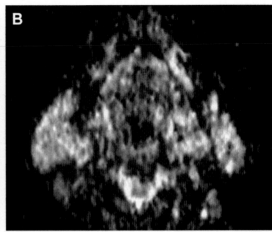

Fig. 8. Sjögren syndrome. (*A*) T2-weighted image shows both bilateral enlarged parotid glands with granular appearance. (*B*) ADC map shows increased diffusion of both salivary glands with high ADC value.

ADC value due to presence of fibrous tissue simulating malignancy.[5,43,63]

SUMMARY

Routine and advanced diffusion imaging modules, including IVIM, DKI, and DTI, may contribute to differentiation of malignant from benign salivary gland tumors and characterization of some benign salivary glands tumors. These advanced modules have a role in the assessment of patients after surgery or after radiotherapy or iodine-induced sialadenitis as well as in early diagnosis and staging of Sjögren syndrome.

ACKNOWLEDGMENTS

The author would like to thank Dr Ann King, Department of Diagnostic Radiology, Prince of Wales Hospital, Chinese University of Hong Kong, Hong Kong, for contributing **Fig. 3**.

REFERENCES

1. Attyé A, Troprès I, Rouchy RC, et al. Diffusion MRI: literature review in salivary gland tumors. Oral Dis 2017;23:572–5.
2. Connolly M, Srinivasan A. Diffusion-weighted imaging in head and neck cancer technique, limitations, and applications. Magn Reson Imaging Clin N Am 2018;26:121–33.
3. Abdel Razek AAK, Mukherji SK. State-of-the-art imaging of salivary gland tumors. Neuroimag Clin N Am 2018;28(2):303–17.
4. Thoeny HC, De Keyzer F, King AD. Diffusion-weighted MR imaging in the head and neck. Radiology 2012;263:19–32.
5. Razek AA. Diffusion-weighted magnetic resonance imaging of head and neck. J Comput Assist Tomogr 2010;34:808–15.
6. Partridge SC, Nissan N, Rahbar H, et al. Diffusion-weighted breast MRI: clinical applications and emerging techniques. J Magn Reson Imaging 2017;45:337–55.
7. Taffel MT, Johnson EJ, Chandarana H. Diffusion quantification in body imaging. Top Magn Reson Imaging 2017;26:243–9.
8. Juan CJ, Chang HC, Hsueh CJ, et al. Salivary glands: echo-planar versus PROPELLER diffusion-weighted MR imaging for assessment of ADCs. Radiology 2009;253:144–52.
9. Yoshino N, Yamada I, Ohbayashi N, et al. Salivary glands and lesions: evaluation of apparent diffusion coefficients with split-echo diffusion-weighted MR imaging–initial results. Radiology 2001;221:837–42.
10. Iima M, Le Bihan D. Clinical intravoxel incoherent motion and diffusion MR imaging: past, present, and future. Radiology 2016;278:13–32.
11. Rosenkrantz AB, Padhani AR, Chenevert TL, et al. Body diffusion kurtosis imaging: basic principles, applications, and considerations for clinical practice. J Magn Reson Imaging 2015;42:1190–202.
12. Koontz NA, Wiggins RH 3rd. Differentiation of benign and malignant head and neck lesions with diffusion tensor imaging and DWI. AJR Am J Roentgenol 2017;208:1110–5.
13. Razek AAKA, El-Serougy L, Abdelsalam M, et al. Differentiation of residual/recurrent gliomas from post-radiation necrosis with arterial spin labeling and diffusion tensor magnetic resonance imaging-derived metrics. Neuroradiology 2017. https://doi.org/10.1007/s00234-017-1955-3.
14. Attyé A, Karkas A, Troprès I, et al. Parotid gland tumours: MR tractography to assess contact with the facial nerve. Eur Radiol 2016;26:2233–41.

15. Brynolfsson P, Nilsson D, Henriksson R, et al. ADC texture–an imaging biomarker for high-grade glioma? Med Phys 2014;41:101903.

16. Pinker K, Shitano F, Sala E, et al. Background, current role, and potential applications of radiogenomics. J Magn Reson Imaging 2017. https://doi.org/10.1002/jmri.25870.

17. Thoeny HC, De Keyzer F, Claus FG, et al. Gustatory stimulation changes the apparent diffusion coefficient of salivary glands: initial experience. Radiology 2005;235:629–34.

18. Habermann CR, Gossrau P, Kooijman H, et al. Monitoring of gustatory stimulation of salivary glands by diffusion-weighted MR imaging: comparison of 1.5T and 3T. AJNR Am J Neuroradiol 2007;28:1547–51.

19. Xu XQ, Su GY, Liu J, et al. Intravoxel incoherent motion MR imaging measurements of the bilateral parotid glands at 3.0-T MR: effect of age, gender and laterality in healthy adults. Br J Radiol 2015;88. 20150646.

20. Becker AS, Manoliu A, Wurnig MC, et al. Intravoxel incoherent motion imaging measurement of perfusion changes in the parotid gland provoked by gustatory stimulation: a pilot study. J Magn Reson Imaging 2017;45:570–8.

21. Karaman Y, Ozgur A, Apaydın D, et al. Role of diffusion-weighted magnetic resonance imaging in the differentiation of parotid gland tumors. Oral Radiol 2016;32:22–32.

22. Razek AAKA. Prediction of malignancy of submandibular gland tumors with apparent diffusion coefficient. Oral Radiol 2017.

23. Abdel Razek AAK, Mukherji SK. Imaging of minor salivary glands. Neuroimag Clin N Am 2018;28(2):295–302.

24. Habermann C, Arndt C, Graessner J, et al. Diffusion-weighted echo-planar MR imaging of primary parotid gland tumors: is a prediction of different histologic subtypes possible? AJNR Am J Neuroradiol 2009;30:591–6.

25. Eida S, Sumi M, Sakihama N, et al. Apparent diffusion coefficient mapping of salivary gland tumors: prediction of the benignancy and malignancy. AJNR Am J Neuroradiol 2007;28:116–21.

26. Yabuuchi H, Matsuo Y, Kamitani T, et al. Parotid gland tumors: can addition of diffusion-weighted MR imaging to dynamic contrast enhanced MR imaging improve diagnostic accuracy in characterization? Radiology 2008;246:909–16.

27. Tao X, Yang G, Wang P, et al. The value of combining conventional, diffusion-weighted and dynamic contrast-enhanced MR imaging for the diagnosis of parotid gland tumours. Dentomaxillofac Radiol 2017;46. 20160434.

28. Yuan Y, Tang W, Tao X. Parotid gland lesions: separate and combined diagnostic value of conventional MRI, diffusion-weighted imaging and dynamic contrast enhanced MRI. Br J Radiol 2016;89. 20150912.

29. Abdel Razek AA, Samir S, Ashmalla GA. Characterization of parotid tumors with dynamic susceptibility contrast perfusion-weighted magnetic resonance imaging and diffusion-weighted Mr imaging. J Comput Assist Tomogr 2017;41:131–6.

30. Takumi K, Fukukura Y, Hakamada H, et al. Value of diffusion tensor imaging in differentiating malignant from benign parotid gland tumors. Eur J Radiol 2017;95:249–56.

31. Yu J, Du Y, Lu Y, et al. Application of DTI and ARFI imaging in differential diagnosis of parotid tumours. Dentomaxillofac Radiol 2016;45. 20160100.

32. Abdel Razek A. Characterization of salivary gland tumors with diffusion tensor imaging. in press.

33. Yu J, Zhang Q, Lu Y, et al. Diffusion kurtosis imaging for differentiating parotid tumors. Int J Clin Exp Med 2017;10:8025–30.

34. Sumi M, Van Cauteren M, Sumi T, et al. Salivary gland tumors: use of intravoxel incoherent motion MR imaging for assessment of diffusion and perfusion for the differentiation of benign from malignant tumors. Radiology 2012;263:770–7.

35. Mikaszewski B, Markiet K, Smugała A, et al. Diffusion-weighted MRI in the differential diagnosis of parotid malignancies and pleomorphic adenomas: can the accuracy of dynamic MRI be enhanced? Oral Surg Oral Med Oral Pathol Oral Radiol 2017;124:95–103.

36. Espinoza S, Felter A, Malinvaud D, et al. Warthin's tumor of parotid gland: surgery or follow-up? Diagnostic value of a decisional algorithm with functional MRI. Diagn Interv Imaging 2016;97:37–43.

37. Mukai H, Motoori K, Horikoshi T, et al. Basal cell adenoma of the parotid gland; MR features and differentiation from pleomorphic adenoma. Dentomaxillofac Radiol 2016;45. 20150322.

38. Kato H, Fujimoto K, Matsuo M, et al. Usefulness of diffusion-weighted MR imaging for differentiating between Warthin's tumor and oncocytoma of the parotid gland. Jpn J Radiol 2017;35:78–85.

39. Abdel Razek AA, Gaballa G, Elhawarey G, et al. Characterization of pediatric head and neck masses with diffusion-weighted MR imaging. Eur Radiol 2009;19:201–8.

40. Kato H, Kanematsu M, Goto H, et al. Mucosa-associated lymphoid tissue lymphoma of the salivary glands: MR imaging findings including diffusion-weighted imaging. Eur J Radiol 2012;81:e612–7.

41. Razek AA, Megahed AS, Denewer A, et al. Role of diffusion-weighted magnetic resonance imaging in differentiation between the viable and necrotic parts of head and neck tumors. Acta Radiol 2008;49:364–70.

42. Freling N, Crippa F, Maroldi R. Staging and follow-up of high-grade malignant salivary gland tumours: the

role of traditional versus functional imaging approaches - a review. Oral Oncol 2016;60:157–66.

43. Abdel Razek AA, Soliman NY, Elkhamary S, et al. Role of diffusion-weighted MR imaging in cervical lymphadenopathy. Eur Radiol 2006;16:1468–77.

44. Abdel Razek AAK, Mukherji SK. Imaging of post-treatment salivary gland tumors. Neuroimag Clin N Am 2018;28(2):199–208.

45. Abdel Razek AA, Kandeel AY, Soliman N, et al. Role of diffusion-weighted echo-planar MR imaging in differentiation of residual or recurrent head and neck tumors and posttreatment changes. AJNR Am J Neuroradiol 2007;28:1146–52.

46. Zhang Y, Ou D, Gu Y, et al. Diffusion-weighted MR imaging of salivary glands with gustatory stimulation: comparison before and after radiotherapy. Acta Radiol 2013;54:928–33.

47. Loimu V, Seppälä T, Kapanen M, et al. Diffusion-weighted magnetic resonance imaging for evaluation of salivary gland function in head and neck cancer patients treated with intensity-modulated radiotherapy. Radiother Oncol 2017;122:178–84.

48. Juan CJ, Cheng CC, Chiu SC, et al. Temporal evolution of parotid volume and parotid apparent diffusion coefficient in nasopharyngeal carcinoma patients treated by intensity-modulated radiotherapy investigated by magnetic resonance imaging: a pilot study. PLoS One 2015;10:e0137073.

49. Zhou N, Guo T, Zheng H, et al. Apparent diffusion coefficient histogram analysis can evaluate radiation-induced parotid damage and predict late xerostomia degree in nasopharyngeal carcinoma. Oncotarget 2017;8:70226–38.

50. Marzi S, Forina C, Marucci L, et al. Early radiation-induced changes evaluated by intravoxel incoherent motion in the major salivary glands. J Magn Reson Imaging 2015;41:974–82.

51. Zhou N, Chu C, Dou X, et al. Early evaluation of irradiated parotid glands with intravoxel incoherent motion MR imaging: correlation with dynamic contrast-enhanced MR imaging. BMC Cancer 2016;16:865.

52. Zhou N, Chen W, Pan X, et al. Early evaluation of radiation-induced parotid damage with diffusion kurtosis imaging: a preliminary study. Acta Radiol 2017. https://doi.org/10.1177/0284185117710051.

53. Shen J, Xu XQ, Su GY, et al. Intravoxel incoherent motion magnetic resonance imaging of the normal-appearing parotid glands in patients with differentiated thyroid cancer after radioiodine therapy. Acta Radiol 2017. https://doi.org/10.1177/0284185117709037.

54. Abdel Razek AA. Imaging of connective tissue diseases of the head and neck. Neuroradiol J 2016;29:222–30.

55. Abdel Razek A, Suresh M. Imaging of sialadenitis. Neuroradiol J 2017;30:205–15.

56. Xu X, Su G, Hu H, et al. Effects of regions of interest methods on apparent coefficient measurement of the parotid gland in early Sjögren's syndrome at 3T MRI. Acta Radiol 2017;58:27–33.

57. Ding C, Xing X, Guo Q, et al. Diffusion-weighted MRI findings in Sjögren's syndrome: a preliminary study. Acta Radiol 2016;57:691–700.

58. Chu C, Zhou N, Zhang H, et al. Correlation between intravoxel incoherent motion MR parameters and MR nodular grade of parotid glands in patients with Sjögren's syndrome: a pilot study. Eur J Radiol 2017;86:241–7.

59. Su GY, Xu XQ, Wang YY, et al. Feasibility study of using intravoxel incoherent motion MRI to detect parotid gland abnormalities in early-stage Sjögren syndrome patients. J Magn Reson Imaging 2016;43:1455–61.

60. Chu C, Zhang H, Zhou N, et al. Diffusional kurtosis imaging of parotid glands in Sjögren's syndrome: initial findings. J Magn Reson Imaging 2017;46:1409–17.

61. Abdel Razek AA, Nada N. Role of diffusion-weighted MRI in differentiation of masticator space malignancy from infection. Dentomaxillofac Radiol 2013;42. 20120183.

62. Ries T, Arndt C, Regier M, et al. Value of apparent diffusion coefficient calculation before and after gustatory stimulation in the diagnosis of acute or chronic parotitis. Eur Radiol 2008;18:2251–7.

63. Razek AA, Castillo M. Imaging appearance of granulomatous lesions of head and neck. Eur J Radiol 2010;76:52–60.

Imaging of Inflammatory Disorders of Salivary Glands

Asim K. Bag, MD*, Joel K. Curé, MD,
Philip R. Chapman, MD, Aparna Singhal, MD,
Atif Wasim Haneef Mohamed, MD

KEYWORDS

- Salivary gland • Sialadenitis • Inflammation • Parotitis • Autoimmune • CT • MR imaging

KEY POINTS

- Sialadenitis is the most common disease of the major salivary glands.
- Sialadenitis typically presents with pain and swelling of the involved glands.
- Infection is the most common cause of the acute sialadenitis; chronic sialadenitis has many different causes.
- Obstructive sialadenitis most commonly involves the submandibular gland, whereas nonobstructive sialadenitis more commonly involves the parotid gland.
- Autoimmune diseases are the most common cause of nonobstructive sialadenitis.
- Imaging often can establish the cause of sialadenitis.

INTRODUCTION

Sialadenitis, inflammation of the salivary glands, is the most common disease involving salivary glands. Inflammation can occur as the common endpoint for a wide variety of conditions. Although the inflammation is sometimes idiopathic, it is often attributable to well-recognized infectious causes or autoimmune conditions (**Box 1**). The most typical presentation of sialadenitis is pain, with or without enlargement of the involved gland. Depending on the cause, the presentation can be acute or chronic exacerbation of a chronic sialadenitis.

IMAGING APPROACH OF SALIVARY GLAND INFLAMMATION

Acute sialadenitis of the major salivary glands is generally easily clinically recognized given the intense pain and swelling localized to the parotid, submandibular, or sublingual gland. Occasionally, clinical presentation can be confusing and precise clinical localization can be difficult. Sialadenitis might be confused with salivary gland tumor, odontogenic disease, facial cellulitis, adenopathy, or otitis externa. Radiologic evaluation can generally provide an accurate diagnosis of sialadenitis, evaluate for obstructive calculus, or evaluate for complications. Many different imaging technologies are available for the evaluation of the salivary glands. Appropriate use of imaging mainly depends on availability of a technique and the clinical questions that need to be answered. A general approach is depicted in **Fig. 1**.

Conventional Radiograph

Conventional radiograph can identify most of the submandibular stones because they are radiopaque

Disclosure Statement: Consultant to ABC MedED LLc (A.K. Bag). No disclosure (J.K. Curé, P.R. Chapman, A. Singhal, and A.W. Haneef Mohamed).
Department of Radiology, University of Alabama at Birmingham, JT N432, 619 19th Street South, Birmingham, AL 35249, USA
* Corresponding author.
E-mail address: abag@uabmc.edu

Neuroimag Clin N Am 28 (2018) 255–272
https://doi.org/10.1016/j.nic.2018.01.006
1052-5149/18/© 2018 Elsevier Inc. All rights reserved.

and relatively large. However, the use of the conventional radiograph has diminished over the years given the availability of cross-sectional imaging, especially computerized tomography (CT) scans.

Conventional sialography is an invasive technique in which contrast is directly injected into the main ducts of the parotid or submandibular glands. When the proper technique is used and the patient is cooperative, this can provide excellent depiction of the morphology of the extra- and intraglandular ductal system. Strictures, ductal dilations, and architecture and arborization pattern of the intraglandular ductal system can be exquisitely detailed with conventional sialography. Over the years, use of conventional sialography has also faded owing to the invasiveness of this technique. If necessary, MR sialography can be performed. This is a noninvasive technique and can reasonably evaluate the ductal system.

Ultrasound

Modern high-resolution ultrasound scanners equipped with high-frequency linear transducers can generate excellent images of the major salivary glands. Superficial locations of the glands also contribute to high-quality images. Ultrasound examination by an experienced sonographer can easily identify ductal dilation, calculus, abscess formation, and alteration of the normal glandular morphology. Ultrasound examination with Doppler technology can also easily identify a vascular lesion and can be used to assess vascularity of a lesion.[1]

Cross-Sectional Imaging

Cross-sectional imaging with CT and MR imaging is more commonly used in the developed countries for evaluation of the salivary glands. Both techniques can generate high-quality images of the major salivary glands with excellent soft tissue details that are usually adequate for management of different salivary gland pathologies. A CT scan is excellent for detection of radiopaque stones and MR imaging is better for evaluation of parenchymal architecture. Short-tau inversion recovery sequence is excellent for detection of edema associated with sialadenitis. Diffusion-weighted MR imaging can be helpful in evaluation abscess and in evaluation of postradiation sialadenitis. MR sialography, a heavily T2-weighted imaging technique, has the potential for evaluation of the ductal system of the major salivary glands.

Imaging Approach

There is no strict guideline describing appropriate use of imaging in evaluation of sialadenitis. This largely depends on the availability of different imaging technologies and local expertise. Modern

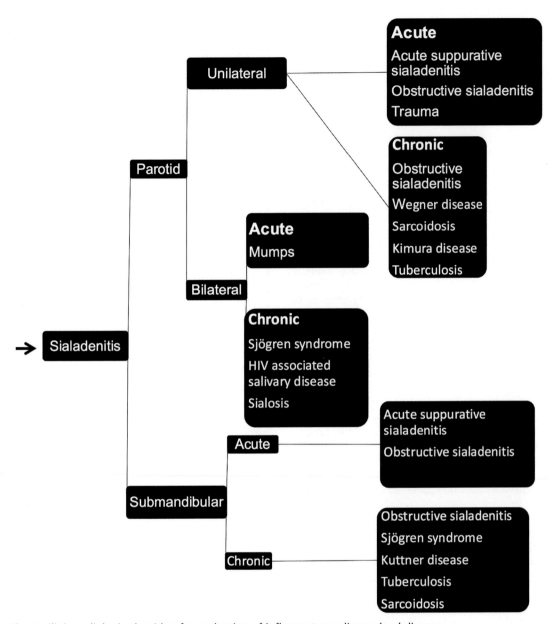

Fig. 1. Clinicoradiologic algorithm for evaluation of inflammatory salivary gland diseases.

ultrasound can generate very high-resolution imaging of the major salivary glands and can be routinely used for evaluation of sialadenitis, particularly for solitary salivary gland involvement.[1] If inadequate, cross-sectional imaging with CT and MR imaging can be contemplated. However, cross-sectional imaging is more frequently used for evaluation of sialadenitis in developed countries, particularly CT scans. At the authors' institution, contrast-enhanced CT scans are preferentially used for evaluation of patients with sialadenitis when imaging is required.

ACUTE SIALADENITIS

Infection of the salivary glands is the most common cause of acute inflammatory sialadenitis. The combination of bacterial and viral infections represents the largest category of sialadenitis.[2]

Acute Infectious Sialadenitis

Acute infections of the salivary glands can be caused by bacterial or viral infections. Rarely, mycobacterial and fungal infections can also affect the parotid gland. Most of these infections occur as a result of ascending infection from the oral cavity or oropharynx.

The predisposing factors of acute bacterial suppurative sialadenitis are salivary stasis in patients with severe dehydration and poor dental hygiene. Disruption to the normal continuous antegrade flow of saliva is the most important factor against bacterial colonization. Impaired salivary flow in ductal obstruction due to calculi, strictures, or injury; alteration of salivary flow by diuretic or anticholinergic medications; and prior irradiation can lead to acute bacterial suppurative sialadenitis. Furthermore, debilitated patients and patients with dehydration and immunodeficiency are also at higher risk of developing acute sialadenitis.

Ascending infection has a predilection for the parotid compared with the submandibular or sublingual gland because of several factors. There is (1) a wider orifice and relatively smaller caliber of the Stensen duct compared to the Wharton duct; (2) a higher incidence of the traumatic injury of the Stensen duct orifice due to its strategic location in the buccal space; (3) easier interruptions of salivary flow due to the smaller caliber of the Stensen duct; (4) more serous saliva produced by the parotid glands with inherent paucity of antibacterial mechanisms, such as low levels of secretory immunoglobulin (Ig)A antibodies, and low specific glycoproteins that inhibit bacterial attachment to the ductal epithelial cells and low level of mucin, which helps to agglutinates bacteria[3]; and (5) a relatively slower resting salivary flow rate in the Stensen compared to the Wharton duct (Box 2).

Acute suppurative sialadenitis

Acute suppurative sialadenitis is an acute, painful disease. The most common bacteria responsible are *Staphylococcus aureus*, *Streptococcus viridans*, *Streptococcus pneumoniae*, *Streptococcus pyogenes*, *Haemophilus influenzae*, and *Escherichia coli*.[1] Acute suppurative sialadenitis is typically a unilateral disease but in rare cases can be bilateral. Although acute suppurative sialadenitis typically involves the parotid gland (see previous discussion), submandibular glands can also be involved. Presence of a sialolith is the major predisposing factor for acute suppurative submandibular sialadenitis. Sialolith can also present with isolated sialodochitis of the Wharton duct or the Stensen duct.

Patients present with signs of acute inflammation, including fever, leukocytosis, pain, and tenderness of the affected gland. Purulent discharge can be seen from the Stensen duct orifice. Hydration and antibiotic treatment typically cure acute suppurative bacterial infections.

Box 2
Reasons acute suppurative sialadenitis is more common in parotid gland

1. Wider orifice of the Stensen duct compared with Wharton duct

2. Relatively small caliber of the Stenson duct compared with Wharton duct

3. Higher incidence of the traumatic injury of the Stensen duct orifice due to its strategic location in the buccal space

4. Easier interruptions of salivary flow due to smaller caliber of the Stenson

5. More serous saliva produced by the salivary glands with inherent paucity of antibacterial mechanisms

   a. Relative paucity of secretory IgA antibodies,

   b. Relative paucity of specific glycoproteins that inhibit bacterial attachment to the ductal epithelial cells

   c. Lower concertation of mucin that, with the help of sialic acid, helps to agglutinates bacteria

6. Relatively slower resting salivary flow rate in the Stensen duct compared with the Wharton duct

---

Acute suppurative sialadenitis can be complicated by intraglandular abscess, especially in cases of delayed or insufficient treatment. Abscesses can be large and can extend into the adjacent subcutaneous and deep neck spaces.

Imaging is usually not necessary in evaluation of all cases of acute suppurative sialadenitis because most cases respond to agent-directed medical management. In prolonged symptomatic cases of acute sialadenitis, ultrasound or CT scan may be warranted to assess for calculi, intraparotid abscesses, deep neck space extension of infection, or other local complications.[4] The appearance of the gland on imaging depends on the stage of the disease. In the early stage, diffuse homogenous enlargement of the gland is noted with varying degrees of stranding of the adjacent soft tissue (Fig. 2). Acutely inflamed gland is typically hypoechoic on ultrasound and hypodense on CT scan due to edema.[1] Parotid infection is often accompanied by ipsilateral upper cervical adenopathy. Enlargement of level 1B lymph nodes is frequently associated with submandibular infection. The gland becomes heterogeneous in the later stage owing to abscess formation (Figs. 3 and 4). Calcified sialolith can be easily seen with both ultrasound

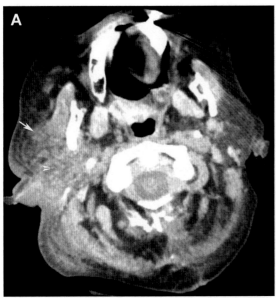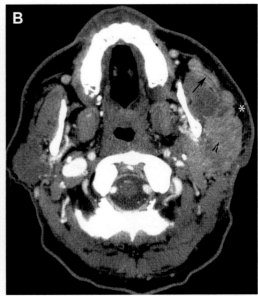

Fig. 2. Acute suppurative sialadenitis. (*A*) A 76-year-old woman with multiple comorbidities presented with right neck swelling for the last 2 days. Noncontrast CT scan through the parotid gland demonstrated diffuse enlargement of the right parotid gland, which is hyperdense (*arrowhead*) compared with the contralateral normal-appearing parotid gland and has an ill-defined margin with stranding of the periparotid tissue (*arrow*). (*B*) A 35-year-old woman who presented with pain and left neck swelling for the last 1 week. The contrast enhanced neck CT scan demonstrated diffuse enlargement of the left parotid gland, which is hyperdense (*arrowhead*) compared with the right gland. There was Stensen duct dilatation (*arrow*) with enhancement of periductular tissue. There was also stranding of the periparotid tissue (*asterisk*) due to extension of inflammation into this space.

and CT scan examination. Noncalcified stones can also be seen on CT scans. Varying degrees of ductal dilation are almost always present with obstructing sialoliths. Ductal enhancement can also be seen on contrast-enhanced CT scans. In addition to the intraglandular involvement, cross-sectional imaging can help to demonstrate extension of the inflammation into the overlying skin and subcutaneous fat and deeper structures, including the masticator, submandibular, and parapharyngeal spaces. Additionally, cross-sectional imaging can help evaluate complications of severe acute pyogenic sialadenitis, which may include mandibular osteomyelitis, or temporomandibular joint septic arthritis, jugular vein thrombosis, abscess, and airway obstruction.[5] Because acute bacterial sialadenitis is associated with significant edema of the gland, typical MR imaging appearances include hypointensity on T1-weighted sequence, hyperintensity on T2-weighted sequences, facilitated diffusion (increased apparent diffusion coefficient [ADC]) on diffusion-weighted MR imaging, and heterogeneous enhancement on contrast-enhanced MR imaging.[6] However, if sialadenitis ultimately leads to abscess formation, the pus in the abscess cavity typically demonstrates diffusion restriction with very low ADC and the wall

typically demonstrates heterogeneous enhancement on postcontrast scans.[1]

Acute viral sialadenitis

Mumps is the most common cause of acute viral sialadenitis and is, in fact, the most common of all salivary gland diseases (SGDs).[2] The incidence of mumps has been dramatically reduced in the developed countries due to widespread use of vaccines. The disease, however, has been reemerging with several outbreaks in the United States in the last decade. Travel to the endemic areas and lack of or inadequate vaccination are common causes for the outbreaks.

Mumps begins with a prodrome of low-grade fever, myalgias, and malaise or anorexia, followed by development of nonsuppurative parotitis, which is the pathognomonic finding associated with acute mumps infection.[7] Although mumps primarily infects the parotid gland, the other major salivary glands can be rarely involved as well. Bilateral parotid involvement is more common and can be seen in up to 75% of patients. Typically, the patients are young adults with 85% of patients younger than 15 years of age. In the acute stage, there is painful enlargement of the involved gland. The acute stage typically lasts about 1 week. During this stage, the saliva is clear

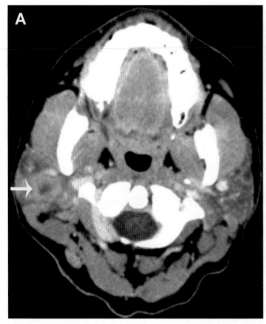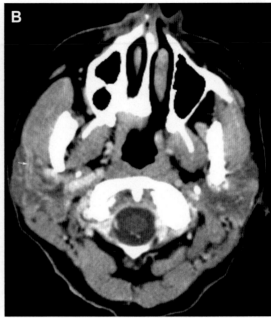

Fig. 3. Salivary gland abscess. A 35-year-old woman presented with painful right neck swelling for 1 week. She had extraction of her right maxillary molar 3 weeks ago. Contrast-enhanced CT scan of neck demonstrated an abscess of the right parotid gland (*arrow*) in (*A*) and dilatation of the Stensen duct (*arrow*) in (*B*). There is no calculus.

and contains the virus. The diagnosis can be confirmed by measuring serum antibody titer. Other common viral causes include Epstein Barr

virus, cytomegalovirus, and human herpesvirus-6B.[8]

There are no specific imaging findings. The involved gland is enlarged and can be hyperdense due to cellular infiltrates. On ultrasound examination, the involved gland appears homogenous and may contain hypoechoic enlarged lymph nodes.[5]

Trauma

Given their superficial location, the parotid glands are susceptible to blunt trauma. Manifestations of trauma include edema, contusion, hemorrhage, or localized hematomas. Blunt trauma is uncommon in submandibular gland owing to protection offered by the mandible. Penetrating injuries can involve either parotid or submandibular glands or their ductal systems. Sialocele, a focal collection of saliva that communicates with the parent ductal system, can complicate a penetrating injury. Sialoceles more commonly occur in parotid glands.

CHRONIC SIALADENITIS
Sjögren Syndrome

Sjögren syndrome (SS) is a chronic autoimmune exocrinopathy affecting salivary and lacrimal glands, which is described in details elsewhere in this edition of Neuroimaging Clinics of North America. Primary SS selectively affects

Fig. 4. Left parotid abscess. Contrast-enhanced CT scan of a patient with a painful left parotid swelling demonstrated a peripherally enhancing (*arrow*) abscess cavity (*asterisk*) within an enlarged and ill-defined left parotid gland. There was thickening of the left platysma (*arrowhead*) with stranding of the subcutaneous fat.

the salivary glands without any extraglandular involvement, whereas secondary SS is associated with another autoimmune disease, such as systemic lupus erythematosus, rheumatoid arthritis, or scleroderma. The most common clinical presentation of SS is sicca syndrome manifesting as xerophthalmia and xerostomia. Parotid glands are predominantly affected. A myriad of radiological findings has been described and depend on the stage of the disease and degree of destruction of the gland by the disease. In the earlier stage, the glands are normal in appearance on imaging. Glandular enlargement followed by honeycomb appearance is noted as the disease progresses. In this stage, a normal main duct and punctate foci of contrast accumulation uniformly scattered throughout the gland are typically seen on conventional sialogram owing to preferential destruction of the peripheral ductal system. Finally, the gland atrophies. Histologically, SS is characterized by periductal CD4-positive T lymphocyte aggregates that extend into and finally destroy the acinar structures of the gland.

Human Immunodeficiency Virus–Associated Salivary Gland Disease

More than half of human immunodeficiency virus (HIV)-infected patients experience head and neck manifestations of their disease.[9] HIV-SGD is a spectrum of diseases that includes isolated parotid gland enlargement and lymphocytic parotid gland enlargement.[10]

Parotid gland enlargement is the most common salivary gland-related presentation of HIV-infected individuals, which can be attributed to acute sialadenitis or benign lymphoepithelial cysts (BLECs). Antiretroviral therapy has also been associated with parotid gland enlargement.[10]

Lymphocytic parotid gland enlargement has been described in the literature with a variety of names, including BLEC, benign lymphoepithelial lesion (BLEL), cystic BLEL, AIDS-related lymphadenopathy, polyglandular disease, diffuse lymphocytosis syndrome, cystic lymphoid hyperplasia, and HIV-associated SGD[11] (Box 3). Histologically, the lymphocytic involvement has 3 distinct subtypes that include reactive follicular hyperplasia manifesting as persistent generalized lymphadenopathy, diffuse lymphocytic infiltration, and intraductal epithelial proliferation with cyst formation. To simplify the nomenclature, lymphocytic sialadenitis in the setting of HIV infection can be classified into (1) persistent generalized lymphadenopathy, (2) HIV-associated BLEL, and (3) HIV-associated BLEC.[11]

Box 3
Terminology describing lymphocytic enlargement of the parotid gland in the setting of human immunodeficiency virus infection

1. BLEC
2. BLEL
3. Cystic BLEL
4. AIDS-related lymphadenopathy
5. Polyglandular disease
6. Diffuse lymphocytosis syndrome
7. Cystic lymphoid hyperplasia
8. HIV-associated SGD

Persistent generalized lymphadenopathy
Persistent generalized lymphadenopathy refers to extensive generalized whole body lymph node enlargement in patients with HIV infection that demonstrate follicular hyperplasia.[11] In the setting of persistent generalized lymphadenopathy, the intraparotid lymph nodes can also be affected and lead to generalized bilateral enlargement of the parotid glands.[11,12]

Human immunodeficiency virus–associated benign lymphoepithelial lesion
A host of terminology has been used to describe the benign lymphoepithelial lesion of the parotid gland, including Mikulicz disease, Godwin tumor, myoepithelial sialadenitis, and so forth[12] (Box 4). Parotid gland BLEL can be seen in many different diseases, including HIV infection, sarcoidosis, chronic sialadenitis, and most commonly in Sjögren disease.[11] To avoid confusion, it has been suggested to use the term BLEL

Box 4
Terminology to describe benign lymphoepithelial lesion of the parotid gland

1. Mikulicz disease
2. Godwin tumor
3. Myoepithelial sialadenitis
4. Chronic lymphoepithelial sialadenopathy
5. Solid adenolymphoma
6. Lymphomatoid adenoma
7. Chronic inflammation
8. Chronic lymphoepithelial sialadenopathy
9. Chronic punctuate parotitis
10. Lymphoepithelioma

as a pathologic diagnosis in connection with a specific disease (ie, Sjögren-associated BLEL). The pathologic triad of BLEL includes lymphocytic infiltration, intraductal epithelial proliferation, and atrophy or destruction of salivary gland acini.[11,13] Clinically, BLEL manifests as diffuse parotid gland enlargement. The BLELs are typically solid lesions.

Human immunodeficiency virus–associated benign lymphoepithelial cyst

HIV-associated BLEC often presents early in the disease process, usually before development of AIDS. Progressive painless enlargement of the bilateral parotid glands is the typical presentation. In up to 90% of cases, BLEC is associated with extensive cervical adenopathy as a part of persistent generalized lymphadenopathy. The cysts are typically multiple, painless, and involve the superficial lobes of both the parotid glands.[11,14] Nevertheless, solitary cyst, intermittent pain, unilateral involvement, and involvement of the deep lobe are not uncommon.[14,15] HIV-associated BLEC can rarely involve the submandibular gland as well.[11] Multiple intraparotid cystic lesions on cross-sectional imaging in the setting of HIV infection may be sufficient for the diagnosis of HIV-associated BLEC (**Fig. 5**). However, fine-needle aspiration cytology is usually recommended in adult patients even when the diagnosis is clear on imaging (≥3 cysts) and should always

be performed in adults with 2 or fewer intraparotid cysts to rule out other salivary gland pathologic complications.[11] BLEC cysts are lined by hyperplastic and metaplastic squamous epithelium and the cyst wall also contains lymphoid aggregates with varying degrees of reactive follicular hyperplasia.

Although Sjögren-associated BLEL and other non–HIV-associated BLEL have an increased risk of simultaneous development or subsequent progression to lymphoma, the association of HIV-associated BLEL and malignant transformation is less well documented.[11] Malignant degeneration of HIV-associated BLEC has not been reported.[11] Because there is higher incidence of developing lymphoma in HIV-infected patients, a close follow-up is generally recommended in all patients with lymphocytic parotid gland enlargement.[11]

Granulomatosis with Polyangiitis (Wegener Granulomatosis)

Wegener granulomatosis (WG) is a potentially lethal disease characterized by aseptic, necrotizing granulomatous vasculitis of small and medium sized blood vessels due to overproduction of anticytoplasmic autoantibodies (ANCAs).[16] In WG, the upper and lower respiratory tracts and kidney are typically involved. Although otolaryngologic involvement can be up to 92% (mainly involvement of

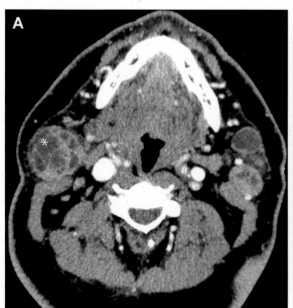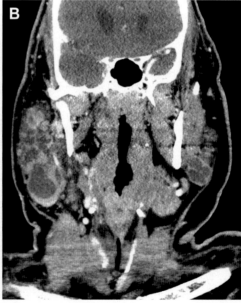

Fig. 5. HIV-associated BLEC. Axial (*A*) and coronal (*B*) contrast-enhanced CT scans of the neck demonstrated multiple cystic lesions within both of the enlarged parotid glands. Multiple enhancing septae were noted within the larger right parotid tail lesion (*asterisk*).

paranasal sinuses), involvement of the salivary glands is relatively unusual. WG can rarely present with isolated salivary gland involvement, the diagnosis of which is challenging owing to nonspecific clinical, radiological, and serologic changes.[17] There is no preferential involvement of the major salivary glands in WG, and involvement can be bilateral, unilateral, or synchronous involvement of both submandibular and parotid glands.[17] Elevated serum ANCA is usually associated with salivary gland involvement; however, its absence does not exclude the diagnosis. There is no specific imaging finding. Swelling of the involved gland with or without intraglandular solid or necrotic lesions has been described with WG. Honeycomb appearance of the gland on CT scan, similar to SS, can also be seen (**Fig. 6**). Histopathological diagnosis is also difficult owing to lack of disease-specific histologic abnormalities.[17]

Sarcoidosis

Sarcoidosis is a systemic disease of unknown cause that manifests by development of noncaseating epithelial granulomas in multiple organ systems. The parotid gland can be involved in up to 30% of sarcoidosis cases, and is primarily seen in African American patients.[2] The incidence of parotid sarcoidosis in the white population is dramatically low, only 2%.[18] Progressive parotid enlargement is the typical presentation, which can be painful or painless.[19] Salivary gland involvement can be unilateral or bilateral, and multiple glands can be involved synchronously and may be the initial presentation of sarcoidosis in some individuals. On occasion, parotid sarcoidosis can be accompanied with uveitis, and facial nerve paralysis (Heerfordt syndrome), which may be mistaken for a parotid malignancy. Imaging findings of salivary gland sarcoidosis are nonspecific. Cross-sectional imaging typically demonstrates enlargement of the involved gland with or without intraglandular solid-appearing lesions (**Fig. 7**). There may be coexistent adenopathy and these findings may incorrectly suggest lymphoma. On gallium-67 scintigraphy, a characteristic Panda sign can be seen due to increased abnormal uptake of bilateral salivary and lacrimal glands and normal physiologic uptake in the nasopharynx.[19]

Eosinophilic Lymphogranuloma (Kimura Disease)

Eosinophilic lymphogranuloma, also known as Kimura disease, is a chronic inflammatory condition of unknown cause that is endemic in Far East Asia with sporadic reports from the western world. The disease typically affects young to middle-aged patients with a strong male predominance.

The cause of the disease is still not known. It is believed to be due to imbalance of type 1 and type 2 T-helper cells resulting in high production of eosinophilotrophic[20] cytokines such as interleukin 4. Patients with Kimura disease demonstrate eosinophilia and high serum and tissue IgEs. The inciting events are still not known.

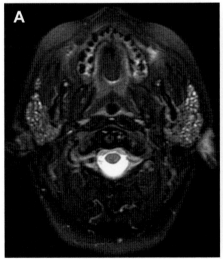 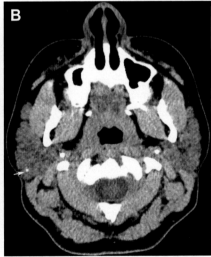

Fig. 6. Wegner granulomatosis. A 56-year-old man with a known diagnosis of ANCA-positive Wegner granulomatosis presented with bilateral parotid pain. An axial T2-weighted image (*A*) demonstrated numerous punctate T2 hyperintense foci, similar to the honeycomb appearance of Sjögren disease. There was no ductal dilatation. (*B*) An axial noncontrast CT scan demonstrated a single punctate focus of calcification (*arrow*) in the right parotid gland. The cysts were less well appreciated.

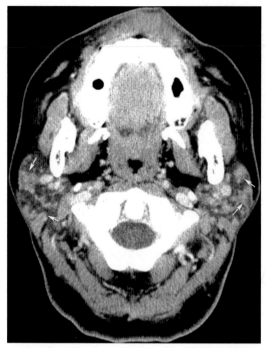

Fig. 7. Sarcoidosis. A 43-year-old man with a known diagnosis of sarcoidosis demonstrated bilateral parotid pain. The contrast-enhanced neck CT scan demonstrated multiple intraparotid ill-defined enhancing lesions (*arrows*) in a relatively normal-sized gland. No biopsy was performed. The lesions were presumed to be intraparotid lymph node enlargement and can be considered as sarcoidosis-associated benign lymphoepithelial lesions.

The triad of Kimura disease includes (1) painless subcutaneous mass with regional cervical lymphadenopathy, (2) blood and tissue eosinophilia, and (3) markedly elevated serum IgE levels. Although any area of head and neck can be involved, the periglandular tissue of the parotid and the submandibular glands are more commonly involved. Renal involvement is seen in about half of the patients, ranging from extramembranous glomerulonephritis to nephrotic syndrome.[20]

Typical histologic features include florid follicular hyperplasia with IgE-containing proteinaceous precipitate and vascularization of the germinal centers. Follicle lysis and eosinophilic abscess are characteristically seen in the germinal center or in the paracortex. Histologically, it can mimic some features of angiolymphoid hyperplasia with eosinophilia.[21]

Chronic Sclerosing Sialadenitis

Chronic sclerosing sialadenitis (CSS), also known as Küttner tumor, is a relatively uncommon and underdiagnosed chronic inflammatory disease of the salivary glands, which is now classified under IgG4-related sialadenitis and has been described in details elsewhere in this edition. CSS characteristically involves the submandibular gland, although parotid gland involvement has been described. CSS typically presents in middle-aged or older patients with a slight male predominance. Clinically, CSS produces a firm glandular swelling of the neck and can be concerning for a tumor. Painful swallowing can be associated. In some cases, CSS can involve both the submandibular glands.[22] Under microscopy, CSS typically demonstrates a well-defined lesion with preservation of lobular architecture, marked IgG4-positive lymphoplasmacytic infiltration, formation of lymphoid follicles, and abundance of cytotoxic T cells. Due to presence of IgG4-positive plasma cells, CSS is now considered an IgG4-associated disease.[23] On ultrasound examination, typically there is diffuse enlargement of the entire gland or part of a gland with maintained gland margin demonstrating either a diffuse, extremely heterogeneous echo pattern or multiple small hypoechoic foci amid extremely heterogeneous echotexture, similar to chronic liver disease.[22] On CT scans, the involved gland is enlarged in size with homogenous enhancement. The adjacent platysma might be thickened with or without stranding of the adjacent fatty tissue, suggesting extension of the inflammation to the periglandular tissue (**Fig. 8**). On MR imaging, typically there is diffuse enlargement of the involved submandibular gland. The enlarged gland is typically hyperintense on T2-weighted sequences.[24] On diffusion-weighted sequence and dynamic contrast-enhanced sequence, this lesion demonstrates diffusion restriction and fast washout similar to the malignant salivary gland tumor. Although the ADC and the wash pattern mimic malignant tumor, diffuse glandular involvement is a diagnostic clue for CSS.[24]

Chronic Granulomatous Infectious Sialadenitis

Tuberculosis

Tuberculosis of the salivary glands can be primary or secondary. Primary tuberculous sialadenitis is extremely rare. Tuberculous sialadenitis typically results from spread of *Mycobacterium tuberculosis* into the salivary glands from the regional lymph nodes. Both primary and secondary tuberculous sialadenitis are far more common in developing countries where tuberculosis is endemic. Tubercular sialadenitis more commonly involves the parotid gland, probably due to presence of intraglandular lymph nodes.[25] The clinical presentation of tuberculous sialadenitis of the parotid glands can be acute sialadenitis with abscess

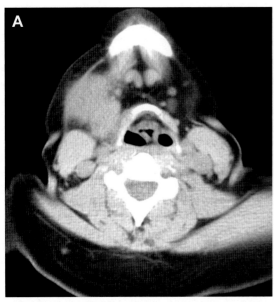
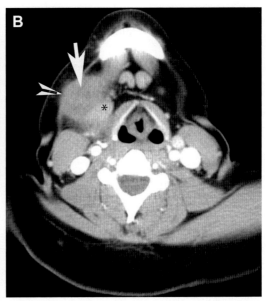

Fig. 8. CSS. Axial noncontrast (*A*) and contrast-enhanced (*B*) CT scan of the neck of a patient with right-sided painless neck swelling demonstrated an exophytic mass extending beyond the inferolateral aspect of the gland margin. The inferolateral pole of the submandibular gland was not involved because it demonstrated normal enhancement pattern (*asterisk*). The exophytic mass (*arrow*) was relatively less enhancing than the uninvolved gland. There was also thickening of the left platysma and stranding of the subcutaneous fat (*arrowhead*) suggestive of inflammatory cause. The biopsy proved to be IgG4-associated SGD.

formation. Presence of asymmetric lymphadenopathy and contiguous necrotic abscess in the soft tissue and skin, with or without a cutaneous fistula, can be a helpful clue to differentiate tuberculous sialadenitis from other acute pyogenic parotitides.[25] A more chronic presentation can also be seen in which the disease may mimic a tumor.[25] In this setting, it is necessary to rule out lymphoma or metastatic disease that also present with single gland enlargement combined with asymmetric lymphadenopathy.[5]

Actinomycosis, cat-scratch disease, and toxoplasmosis can rarely involve the major salivary glands as a part of systemic involvement without any specific tropism to the glands.

Postirradiation Sialadenitis

Postirradiation sialadenitis has also been described in details elsewhere in this edition. Acute presentation is typically associated with very high local radiation which is not used in modern radiation treatment. The chronic form develops when a salivary gland is included in the radiation treatment volumes, typically for treatment of mucosal cancers. The early response is decreased salivary flow, which is measured by sialometry.[26] The parotid gland is more sensitive to radiation compared with submandibular gland.[1] If the entire gland receives the tumoricidal dose, it usually atrophies

with resulting xerostomia. If part of the gland receives the tumoricidal dose, the rest of the acinar structures demonstrate hyperplasia and xerostomia, which is temporary. Imaging appearance varies. In the early stage, the irradiated gland might demonstrate homogenous enhancement on cross-sectional imaging. Fatty replacement of the gland is noted when it atrophies.

OBSTRUCTIVE SIALADENITIS
Sialolithiasis

Salivary stones (sialolithiasis) are the most common benign pathologies of the salivary glands. Up to 90% of the salivary gland stones involve the submandibular gland, up to 20% involve the parotid gland, and up to 7% occur in the sublingual glands. Minor salivary gland calculi are rare. Most salivary gland stones are solitary. Multiple stones can be seen in up to 32% of cases, more commonly in the parotid glands.

Stones in the submandibular gland are far more common than in the parotid gland (1) because the saliva produced by the submandibular gland is more mucinous, more viscous, and has alkaline pH that helps easy precipitation of higher concentrations of hydroxyapatite salts; (2) because of the narrower orifice compared to the wider caliber of the Wharton duct; and (3) because of the uphill direction of the terminal duct (**Box 5**). Most submandibular gland stones occur in the duct, approximately 30% near to the orifice, 35% at the bend in the duct where it changes its direction, and 20% in the midportion of the duct.[2] The remaining 15% of the stones occur within the gland proper. Symptomatic stones in the parotid gland are primarily located within the Stensen duct.

The interval of initial presentation to diagnosis is longer (12 months vs 2 months) in submandibular stones compared with parotid stones because of the wider caliber of the Wharton duct, which also has pseudodiverticuli.[2] Typical presentation includes colicky preprandial pain and salivary gland swelling, which is frequently recurrent.[4] The gland may be tender.

A radiograph can easily identify larger stones because the stones are usually radiopaque. Ultrasound may detect 90% of stones larger than 2 mm in diameter[27] and can be tried, particularity if sialolithiasis is suspected in children. A cross-sectional imaging may be warranted n cases of infected sialolithiasis (**Figs. 9** and **10**). MR imaging is less sensitive for calcified stones but stone-related complications can be better demonstrated with MR imaging. Additionally, nonradiopaque stones can also be easily identified in MR imaging, particularly with MR sialography techniques.[25]

Chronic Sialadenitis of the Parotid Gland

Chronic sialadenitis of the parotid gland is a common clinical condition characterized by recurrent, diffuse or localized, often painful swelling and inflammation of the parotid gland with or without discharge of pus,[28] which may develop as a consequence of repeated infections of the parotid gland. With recurrent sialadenitis, the glandular architecture is destroyed and over time global glandular dysfunctions sets in. On sialogram, the typical findings include stricture of the main ducts with central ductal dilatation (sialectasis). The intraglandular acini can be normal in the early stage and the gland can function normally if the main ductal obstruction is relieved. If the acini are not visualized in an otherwise good-quality sialogram, or if the normal architecture of the acini is lost, a partial glandular resection might be required. On cross-sectional imaging, there is enlargement of the gland with heterogeneous enhancement. Punctate intraglandular calcification is a common finding (**Fig. 11**).

Chronic sialadenitis of the parotid gland is known to clinicians by many names, including recurrent parotitis, nonobstructive parotitis, recurrent pyogenic parotitis, and recurrent parotitis of childhood (when it presents in the children). A simple and practical classification of chronic sialadenitis of the parotid gland has been suggested by Wang and colleagues[28]: (1) recurrent parotitis of childhood, if it presents before 15 years of age with parotid swelling and focal or diffuse sialectasis; (2) recurrent parotitis of adulthood, if it is recurrent parotitis of childhood lasting into adulthood; and (3) chronic obstructive parotitis, if it presents with recurrent parotid gland enlargement attributed to any obstructive causes, including stone, stricture, foreign body, and so forth.

Sialodochitis Fibrinosa

Sialodochitis fibrinosa, also known as Kussmaul disease, is caused by obstruction of the Wharton or Stensen duct by mucofibrinous plug.[29] The cause of this disease is unknown. An allergic cause is suspected (1) because this disease is more common in patients with asthma or chronic allergic rhinitis and (2) because of the high serum IgE level in the patients.[29] In the reported cases, the disease more frequently involves women older than 45 years of age. There is also preferential involvement of the parotid gland.

Typically, patients present with recurrent acute painful or painless swelling of 1 of the major salivary glands. The diagnosis can be difficult because salivary gland swelling is nonspecific and is more commonly caused by other salivary gland-specific diseases, such as Sjögren disease or sialolith, or by other causes of sialadenitis. A high level of suspicion is necessary for this diagnosis. Presence of a mucofibrinous plug at the orifice might be a clue. Elevated serum IgE

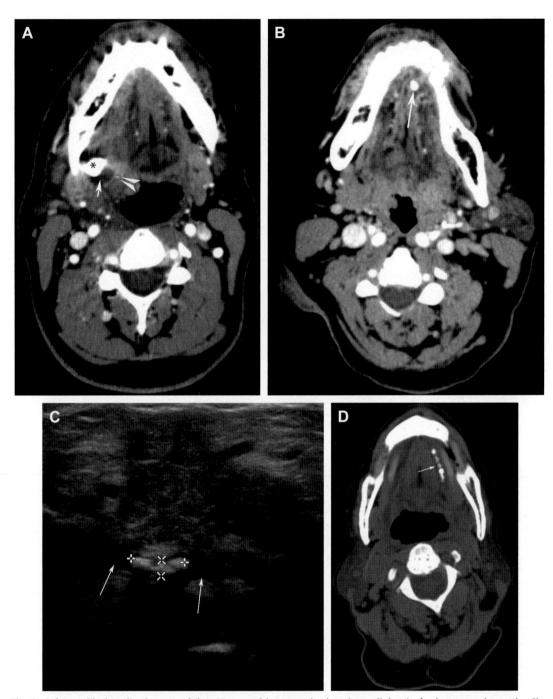

Fig. 9. Submandibular gland stones. (*A*) A 45-year-old woman had periprandial pain for last several months. She presented to the emergency department with fever and severe pain in the back of the mouth. A contrast-enhanced CT scan demonstrated a large calcified stone (*asterisk*) at the junction of the Wharton duct and the right submandibular gland, which was significantly enlarged in size. There was a fluid collection (*arrow*) immediately posterior to the stone that demonstrated subtle peripheral enhancement (*arrowhead*) suggestive of stone-associated right submandibular gland abscess. (*B*) A left Wharton duct stone (*arrow*) was incidentally identified on a CT angiogram of the neck of a patient without any stone-associated complication. (*C*) An ultrasound image of an 83-year-old woman with an enlarged painful submandibular gland demonstrated hyperechoic stones (*electronic calipers*) with strong acoustic shadowing within the dilated Wharton duct (*arrows*). Subsequent CT scan (*D*) of this subject demonstrated multiple stones were arranged along the dilated Wharton duct (*arrow*).

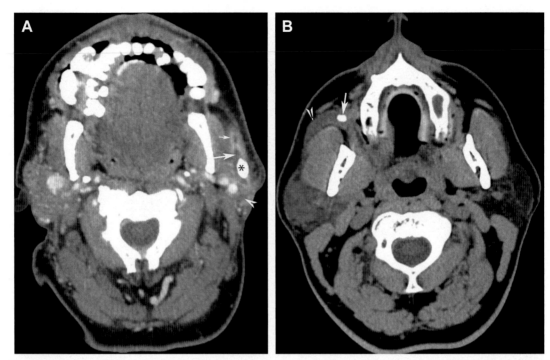

Fig. 10. Parotid stones. (*A*) A relatively large stone (*asterisk*) is noted at the junction of the dilated (*larger arrow*) left Stensen duct and the atrophic left parotid gland (*arrowhead*) in a 75-year-old debilitated patient. There is enhancement of the duct wall (*smaller arrow*) suggesting superimposed infection. (*B*) A stone (*arrow*) at the orifice of the dilated (*arrowhead*) right Stensen duct is noted on a noncontrast CT scan of a young woman with painful right parotid. The right parotid gland is inflamed because it is hyperdense compared with the left gland.

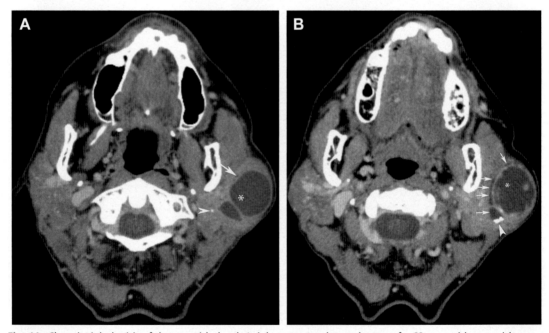

Fig. 11. Chronic sialadenitis of the parotid gland. Axial contrast-enhanced scans of a 62-year-old man with recurrent painful left parotid gland selling. (*A*) A large septated cystic lesion (*asterisk*) within the left parotid gland. A punctate calcification is partly included in this plane (*arrowhead*). Dilated intraglandular ductal system (*arrow*) is also partially included. (*B*) A septated large left parotid cyst (*asterisk*), and another focus of relatively large calcification (*arrowhead*). Dilatation of the intraglandular ductal system (*arrows*) is better demonstrated in this image.

and/or eosinophilia are frequently associated. On imaging, there is irregular dilation of the main salivary ducts. Filling defects can be seen within the ducts on sialogram (**Fig. 12**). Lymphocytic infiltrates and abundant eosinophils within the interstitial tissue surrounding the salivary ducts are typically seen on biopsy.

Treatment of the disease depends on the severity of the symptoms. Initial therapy includes compression massaging of the involved gland, proper hydration, and antihistamines with or without corticosteroids.

Ductal Foreign Bodies

Ductal foreign bodies are rare. The exact mechanism by which the foreign bodies gain access to the ductal system is not known. Vegetable remnants are the most common. It can cause ductal obstruction, resulting in ductal dilation, chronic recurrent sialadenitis, and stone formation.

SALIVARY GLAND DISEASES DUE TO UNIQUE REPARATIVE PROCESS
Necrotizing Sialometaplasia

Necrotizing sialometaplasia (NS) is a benign self-limited lesion of the salivary glands that predominantly involves the minor salivary glands of the palate, although it can involve any mucoserous surface containing minor salivary glands.[30] Only about 10% of the reported cases involved

major salivary glands. The age of presentation is usually older than 40 years of age and men are affected 2 to 3 times more commonly than women.[30]

The generally accepted cause of NS is a unique reparative process secondary to ischemic necrosis of the salivary tissue. In addition to ischemia, prior surgery, trauma including dental procedures, and tobacco and alcohol can induce NS.[30,31] More recently, NS has been associated with bulimia.[32] Induction of vomiting by a mechanical gag reflex or by ingestion of ipecac is likely to induce the injury of the salivary glands of the palate. Although male patients are more commonly affected by NS, all the NS cases reported in the setting of bulimia were white adult women between the ages of 29 and 32 years, and the typical site of involvement was palate.

The lesion is typically well-circumscribed, approximately 1 to 3 cm, and ulcerating. It typically arises from the posterior hard palate or from the hard palate and soft palate junction. The lesion can be painful or painless. It can arise as a spontaneous lesion or as a reaction to the mucoserous surface. Squamous metaplasia and pseudoepitheliomatous hyperplasia are the dominant histopathologic findings. On imaging, a nonspecific, focal soft tissue swelling may be seen at the posterior hard palate or from the hard palate and soft palate junction without any associated bone erosion.

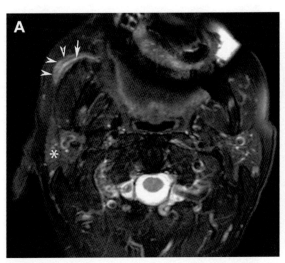 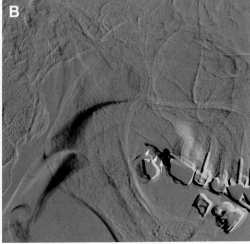

Fig. 12. Sialodochitis fibrinosa. A 55-year-old woman presented with recurrent painful swelling of the right parotid gland. An axial T2-weighted MR imaging (*A*) demonstrated relative normal appearance of the main gland (*asterisk*). There was dilatation of the terminal Stensen duct (*arrow*) with edema of the periductal tissues (*arrowheads*). (*B*) The early phase of digital subtraction sialogram demonstrated multifocal filling defects (*arrows*) close to the orifice of the Stensen duct. In retrospect, there was no identifiable intraductal abnormality on the prior MR imaging.

Adenomatoid Hyperplasia

Adenomatoid hyperplasia is typically a disease of minor salivary glands that presents as an asymptomatic, nonulcerated soft tissue mass either in the palate or in the retromolar trigone area.[33,34] The cause of adenomatoid hyperplasia has remained idiopathic; however, recurrent local trauma has been suggested as an important factor for its development.[34] This is more commonly seen in male patients with no age predilection.[35] A soft tissue mass with intact overlying mucosa is the typical macroscopic examination, and can be frequently mistaken as a salivary gland neoplasm or a fibroma. An increased number of mucinous acini within abundant normal lobules in the submucosa are a typical histopathological finding.[36] Cellular proliferation or inflammatory infiltrates are typically absent. The lesions are typically treated with local excision. Recurrence has not been reported. This lesion is not well known in the radiology community because it is usually biopsied and excised without any imaging.

Sclerosing Polycystic Adenosis

Sclerosing polycystic adenosis is a recently described, rare, reactive inflammatory lesion of salivary glands that can simulate neoplasia both clinically and histologically.[37] This pseudoneoplastic lesion mimics the histopathological findings of a benign fibrocystic disease of the breast. The lesion typically arises within the parotid gland although other major salivary glands and minor salivary glands can also be involved.[38] The reported age at presentation can be varied between 9 and 80 years, with the average age at presentation of 40 years.[39] Typical clinical manifestation is a slow-growing painless mass of less than 2 years duration.[37] Rarely, the presentation can be painful. Macroscopically, most lesions were well circumscribed although without any clearly defined capsule, with a minority forming multifocal nodules. Microscopically, lesions are characterized by abundance of collagen, sparsely cellular with fibrous tissue surrounding ill-defined hyperplastic salivary gland ducts, and acinar lobules with occasional cystic ductal dilatation and structures.[37] On imaging, the lesion is hypointense on T1-weighted sequence and shows slight hyperintensity on T2-weighted sequence, with moderate homogenous enhancement, mimicking a pleomorphic adenoma.[40] Treatment is total surgical excision.

NONINFLAMMATORY NONNEOPLASTIC SALIVARY GLAND DISEASES
Sialosis

Sialosis or sialadenosis is a chronic, bilateral, diffuse, noninflammatory, and nonneoplastic nontender enlargement of the parotid glands. Although sialosis has been associated with numerous systemic diseases, diabetes is most commonly associated. Other causes include alcoholism, obesity, starvation, endocrinological abnormalities, and numerous medications. Sialosis can also be idiopathic. The condition typically reverses when the underlying cause is treated, unless there is fatty replacement of the gland, which is the usual outcome of longstanding sialosis. Acinar hypertrophy with zymogen granulation is an early histopathologic finding, whereas fatty atrophy and/or fibrosis dominate the histopathological findings at the later stages of the disease.

Due to extreme variability of the normal size of parotid gland, it is often difficult to assess gland enlargement in mild cases. On CT and on MR imaging, typically there is enlargement of both the parotid glands without any focal intraglandular lesion (**Fig. 13**). Typically, the glands are not hyperintense on fat-suppressed T2-weighted sequence. The density on CT scan and the signal intensity on MR imaging depends on the stage of the disease and the degree of fibrosis or fatty atrophy. Imaging is mostly used to exclude other

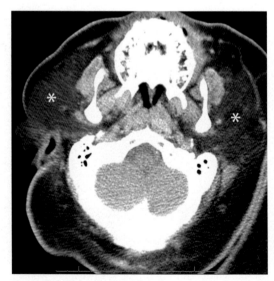

Fig. 13. Sialosis. A morbidly obese patient had a CT scan of the neck for evaluation of tracheal narrowing. Diffuse bilateral parotid swelling (*asterisks*) was incidentally identified, which was presumed to be due to sialosis.

organic diseases that commonly affect the parotid glands, such as autoimmune inflammatory diseases, HIV infection, sarcoidosis, and lymphoepithelial disease.[41]

REFERENCES

1. Abdel Razek AAK, Mukherji S. Imaging of sialadenitis. Neuroradiol J 2017;30(3):205–15.
2. Som PM, Brandwein-Gensler MS. Anatomy and pathology of the salivary glands. In: Som PM, Curtin H, editors. Head and neck imaging, vol. 2, 5th edition. Missouri: Mosby; 2011. p. 2449–610.
3. McQuone SJ. Acute viral and bacterial infections of the salivary glands. Otolaryngol Clin North Am 1999; 32(5):793–811.
4. Bag AK, Cure JK, Chapman PR, et al. Practical imaging of the parotid gland. Curr Probl Diagn Radiol 2015;44(2):167–92.
5. Zenk J, Iro H, Klintworth N, et al. Diagnostic imaging in sialadenitis. Oral Maxillofac Surg Clin North Am 2009;21(3):275–92.
6. Terra GT, Oliveira JX, Hernandez A, et al. Diffusion-weighted MRI for differentiation between sialadenitis and pleomorphic adenoma. Dentomaxillofac Radiol 2017;46(1):20160257.
7. Koenig KL, Shastry S, Mzahim B, et al. Mumps virus: modification of the identify-isolate-inform tool for frontline healthcare providers. West J Emerg Med 2016;17(5):490–6.
8. Barskey AE, Juieng P, Whitaker BL, et al. Viruses detected among sporadic cases of parotitis, United States, 2009-2011. J Infect Dis 2013;208(12):1979–86.
9. Yengopal V, Naidoo S. Do oral lesions associated with HIV affect quality of life? Oral Surg Oral Med Oral Pathol Oral Radiol Endod 2008;106(1):66–73.
10. Shanti RM, Aziz SR. HIV-associated salivary gland disease. Oral Maxillofac Surg Clin North Am 2009; 21(3):339–43.
11. Dave SP, Pernas FG, Roy S. The benign lymphoepithelial cyst and a classification system for lymphocytic parotid gland enlargement in the pediatric HIV population. Laryngoscope 2007;117(1):106–13.
12. DiGiuseppe JA, Corio RL, Westra WH. Lymphoid infiltrates of the salivary glands: pathology, biology and clinical significance. Curr Opin Oncol 1996; 8(3):232–7.
13. Sujatha D, Babitha K, Prasad RS, et al. Parotid lymphoepithelial cysts in human immunodeficiency virus: a review. J Laryngol Otol 2013;127(11):1046–9.
14. Uccini S, D'Offizi G, Angelici A, et al. Cystic lymphoepithelial lesions of the parotid gland in HIV-1 infection. AIDS Patient Care STDS 2000;14(3):143–7.
15. Marcus A, Moore CE. Sodium morrhuate sclerotherapy for the treatment of benign lymphoepithelial cysts of the parotid gland in the HIV patient. Laryngoscope 2005;115(4):746–9.
16. Razek AA, Castillo M. Imaging appearance of granulomatous lesions of head and neck. Eur J Radiol 2010;76(1):52–60.
17. Barrett AW. Wegener's granulomatosis of the major salivary glands. J Oral Pathol Med 2012;41(10): 721–7.
18. Ungprasert P, Crowson CS, Matteson EL. Clinical characteristics of parotid gland sarcoidosis: a population-based study. JAMA Otolaryngol Head Neck Surg 2016;142(5):503–4.
19. Chapman MN, Fujita A, Sung EK, et al. Sarcoidosis in the head and neck: an illustrative review of clinical presentations and imaging findings. AJR Am J Roentgenol 2017;208(1):66–75.
20. Mrowka-Kata K, Kata D, Kyrcz-Krzemien S, et al. Kikuchi-Fujimoto and Kimura diseases: the selected, rare causes of neck lymphadenopathy. Eur Arch Otorhinolaryngol 2010;267(1):5–11.
21. Kuo TT, Shih LY, Chan HL. Kimura's disease. Involvement of regional lymph nodes and distinction from angiolymphoid hyperplasia with eosinophilia. Am J Surg Pathol 1988;12(11):843–54.
22. Ahuja AT, Richards PS, Wong KT, et al. Kuttner tumour (chronic sclerosing sialadenitis) of the submandibular gland: sonographic appearances. Ultrasound Med Biol 2003;29(7):913–9.
23. Geyer JT, Ferry JA, Harris NL, et al. Chronic sclerosing sialadenitis (Kuttner tumor) is an IgG4-associated disease. Am J Surg Pathol 2010;34(2): 202–10.
24. Abu A, Motoori K, Yamamoto S, et al. MRI of chronic sclerosing sialoadenitis. Br J Radiol 2008;81(967): 531–6.
25. Ugga L, Ravanelli M, Pallottino AA, et al. Diagnostic work-up in obstructive and inflammatory salivary gland disorders. Acta Otorhinolaryngol Ital 2017; 37(2):83–93.
26. Cheng SC, Wu VW, Kwong DL, et al. Assessment of post-radiotherapy salivary glands. Br J Radiol 2011; 84(1001):393–402.
27. Armstrong MA, Turturro MA. Salivary gland emergencies. Emerg Med Clin North Am 2013;31(2): 481–99.
28. Wang S, Marchal F, Zou Z, et al. Classification and management of chronic sialadenitis of the parotid gland. J Oral Rehabil 2009;36(1):2–8.
29. Flores RBJ, Brea AB, Sanabria SAA, et al. Sialodochitis fibrinosa (kussmaul disease) report of 3 cases and literature review. Medicine (Baltimore) 2016; 95(42):e5132.
30. Carlson DL. Necrotizing sialometaplasia: a practical approach to the diagnosis. Arch Pathol Lab Med 2009;133(5):692–8.
31. Brannon RB, Fowler CB, Hartman KS. Necrotizing sialometaplasia. A clinicopathologic study of sixty-nine cases and review of the literature. Oral Surg Oral Med Oral Pathol 1991;72(3):317–25.

32. Solomon LW, Merzianu M, Sullivan M, et al. Necrotizing sialometaplasia associated with bulimia: case report and literature review. Oral Surg Oral Med Oral Pathol Oral Radiol Endod 2007;103(2): e39–42.

33. Chen YK, Lin CC, Lin LM, et al. Adenomatoid hyperplasia in the mandibular retromolar area. Case report. Aust Dent J 1999;44(2):135–6.

34. Buchner A, Merrell PW, Carpenter WM, et al. Adenomatoid hyperplasia of minor salivary glands. Oral Surg Oral Med Oral Pathol 1991;71(5):583–7.

35. Barrett AW, Speight PM. Adenomatoid hyperplasia of oral minor salivary glands. Oral Surg Oral Med Oral Pathol Oral Radiol endodontics 1995;79(4): 482–7.

36. Dereci O, Cimen E. Adenomatoid hyperplasia of the minor salivary glands on the buccal mucosa: a rare case report. Int J Surg Case Rep 2014;5(5):274–6.

37. Smith BC, Ellis GL, Slater LJ, et al. Sclerosing polycystic adenosis of major salivary glands. A clinicopathologic analysis of nine cases. Am J Surg Pathol 1996;20(2):161–70.

38. Gnepp DR. Sclerosing polycystic adenosis of the salivary gland: a lesion that may be associated with dysplasia and carcinoma in situ. Adv Anat Pathol 2003;10(4):218–22.

39. Noonan VL, Kalmar JR, Allen CM, et al. Sclerosing polycystic adenosis of minor salivary glands: report of three cases and review of the literature. Oral Surg Oral Med Oral Pathol Oral Radiol Endod 2007; 104(4):516–20.

40. Perottino F, Barnoud R, Ambrun A, et al. Sclerosing polycystic adenosis of the parotid gland: diagnosis and management. Eur Ann Otorhinolaryngol Head Neck Dis 2010;127(1):20–2.

41. Scully C, Bagan JV, Eveson JW, et al. Sialosis: 35 cases of persistent parotid swelling from two countries. Br J Oral Maxillofac Surg 2008;46(6): 468–72.

Routine and Advanced Ultrasound of Major Salivary Glands

Kunwar Suryaveer Singh Bhatia, B Med Sci, MBBS, MRCS, DLO, FRCR[a],*,
Yuk-Ling Dai, MBBS, MRes (Med), FRCR[b]

KEYWORDS

- Salivary gland • Salivary ultrasound • Salivary neoplasm • Contrast-enhanced ultrasound
- Ultrasound elastography • Sialolithiasis • Sialadenitis

KEY POINTS

- Ultrasound (US) is suitable for initial evaluation of suspected major salivary gland diseases, including sialadenitis, ductal obstruction, neoplasms, non-neoplastic masses, and other inflammatory diseases.
- US can be performed first line in patients with obstructive symptoms and is sensitive for stones, strictures, and complications that influence treatment options.
- The 2 most common salivary neoplasms, pleomorphic adenomas and Warthin tumors, have typical sonographic features but these are not sufficiently discriminatory to avoid fine-needle aspiration for cytology.
- Salivary neoplasms with irregular margins on US are suggestive of aggressive high-grade malignancies, whereas those with smooth margins can be benign or malignant.
- Limited evidence available for US elastography in salivary tumors suggests that it is suboptimal for differentiating benign and malignant neoplasms.

 Video content accompanies this article at http://www.neuroimaging.theclinics.com/.

INTRODUCTION

The major salivary glands are predominantly superficial structures that are readily accessible to ultrasound (US) assessment. US has several qualities making it an ideal first-line technique for salivary gland evaluation, including wide availability, low cost, safety, excellent spatial resolution, real-time assessment, and image guidance for needle biopsies and therapeutic aspirations.[1] Both US and US-guided procedures, however, are dependent on operator experience. In addition, US cannot assess tissues that are deeply sited or obscured by bone, including deep lobe of parotid and deeply sited lymph nodes, or evaluate specific features of malignancy, including perineural spread and bony invasion. Nevertheless, a vast major salivary diseases are suitable for assessment by US initially, with complementary information provided by other modalities as required, including sialography, cross-sectional imaging, and nuclear medicine. Ultimately, the choice between US and cross-sectional imaging as the initial technique depends on several factors, and it is

The authors have no disclosure to make in relation to the submission, including financial or other competing interests.
[a] Imaging Department, Imperial College Healthcare NHS Trust, St Mary's Hospital, 3rd Floor, QEQM Building, Praed Street, London W2 1NY, UK; [b] Department of Imaging and Interventional Radiology, Prince of Wales Hospital, The Chinese University of Hong Kong, Ngan Shing Street, Sha Tin, Hong Kong
* Corresponding author.
E-mail address: kunwar.bhatia@nhs.net

Neuroimag Clin N Am 28 (2018) 273–293
https://doi.org/10.1016/j.nic.2018.01.007

widely used first line in Europe and Asia and under-used in the United States.

This article reviews the US scanning technique and normal sonographic anatomy of major salivary glands, overviews US appearances of salivary diseases in adults, and summarizes evidence for advanced techniques, including contrast-enhanced (CE) US and US elastography (USE). Salivary US has an important role in children although the range of pediatric conditions is not discussed.[2]

ULTRASOUND SCANNING TECHNIQUE
Routine Ultrasound Technique

The major salivary glands are optimally examined by gray-scale and Doppler US (color or power Doppler) using high-frequency linear transducers, historically 5 MHz to 12 MHz, although currently multiband transducers up to 18 MHz can be used. Advances in US hardware and postprocessing enable even greater spatial resolution, speckle (noise) reduction, compounding, and other image optimizations for clearer display of edges, cyst content, and microvascularity. Curvilinear 5-MHz transducers are also useful to assess large salivary masses, the anterior floor of mouth, and deep lobe parotid lesions.[1] Color Doppler and power Doppler are used for qualitative evaluation of vascularity, which is useful for characterizing focal salivary gland neoplasms and sialadenitis, whereas quantitative analysis of peak systolic velocity, pulsatility indices (PIs), and resistive indices (RIs) of salivary neoplasms using spectral doppler is documented but not commonly practiced.

Oral sialagogues (citric acid containing fluid or lemon sticks) should be used if a clinical history is suggestive of obstructive sialadenitis (eg, peri-prandial swelling) but initial sonographic findings are negative or equivocal for ductal obstruction. They produce minimal distension of normal ducts but obvious distension of obstructed ducts, which may reveal subtle strictures and intraluminal calculi.

Ultrasound-Guided Fine-Needle Aspiration/Biopsy

US-guided fine-needle aspiration for cytology (FNAC) is simple to perform, safe, and cost effective. It has a variably reported sensitivity of 55.0% to 98.0% (average 81.9%) and specificity from 92.0% to 99.0% (average 97.1%) for malignancy.[3] Its lowered sensitivity is well recognized and reflects sampling issues, interpretative experience, and cytologic overlap. Furthermore, nondiagnostic specimens occur in up to 10% of FNACs despite repeated attempts.[4] US-guided core needle biopsy increases the diagnostic accuracy but is not widely adopted at present.[5] Its accuracy and safety record is excellent; a recent meta-analysis of 1315 US-guided core needle biopsies reported a pooled sensitivity of 94% and specificity of 98%, 1 case of transient facial palsy attributed to local anesthetic administration, and no cases of permanent facial palsies or tumor seeding.[6]

NORMAL ANATOMY OF SALIVARY GLANDS

A systematic US evaluation includes all paired major salivary glands (sublingual, submandibular, and parotid) as well as regional lymph nodes. Patients are positioned supine or semirecumbent, with the neck either rotated to 1 side or in the midline with the chin slightly elevated depending on the gland examined. Salivary glands are examined in at least 2 orthogonal planes and have homogeneous bright echotexture (**Figs. 1–5**) with several fine echogenic lines representing collapsed intraglandular ducts and a couple of small named and unnamed arteries and veins. Parenchymal echogenicity is much higher than muscle and similar to subcutaneous adipose tissue but can vary depending on fat content, and submandibular

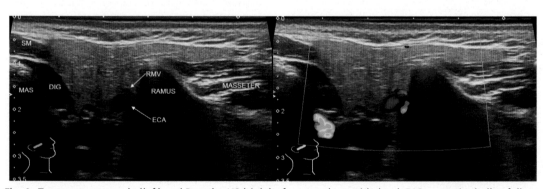

Fig. 1. Transverse gray-scale (*left*) and Doppler US (*right*) of a normal parotid gland. DIG, posterior belly of digastric muscle; ECA, external carotid artery; MAS, mastoid; RMV, retromandibular vein; SM, sternocleidomastoid muscle.

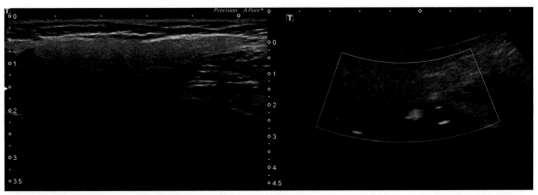

Fig. 2. Transverse gray-scale US of parotid gland using a 12-MHz transducer (*left*) showing suboptimal visualization of the deep lobe due to high fat content; whereas using a 5-MHz transducer (*right*), more of the deep lobe and external carotid artery can be visualized.

and sublingual parenchyma can be slightly less echogenic than parotid parenchyma.

Parotid Glands

The parotid glands, which are located in the retromandibular region, are evaluated in transverse (axial) and coronal planes (see **Fig. 1**; Videos 1 and 2), extending craniocaudally from the zygomatic arch to below the angle of mandible, and posteroanteriorly from the preauricular region, over the ramus of mandible and the superior aspect of masseter muscle. The retromandibular vein and maxillary artery traverse the gland vertically, with the vein slightly more lateral. The facial nerve cannot be identified on US although its position is inferred by the sagittal plane just lateral to the retromandibular vein, which therefore divides the gland into superficial and deep lobes.[7] The deep lobe cannot be completely visualized due to US attenuation as well as obscuration of the anterior portion by the mandible (see **Fig. 2**). A small number of intraparotid lymph nodes are

present, concentrated in the upper and lower poles. The parotid duct (Stensen duct) is traced as it emerges from the anterior surface of the gland, passes horizontally over the surface of the masseter muscle below the zygomatic arch, turns medially to pierce the buccinator muscle, and reaches its orifice in the buccal cavity opposite the upper second molar tooth. Parotid ducts are normally invisible or barely visible as a narrow anechoic tube measuring less than 1 mm diameter, with thin echogenic walls. Minimal pressure should be applied to avoid effacing a mildly dilated duct. Accessory parotid glands, present in 20%, appear as a separate ovoid uniformly echogenic mass along the course of the duct.

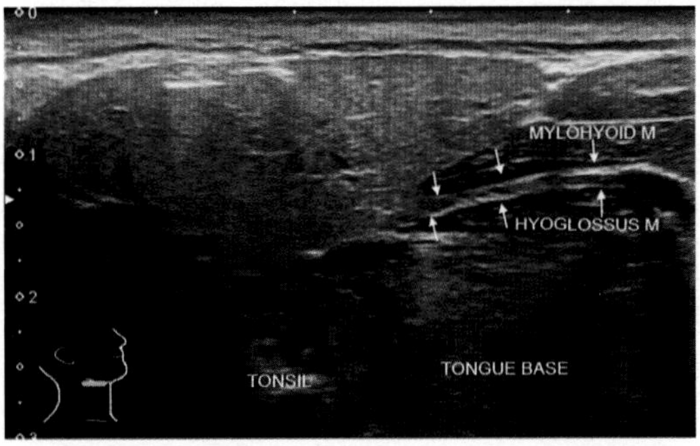

Submandibular Glands

The submandibular glands are located in the posterior aspect of the submandibular space, posterior to the mylohyoid muscle, which partially indents it and divides it into superficial and deep portions, and the facial artery and vein course obliquely along its lateral aspect. Each gland is examined transversely with the probe parallel to the mandibular body (see **Fig. 3**; Video 3) and sweeping inferiorly over the mandible and onto the upper neck. They are also examined coronally with the probe perpendicular to the body of mandible and sweeping from posterior to anterior (see **Fig. 4**; Video 4). The submandibular duct (Wharton duct) exits the gland from the anterior aspect of the deep portion, passes between the mylohyoid muscle on its lateral aspect and hyoglossus muscle on its medial aspect, and courses medially to its orifice at the sublingual caruncle medial to the sublingual gland. This duct is normally collapsed or sometimes visible as a narrow thin-walled anechoic tube. The lingual vein has a similar course between the mylohyoid and

Fig. 3. Transverse gray-scale US of a submandibular gland. Arrows signify the course of the submandibular duct. M, muscle.

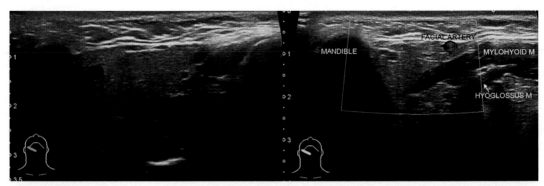

Fig. 4. Coronal gray-scale and Doppler US of submandibular gland; left image is more anterior and right image is more posterior section. The right image shows how the gland is indented by the free edge of the mylohyoid muscle. M, muscle.

hyoglossus muscles but is distinguished from the submandibular duct by identifying its branching pattern and internal flow on Doppler US.

Sublingual Glands

The sublingual glands are located in the anterior aspect of the sublingual space lateral to the genioglossus and geniohyoid muscles and anteromedial to the mylohyoid muscle (see **Fig. 5**; Videos 5 and 6). The sublingual gland and terminal portion of the submandibular duct are visualized in the transverse plane by orientating the probe upwards in the coronal plane, sweeping posteriorly from beneath the chin toward the hyoid bone. These structures are then examined in the sagittal plane, and curvilinear sector probes are additionally useful to assess the most anterior component behind the mandibular symphysis. Focal mylohyoid muscle dehiscences are extremely common, through which accessory salivary tissue or sublingual gland may prolapse, which is seldom symptomatic. Frequently, ipsilateral sublingual and submandibular glands may be contiguous in the sublingual space.

Lymph Nodes and Lacrimal Glands

US examination of regional cervical lymph nodes includes intraparotid and periparotid lymph nodes, submental and submandibular lymph nodes, and other cervical nodes as indicated. Due to timing differences in glandular encapsulation embryologically, parotid lymph nodes are both intraglandular and extraglandular, whereas other nodes are extraglandular. These appear as small, smooth oval, or reniform hypoechoic structures measuring up to 6-mm and 8-mm short-axis diameter in the parotid and submandibular regions, respectively, although they may also be round in these locations.[8] Depending on nodal size, a normal echogenic hilum and hilar pattern of vascularity is identified, although both features may be absent in tiny nodes (**Fig. 6**). The lacrimal glands are simultaneously involved in several diseases affecting the salivary glands, including Sjögren syndrome (SS), IgG4-related disease (RD), and mucosa-associated lymphoid tissue (MALT) lymphoma. The authors also assess lacrimal glands sonographically if these pathologies are suspected, by applying the transducer lightly to the superolateral quadrant of each orbit with the patient's eyes closed.[9] Lacrimal glands normally

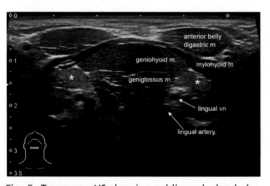

Fig. 5. Transverse US showing sublingual glands (asterisks). m, muscle.

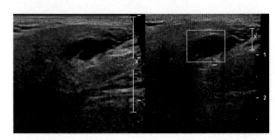

Fig. 6. Gray-scale (*left*) and Doppler US (*right*) of normal parotid lymph node with an echogenic hilum and hilar vascularity.

appear as smooth triangular homogenously echogenic structures, but if involved by the aforementioned diseases, they appear diffusely or partially hypoechoic and have variable size (**Fig. 7**).

DIAGNOSTIC APPROACH AND ROLE OF ULTRASOUND

Salivary US examination is reliant on a relevant clinical history to narrow the differential diagnoses of similar US appearances and tailor the examination, for example, use of sialagogues. Diagnostic clues include pain; swelling, including precipitants (eg, periprandial exacerbations); other neck masses; comorbidities; smoking history; other ear, nose, and throat symptoms (eg, dry eyes and mouth); and constitutional symptoms. Palpation of the salivary glands and their ducts, including intraorally as required, is quick to perform and assists in lesion localization. Palpation can also be reassuring because many swellings may be normal structures, including lymph nodes and senescent prolapsed glands (ptosis).

US examination should first determine whether an abnormality is salivary because many extrasalivary masses, such as epidermal (sebaceous) cysts and enlarged upper cervical lymph nodes, commonly mimic salivary masses clinically. If a salivary abnormality is identified, its precise sonographic features in conjunction with the clinical presentation usually permit classification into one of several diagnostic categories, which include inflammatory conditions (including infections, obstructive sialadenitis, and autoimmune disease), neoplasms, and other non-neoplastic masses.

Inflammatory conditions usually affect the entire gland parenchyma, either diffusely or inhomogeneously, and can be unilateral or bilateral depending on the underlying etiology. US is excellent at depicting solid, cystic, and ductal components of parenchymal abnormalities, which are important to assist in differentiating these conditions. For example, in nonviral infective sialadenitis, typically the parenchyma of a single gland appears heterogeneously hypoechoic with increased parenchymal vascularity, whereas SS usually is bilateral and characterized by presence of multiple microcysts and macrocysts. Autoimmune sialadenitis usually affects glands bilaterally, with different glands affected more severely depending on the disease.

US can readily detect salivary masses, which may be neoplasms, cysts, enlarged intraglandular lymph nodes, and other non-neoplastic conditions. Primary salivary neoplasms are usually unilateral with a couple of exceptions, notably Warthin tumors (WTs) and acinic cell tumors, which can be bilateral. For suspected salivary neoplasms, US fulfills several functions, including localization, characterization, staging, and image-guided biopsy. Fortunately, most salivary tumors are accessible to US, and, in this respect, a vast majority of parotid neoplasms are in the superficial lobe.[10] For parotid tumors, 1 study documented that a distance of 3 mm or greater between the lateral margin of the tumor and lateral parotid capsule (parotideomasseteric fascia) on preoperative US can differentiate deep from superficial lobe tumors, with a sensitivity of 85% and accuracy of 89%.[11] The ability of US to characterize different salivary neoplasms is discussed later.

INFLAMMATORY CONDITIONS
Infective Sialadenitis

Acute sialadenitis is most commonly of viral etiology and self-limiting, although imaging may be performed to exclude other pathologies. Bacterial sialadenitis, which is due to retrograde infection via ducts, stones, or spread from adjacent suppurative nodes, tends to produce unilateral symptoms. Sonographically, infected glands are enlarged and diffusely or inhomogeneously hypoechoic with increased vascularity (**Figs. 8** and **9**).[12] Additionally, hypoechoic streaky bands in the surrounding fascia representing edema can be present as well as adjacent lymphadenopathy. If infections progress, abscesses may develop, appearing as irregular anechoic avascular regions (**Fig. 10**), for which US has an important role in terms of image-guided diagnostic and therapeutic aspiration of pus. In chronic sialadenitis, affected glands appear normal in size or atrophic, coarse, and with mixed or increased echogenicity and may contain tiny cystic foci due to duct ectasia (**Fig. 11**). A variant of chronic sialadenitis, chronic sclerosing sialadenitis, is described separately.

Obstructive Sialadenitis

In centers with US expertise, including that of the authors, US is the initial investigation for

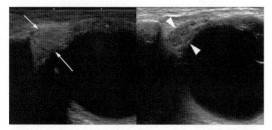

Fig. 7. Gray-scale sonograms of lacrimal glands in a healthy individual (*left, arrows*) which is homogeneously echogenic, and individual with Sjögren syndrome (*right, arrowheads*) which is heterogeneously hypoechoic.

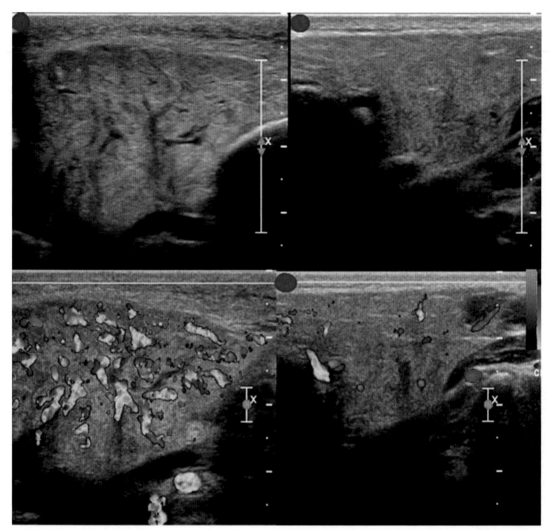

Fig. 8. Acute sialadenitis. Gray-scale (*upper panel*) and Doppler US (*lower panel*) of parotid glands showing acute sialadenitis in 1 gland (*left images*) and a normal contralateral gland (*right images*). Acute radiation sialadenitis can produce a similar appearance.

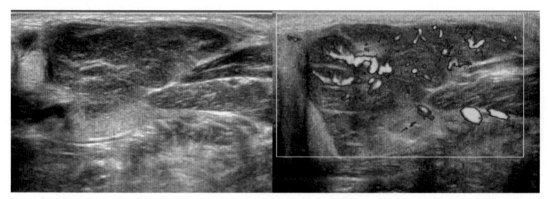

Fig. 9. Acute viral submandibular sialadenitis. Transverse gray-scale (*left*) and power Doppler US (*right*) of acute viral submandibular sialadenitis showing inhomogenous hypoechoic areas and increased vascularity.

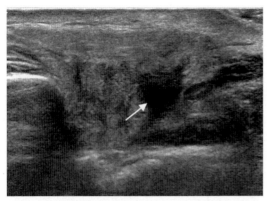

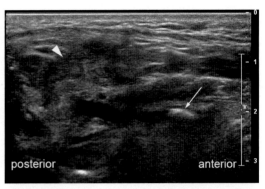

Fig. 12. Sialolithiasis and sialadenitis. Gray-scale US showing a stone in the proximal submandibular duct (*arrow*) associated with sialadenitis (*arrowhead*).

Fig. 10. Acute bacterial parotitis. Transverse gray-scale US of acute bacterial parotitis with a markedly hypoechoic region (*arrow*) compatible with an abscess. US-guided aspiration yielded pus.

suspected obstructive sialadenitis. Salivary calculi (sialolithiasis) account for 75% of cases, which are more common in the submandibular (80%–90%) (**Figs. 12** and **13**) than parotid (5%–20%) (**Fig. 14**) ducts and are multiple in one-quarter.[13,14] Submandibular calculi are located in the distal main duct (50%), followed by gland hilum (31%) and proximal main duct (19%). Sonographically, calculi appear as linear, curvilinear, or rounded echogenic foci with posterior acoustic shadowing, often within a dilated duct. Calculi

3 mm or larger are usually detectable, although with experience, calculi and mucus plugs 1 mm to 2 mm in size may be detected within dilated ducts as shadowing or nonshadowing echogenic foci. Calculi should not be confused for normal echogenic structures, including air in folded floor of mouth mucosa and the greater cornua of the hyoid bone. The size, number, and position of calculi should be documented as well as complications, including acute and chronic sialadenitis, stone erosion through the duct, abscesses, and strictures, because these influence treatment options.

Benign ductal strictures without sialolithiasis account for a quarter of symptomatic ductal obstructions and mostly likely result from retrograde infections[14] (**Fig. 15**). They are more common in the parotid duct (75%) and one-third are multiple. They appear as a focal abrupt tapering of a dilated duct with or without wall thickening (sialodochitis). Sialagogues can unmask subtle strictures (**Fig. 16**). Ductal dilatation due to neoplasm is uncommon but should not be overlooked, especially because small sublingual neoplasms and oral squamous cell carcinomas can present as submandibular sialadenitis due to obstruction at the duct orifice.

Radiation-Induced Sialadenitis

Radiation-induced sialadenitis occurs after radiotherapy for head and neck neoplasms, producing xerostomia with variable recovery depending on the degree of glandular destruction and hyperplasia of any surviving acini. The parotid glands are usually more severely affected than the submandibular glands. In the acute phase, the salivary glands are enlarged and hypoechoic due to edema (see **Fig. 8**). In the chronic phase, the affected glands become atrophic and

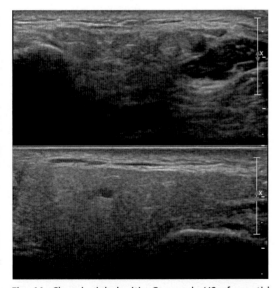

Fig. 11. Chronic sialadenitis. Gray-scale US of parotid gland (*top*) showing a small heterogeneous hypoechoic gland compatible with chronic sialadenitis. Compare this with the normal contralateral gland (*bottom*).

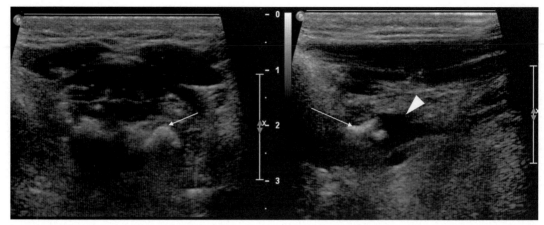

Fig. 13. Sialolithiasis. Gray-scale transverse (*left*) and longitudinal (*right*) US of sublingual space showing a large irregular stone in the distal submandibular duct (*arrows*) causing ductal dilatation (*arrowhead*). (*Courtesy of* Rhian Rhys, FRCR, United Kingdom.)

heterogenous with a coarsened echotexture and intraglandular ducts may become prominent or mildly dilated.[15] The heterogeneous hypoechoic and hyperechoic areas in the irradiated glands have been attributed to inflammatory infiltrates and fibrosis, respectively.

Sjögren Syndrome

Sjögren syndrome is a chronic autoimmune exocrinopathy involving the lacrimal and salivary glands causing keratoconjunctivitis sicca and xerostomia. Bilateral symmetric multiglandular involvement is common, initially involving the parotid glands but progressing to other glands.[16] US findings in SS correlate with histologic changes. In early disease, glands appear inhomogeneously hypoechoic and hypervascular, followed by development of multiple tiny discrete round or ovoid hypo/anechoic foci measuring

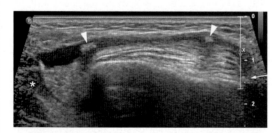

Fig. 14. Sialolithiasis and ductal stricture. Transverse gray-scale US showing 2 stones within a dilated right parotid duct (*arrowheads*) associated with parotitis (*asterisk*). The distal duct near the orifice is also dilated without a stone (*arrow*), which was due to a benign stricture. (*Courtesy of* Anil Ahuja, FRCR, Hong Kong.)

2 mm to 5 mm, reflecting dilatation of small ducts (punctate sialectasis) and lymphoid aggregates (**Fig. 17**).[17] Later, larger cystic cavities and solid masses occur, reflecting cavitary sialadenitis, larger lymphoid aggregates, and lymphadenopathy. In advanced disease, glands are irregular, diffusely hypoechoic, and atrophic. Sialolithiasis and infective sialadenitis can also occur in SS due to salivary stasis (sialectasis). US can increase the sensitivity of SS detection although at present sonographic features are not part of the diagnostic criteria for SS.[18] Monitoring in SS is important due an increased risk of developing salivary gland lymphoma,[19] and disproportionately enlarged or rapidly growing masses on US should be biopsied.[20]

IgG4-Related Disease

IgG4-RD is a chronic systemic inflammatory disease that can affect 1 or many salivary glands.[21] Many cases previously described as chronic sclerosing sialadenitis are now considered part of the salivary gland manifestation of the IgG4-RD spectrum.[22] Differing from Sjögren syndrome, xerostomia is not a predominant feature of IgG4-RD and the submandibular glands are most severely affected. Bilateral albeit asymmetric glandular involvement is common. Sonographically, salivary IgG4-RD appears as inhomogeneous parenchymal hypoechogenicity with a coarsened echotexture and minimal distortion of the parenchymal vascularity. IgG4-RD may affect glands diffusely, producing bilateral painless salivary and lacrimal gland enlargement, which sonographically comprises multiple inhomogeneous hypoechoic regions separated by hyperechoic bands,

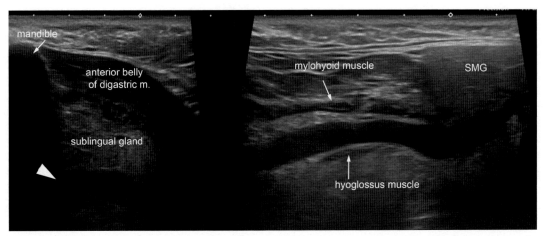

Fig. 15. Ductal stricture. Sagittal oblique gray-scale US showing gross submandibular duct dilatation. This reaches the duct orifice (*arrowhead [left image]*) where no filling defect or extrinsic mass is found. This was later confirmed to be due to a benign stricture. m, muscle; SMG, submandibular gland.

resembling liver cirrhosis (**Fig. 18**).[23] A localized form of the disease in the submandibular glands can produce a mass, which is termed a *Küttner pseudotumor* (**Fig. 19**). The differential diagnosis of Küttner pseudotumor includes primary epithelial neoplasms and lymphoma. US features favoring pseudotumor include undisplaced vascularity and a dilated duct in the hypoechoic region.

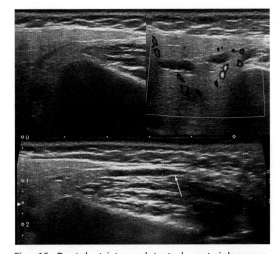

Fig. 16. Ductal stricture detected post-sialogogue. Transverse US image showing a midparotid duct benign stricture (*arrow in lower image*) that was detected only after using oral sialagogue. The duct diameter measures 1.2 mm and 0.6 mm between calipers A and B, respectively. Top left image shows parotid gland in same patient before sialagogue showing no convincing ductal dilatation. Top right image shows the same region several minutes after sialagogue, when dilated ducts were clearly visualized.

Sialadenosis

Sialadenosis or sialosis is a non-neoplastic, noninflammatory condition causing painless enlargement of 1 or more major salivary glands, especially the parotid glands, and has several etiologies, including diabetes mellitus. alcoholism, endocrinopathy, and medications. US is useful to exclude other causes of glandular enlargement, shows the parenchyma is uniformly isoechoic or slightly hyperechoic, and has normal vascularity on Doppler (**Fig. 20**).

Miscellaneous Inflammatory Conditions

Five percent of HIV-positive patients develop single or multiple salivary lesions, termed *benign lymphoepithelial lesions* (*BLELs*), which have variable

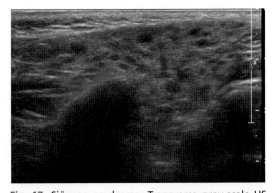

Fig. 17. Sjögren syndrome. Transverse gray-scale US of a parotid gland in a patient with early Sjögren syndrome showing multiple small ovoid hypoechoic foci, which are compatible with punctate sialectasis. A similar appearance was present in all the major salivary glands.

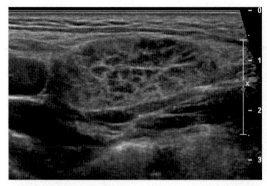

Fig. 18. IgG4-RD. Transverse US of a submandibular gland in a patient with confirmed IgG4-RD showing multiple subtle small hypoechoic regions. Both submandibular glands were involved.

appearances, including well defined anechoic cysts, hypoechoic parenchymal solid or partially cystic masses, and lymphadenopathy[24] (**Fig. 21**). Parotid glands are most severely involved. Solitary BLELs are indistinguishable from other cysts or neoplasms. BLEL transformation into lymphomas are rarely reported.[24]

Granulomatous diseases of salivary glands are rare with numerous heterogeneous causes, which include infections (eg, mycobacteria, cat scratch disease, actinomycosis, toxoplasmosis, and fungi) and noninfective conditions, including amyloidosis, granulomatosis with polyangiitis, and sarcoidosis.[25] Their imaging appearances are beyond the scope of this article but they often present with insidious painless glandular enlargement and have variable sonographic appearances, including hypoechoic infiltrates and masses that can mimic neoplasms.[26] Other diseases with salivary manifestations, including Kimura disease, are extremely rare.[27]

NEOPLASMS AND TUMOR-LIKE MASSES

Salivary neoplasms are uncommon and occur with decreasing frequency in the parotid glands (70%) and submandibular glands (8%), followed by sublingual and minor salivary glands. The risk of malignancy rises as the gland size decreases, equating to 20% to 25% in parotid glands, 40% to 50% in submandibular glands, and 50% to 81% in sublingual and minor salivary glands.[28]

In general, benign tumors appear well circumscribed, with or without lobulated margins, whereas some but not all malignancies have irregular microlobulated or infiltrative borders. Differentiation between benign and malignant neoplasms on US is possible in approximately 80% of cases although there is appreciable overlap mainly because malignancies can also appear benign, especially if they are well differentiated.[29] This limitation, however, affects all imaging modalities. Consequently, US-guided sampling should be performed on all accessible masses with a few exceptions. Recently, an US parotid imaging reporting and data system (PIRADS)[30] has been proposed for focal parotid lesions, which stratifies lesions based on 9 US patterns into 5 categories with different risks of malignancy. Even if US can be performed, MR imaging is also required if a neoplasm is suspected of being malignant, which automatically includes all sublingual tumors, or if its margins cannot be assessed completely, which includes very large and deep lobe parotid tumors.

Benign Epithelial Neoplasms

Benign epithelial salivary neoplasms are histologically diverse and overlap sonographically. Nevertheless, a vast majority are pleomorphic adenomas (PAs) and WTs, which can have typical but

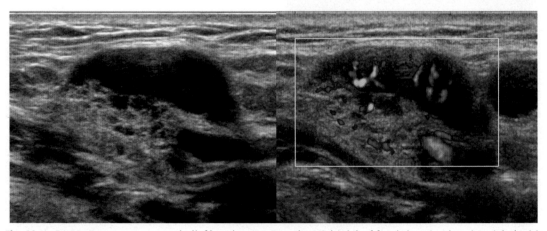

Fig. 19. IgG4-RD. Transverse gray-scale (*left*) and power Doppler US (*right*) of focal chronic sclerosing sialadenitis in the submandibular gland producing a mass, also known as a Kuttner pseudotumor. The lesion does not displace the parenchymal vascularity, which favors this diagnosis over neoplasm.

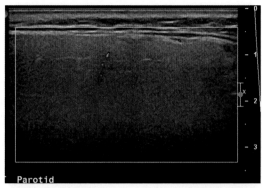

Fig. 20. Sialadenosis. Power Doppler US of a parotid gland in a diabetic patient with progressive smooth parotid enlargement, diagnosed as sialadenosis. It shows a homogeneously echogenic gland with no increased vascularity.

not pathognomonic appearances.[28] PAs are the most common and typically appear as well-circumscribed, smooth, round, or lobulated hypoechoic masses with posterior acoustic enhancement (Fig. 22). They are historically described as homogeneously hypoechoic although intratumoral heterogeneity is frequently seen with modern transducers. PAs usually appear as hypovascular, with relatively sparse vascularity with peripheral distribution on power Doppler for their size in comparison to WTs and malignant neoplasms.[31] Less commonly, PAs may contain cystic areas and occasionally dystrophic calcifications, the latter

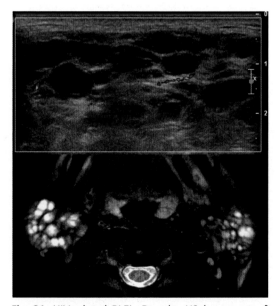

Fig. 21. HIV-related BLEL. Doppler US (upper panel) and axial T2-weighted MR image with fat saturation (lower panel) in an HIV-positive patient showing multiple hypoechoic cysts compatible with BLELs.

suggestive of chronicity. WTs (cystadenolymphomas) are almost exclusively found in the parotid gland or periparotid region, frequently involving the lower pole, and 20% are multicentric or bilateral.[10] They are typically well circumscribed, oval or round, hypoechoic, and solid or partially cystic, with a slightly heterogeneous echopattern (Figs. 23 and 24). WTs have prominent vascularity on power Doppler, which tends to have central or mixed (central and peripheral) distribution. Although spectral Doppler is not routinely performed, intratumoral vessels have reportedly low RIs (<0.8) and PIs (<2.0).[28] Occasionally, internal hemorrhage and infections of WTs can occur, which may result in imaging appearances overlapping with abscesses and malignancy. Other benign epithelial tumors are not described herein, although a smooth margin is the most consistent feature. If a superficial parotid or submandibular tumor displays benign sonographic appearances and has an FNAC result compatible with a benign salivary neoplasm, usually no additional salivary imaging is necessary before surgery.

Other Benign Neoplasms or Masses

Nonepithelial neoplasms and tumor-like lesions can involve salivary glands. Intraparotid lipomas are smooth, ovoid, mildly echogenic masses with echogenic striations producing a feathered appearance resembling subcutaneous fat (Fig. 25). Venolymphatic malformations, which include venous vascular malformations and lymphangiomas, typically appear as loose or tightly arranged clusters of thin-walled anechoic cysts with absent or sluggish internal flow on Doppler (Fig. 26). Other lesions include arteriovenous malformations, hemangiomas (more common in children), and intraparotid facial nerve sheath tumors. These lesions can be diagnosed or suggested sonographically and avoid biopsy, although, apart from confined lipomas, MR imaging is usually performed in adults for confirmation, further characterization, and mapping.

Malignant Epithelial Neoplasms

Primary salivary malignancies are histologically diverse and the 2 most common subtypes in adults are mucoepidermoid carcinoma and adenoid cystic carcinoma.[28] Their sonographic features are even more varied than benign tumors, partly reflecting the range of histologic grades. High-grade malignancies frequently have irregular or ill-defined margins (Figs. 27 and 28), although a significant proportion of malignancies have smooth margins on US, which is more common but not exclusive to low-grade types (Fig. 29).

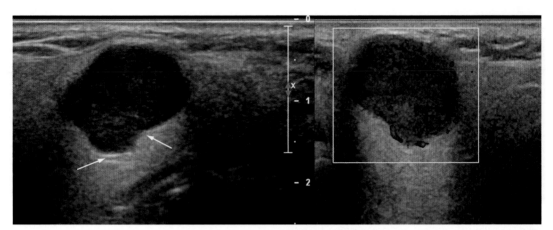

Fig. 22. PA. Gray-scale (*left*) and power Doppler US (*right*) of a parotid tumor with smooth lobulated, margins, homogeneous hypoechoic echogenicity, posterior acoustic enhancement (*arrows*), and minimal peripheral vascularity. Histology revealed PA.

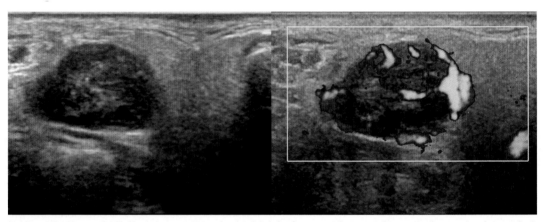

Fig. 23. WT. Gray-scale (*left*) and power Doppler US (*right*) of a parotid mass. It has smooth margins, hypoechoic, slightly reticulated echotexture, and prominent central and peripheral vascularity. Histology revealed WT.

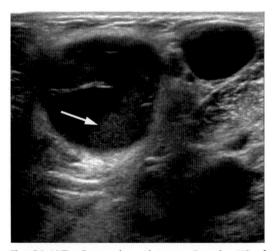

Fig. 24. WTs. Gray-scale and power Doppler US of 2 smooth predominantly cystic intraparotid masses, one with internal debris layering (*arrow*), which were WTs on histology. Internal hemorrhage and cystic change are common in WTs.

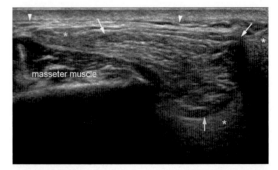

Fig. 25. Lipoma. Transverse gray-scale US of a smooth mildly hypoechoic mass in the parotid (*arrows*), with multiple echogenic linear striations producing a feathered appearance. This resembles the overlying subcutaneous fat (*arrowheads*). Adjacent normal parotid parenchyma is identified (*asterisks*). This is classic appearance for lipoma and does not require biopsy.

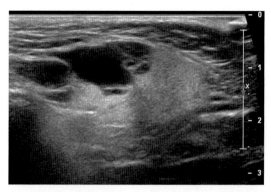

Fig. 26. Venolymphatic malformation. Transverse gray-scale US of parotid gland showing a thin-walled multiloculated anechoic cystic lesion, which has very lobulated margins and thin septations. No vascularity was demonstrated on Doppler US. The lesion is compatible with a venolymphatic malformation, which was also confirmed on MR imaging.

Accordingly, it is appropriate to state a smoothly defined tumor in the parotid and submandibular glands is likely to be a nonaggressive neoplasm, which includes malignancies, rather than stating that it appears benign. Other features of malignancy are also described although less reliable, including heterogeneous echotexture, chaotic and increased vascularity, and high resistive vascular indices on spectral Doppler (RI >0.8, PI >2.0).[28] Furthermore, malignancies can be cystic, especially well-differentiated mucoepidermoid carcinomas; hence, it is important to scrutinize cystic lesions carefully and sample any nodular components.[10] In addition, acinic cell

carcinomas, which typically have benign appearances, can be multifocal and bilateral (3%).[28] If a salivary malignancy is suspected, US can provide information regarding invasion of the skin and adjacent muscles and suspicious metastatic lymph nodes.

Lymphoma

Major salivary gland lymphomas are rare and usually represent parotid nodal involvement as part of disseminated lymphoma, notably of B-cell lineage.[28] Primary salivary involvement is classified as MALT lymphoma and arises in sites of chronic lymphoid hyperplasia, which can develop as a result of chronic antigenic stimulation in any salivary gland. Sonographically, lymphomatous nodes appear smoothly enlarged, rounded, and markedly hypoechoic with thin internal reticulations and posterior acoustic enhancement. Nodal vascularity is usually increased with a preserved hilar pattern, with or without abnormal pericapsular vessels (**Fig. 30**). Parenchymal involvement varies from focal masses (**Fig. 31**) to diffuse areas of irregular heterogeneous hypoechoic parenchyma with increased vascularity, which may resemble cobblestones or tortoiseshell (**Fig. 32**).[32] Depending on the predominant pattern, these can mimic epithelial tumors and sialadenitis sonographically (**Fig. 33**).

Metastases

Intraparotid nodal metastases are usually from cutaneous malignancies of the anterior face, lateral scalp, and external ear, including squamous

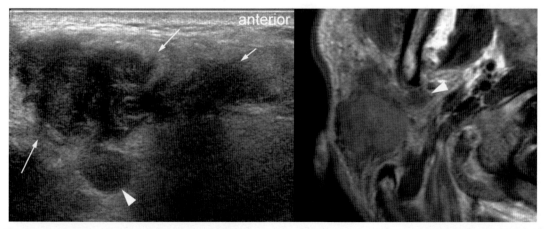

Fig. 27. Mucoepidermoid carcinoma. Transverse gray-scale US (*left*) and axial T1-weighted MR image (*right*) of parotid gland showing a heterogenous, hypoechoic mass with irregular infiltrative margins (*arrows*), highly suggestive of malignancy. A separate deeper nodule (*arrowheads*) is suspicious for metastatic intraparotid node. Cytology and histology showed high-grade mucoepidermoid carcinoma with multiple intraparotid nodal metastases.

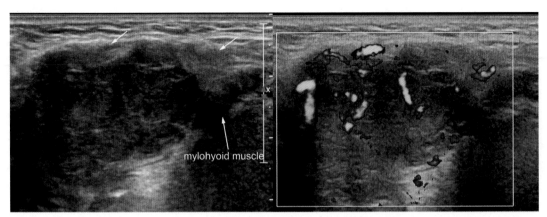

Fig. 28. Adenoid cystic carcinoma. Transverse gray-scale (*left*) and Doppler US (*right*) showing an irregular sub-mandibular hypoechoic mass with chaotic vascularity and a small amount of preserved parenchyma in the lateral aspect of the gland (*arrows*), which suggest an aggressive neoplasm rather than chronic sialadenitis. Histology confirmed adenoid cystic carcinoma. There is suspicious invasion of the posterior free edge of the mylohyoid muscle, which was also suspected on MR imaging and confirmed at surgery.

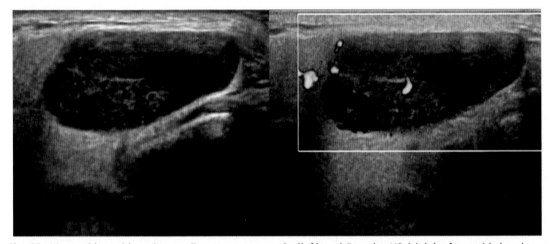

Fig. 29. Mucoepidermoid carcinoma. Transverse gray-scale (*left*) and Doppler US (*right*) of parotid showing a smooth hypoechoic nodule with reticulations and partial vascularity. The appearance is suggestive of a nonaggressive neoplasm. Histology confirmed a well-differentiated mucoepidermoid carcinoma.

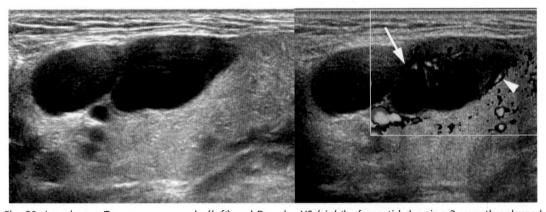

Fig. 30. Lymphoma. Transverse gray-scale (*left*) and Doppler US (*right*) of parotid showing 2 smooth enlarged markedly hypoechoic masses in a patient with known non-Hodgkin lymphoma, compatible with lymphomatous nodes. Note the enhanced hilar pattern of vascularity (*arrow*) as well as mild capsular vascularity (*arrowhead*), which is commonly seen in lymphomatous nodes.

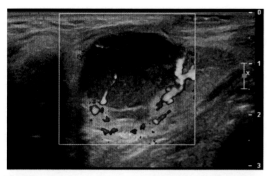

Fig. 31. MALToma. Transverse Doppler US of submandibular gland showing a solid hypoechoic mass, histologically confirmed to be a MALT lymphoma. The imaging features are of neoplasm but nonspecific and overlap with benign and malignant epithelial neoplasms.

cell carcinomas and malignant melanoma,[33] although primaries from other intra- and extra-head and neck sites can also metastasize to any node.[10] Their sonographic appearances are nonspecific and include pathologic nodes (eg, distorted hilum and pathologic capsular vascularity) or irregular, infiltrative parenchymal masses (**Fig. 34**).

Salivary Cysts

Mucus retention cysts can affect any major salivary gland, although are more commonly intraparotid. Sonographically, they appear as thin-walled cysts with anechoic or hypoechoic contents, often with low-level echoes that can be agitated on power Doppler (**Fig. 35**). If cysts have been recently infected, they have thicker albeit smooth walls that can show moderate mural vascularity, and the contents can become echogenic due to debris

(**Fig. 36**). Retention cysts arising in the sublingual space are termed *ranulas*, which are prefixed as *simple* if confined to this space (**Fig. 37**) or as *diving* if they also herniate into the submental or submandibular space through a dehiscent mylohyoid muscle or from around its posterior free edge (**Fig. 38**). First branchial arch anomalies may present as a preauricular intraparotid cyst that is typically indistinguishable from a mucus retention cyst sonographically but may be suspected in terms of location and associated aural or cutaneous symptoms (eg, discharge), reflecting persistence of their embryologic tracts.

ADVANCED TECHNIQUES
Ultrasound Elastography

In the past decade, a growing number of USE modes have appeared on clinical US machines that measure and display tissue elasticity or other biomechanical properties noninvasively. These use US-based tracking methods to measure tissue responses to mild transient deformations, which are either produced mechanically by the operator (termed *freehand compression*), by physiologic compressive sources (eg, adjacent arterial pulsations), or acoustically using highly focused acoustic impulses from a specialized transducer. USE technologies are still evolving and use proprietary technologies but are broadly subdivided into compression strain elastography and shear-wave imaging based on the fundamental waveform measured.[34] USE output also varies considerably but can be displayed dynamically alongside gray-scale images as a color-coded opacity layer, called an *elastogram* (**Fig. 39**). The firmness of a tissue or lesion in the elastogram can be graded visually by examining the relative proportions of

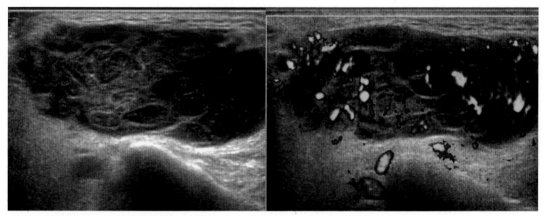

Fig. 32. MALToma. Transverse gray-scale (*left*) and Doppler US (*right*) of parotid showing a large lobulated hypoechoic mass with increased vascularity, which was MALT lymphoma histologically. The mass contains internal echogenic septations, giving a cobblestone appearance.

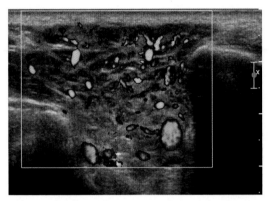

Fig. 33. MALToma. Transverse Doppler US of parotid gland showing a diffuse involvement by MALT lymphoma. The gland is enlarged, heterogeneously hypoechoic and has increased vascularity. (*Courtesy of Anil Ahuja, FRCR, Hong Kong.*)

the colors displayed, semiquantitatively, or quantitatively, including numeric estimates of its elastic modulus (stiffness). The evidence for USE for salivary tissue characterization is controversial.

Approximately a dozen pilot studies of USE in parotid or submandibular neoplasms have been published, most of which suggest that salivary malignancies have higher mean stiffness indices than benign neoplasms although there is marked overlap (**Fig. 40**).[35–37] In this regard, although WTs are generally soft, PAs have a wide range of elasticities (stiffness) that overlap with malignancies.[35,38–40] One study documented mean ±SD stiffness values of 88.7 kPa ± 48 kPa and 146.3 kPa ± 104.7 kPa for benign and malignant neoplasms, respectively.[35] A recent meta-analysis of strain USE comprising 366 masses also reported disappointing results, with pooled sensitivity of 63% and specificity of 59%.[37] Qualitative differences in elastographic patterns of

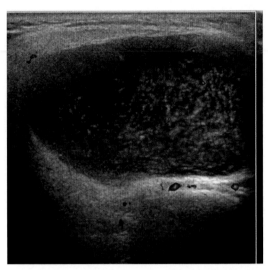

Fig. 35. Mucus retention cyst. Gray-scale US of a parotid mucus retention cyst displaying thin walls and multiple internal echoes, which were mobile.

salivary tumors have also been reported, although these are subjective and have poor predictive value.[41] In the authors' experience of salivary USE, there are other inherent challenges, such as many tumors lacking sufficient acoustic backscatters (ie, are too hypoechoic) for reliable USE measurements (see **Fig. 40**) and salivary masses that can be protuberant, such that it may not be possible to apply a flat transducer evenly onto the skin surface without causing inhomogeneities to the applied stress field, which in turn can produce spuriously high USE measurements (see **Fig. 40**). Based on the available evidence, a definitive role for USE in salivary masses has not emerged.

There are sparse reports of USE in diffuse salivary diseases with variable results, although higher stiffness indices in parenchyma have been documented in patients with primary Sjögren syndrome compared with those with sicca symptoms without established disease, which alludes to a potential role for USE to predict early Sjögren syndrome.[42–44] Another report documents higher stiffness indices in irradiated compared with nonirradiated salivary glands.[45] More evidence is required although USE could become an ancillary diagnostic and monitoring tool for diffuse diseases.[46]

Contrast-Enhanced Ultrasound

CEUS uses microbubble agents as acoustic signal enhancers and is still under evaluation in salivary tissues. Most salivary CEUS has usually been performed intravascularly by injecting intravenously a small volume (4.8 mL) of microbubbles

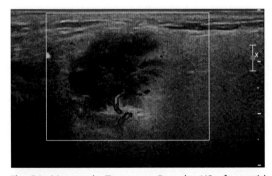

Fig. 34. Metastasis. Transverse Doppler US of parotid gland showing an infiltrative parenchymal nodule, subsequently confirmed to be a metastasis from undifferentiated nasopharyngeal carcinoma. Sonographically, this is indistinguishable from high-grade primary salivary malignancies.

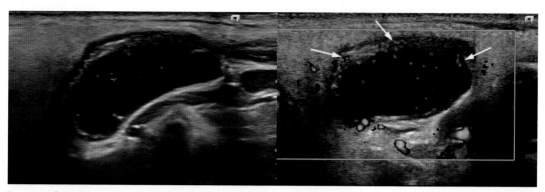

Fig. 36. Infected mucus retention cyst. Gray-scale (*left*) and Doppler US (*right*) images of an infected parotid retention cyst acquired at slightly different planes. It has mild smoothly thickened walls displaying increased vascularity (*arrows*), which can mimic cystic neoplasms.

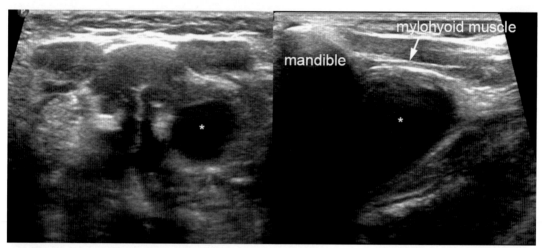

Fig. 37. Simple ranula. Gray-scale US transverse (*left*) and longitudinal (*right*) views of a thin-walled anechoic cystic lesion in anterior sublingual space deep to the mylohyoid muscle, compatible with a simple ranula (*asterisks*). (*Courtesy of* Rhian Rhys, FRCR, United Kingdom.)

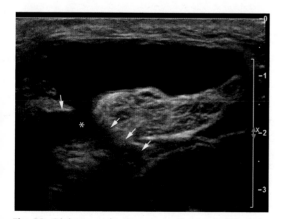

Fig. 38. Diving ranula. Transverse Grayscale US of the sublingual space showing a diving ranula. It has a small component in the sublingual space (*asterisk*) and has herniated through a dehiscence in the mylohyoid muscle (*arrows*) into the submandibular space. (*Courtesy of* Jackie Brown.)

(SonoVue, Bracco, Milan, Italy) into a peripheral vein, with continuous evaluation of the passage of microbubbles through the region of interest for at least 120 seconds. CEUS parameters can be qualitative, for example, enhancement patterns and time-intensity curves (TIC), or (semi) quantitative, for example, area-under time-intensity curve (AUC), mean transit time (MTT), and time to peak (TTP).[47] Evidence for salivary CEUS is preliminary. With respect to salivary neoplasms, some evidence suggests that benignity is suggested by diffuse homogenous enhancement (type 1 TIC) or no enhancement/isoenhancement (type 3 TIC), whereas malignancy is suggested by heterogeneous enhancement (type 2 TIC).[48] Malignant tumors are also associated with high MTTs and AUCs, reflecting prolonged intravascular dwell time of microbubbles, presumably as a result of their more disorganized angioarchitecture.[49,50] WTs have marked enhancement on

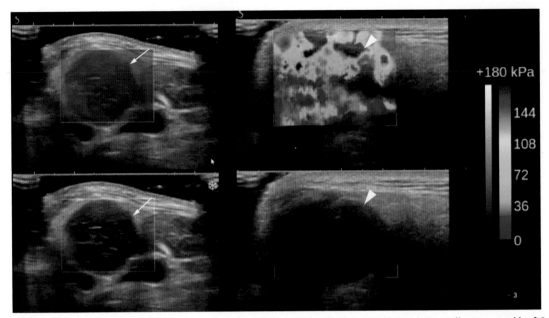

Fig. 39. Transverse shear-wave USE (*upper panels*) and corresponding gray-scale US images (*lower panels*) of 2 hypoechoic parotid tumors in different patients. The elastogram scale is quantitative, ranging from 0 kPa to 180 kPa, and chromatically displays soft and stiff regions as blue and red, respectively. The tumor on the left appears homogeneously blue and soft, with a maximum stiffness of 20 kPa. This soft tumor was a WT histologically. The tumor on right is heterogenous with areas and has maximum stiffness of 172 kPa. This was a high-grade mucoepidermoid carcinoma histologically. USE seems to discriminate the benign and malignant nature of these tumors based on their different stiffness.

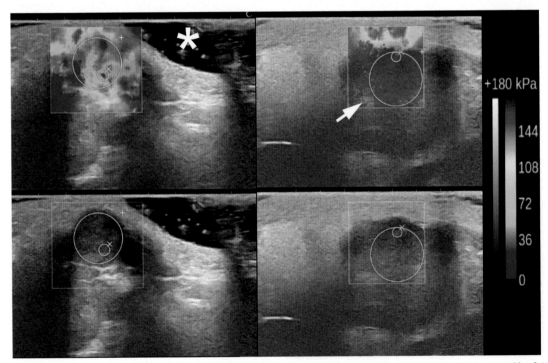

Fig. 40. Transverse shear-wave USE (*upper panels*) and corresponding gray-scale US images (*lower panels*) of 2 hypoechoic parotid tumors in different patients, histologically confirmed as PA (*left*) and high-grade mucoepidermoid carcinoma (*right*). The benign and malignant tumor appeared stiff and soft, measuring 137 kPa and 38 kPa maximum stiffness, respectively, and would be misclassified on USE. Additional challenges to USE of salivary masses, including the frequently protuberant nature of masses (illustrated by the ample US gel layer required beside the protuberance [*asterisk*]) and areas in tumor, may not display USE signal (*arrow*).

CEUS as well as significantly shorter TTP and MTT (usually normalized MTT <1) compared with PAs or malignant tumors. Conversely, PAs appear hypovascularized with slow perfusion indices although there is overlap in MTT and TTP values with malignant tumors. One study evaluated the utility of a multimodal US evaluation pathway using color Doppler, CEUS, and elastography in addition to conventional gray-scale US to differentiate benign and malignant parotid gland lesions and found combined assessment increased the sensitivity of malignancy from 77% to 91%, whereas the specificity decreased from 98% to 81%.[51]

With respect to CEUS for diffuse salivary disease, 1 report documented that anechoic apparently cystic areas in SS may be separated on CEUS into nonenhancing and slowly perfused areas, suggesting lymphoepithelial cysts and myoepithelial inflammation respectively,[49] although at present the clinical utility of this observation is unclear. Intraductal injection of microbubbles has also been anecdotally reported and has potential to assist evaluations of various diseases, including obstructive sialadenitis and SS.[52]

SUMMARY

US is ideally placed as the initial imaging technique for the evaluation of major salivary glands because it is safe and a sensitive and cost-effective imaging gatekeeper for a range of conditions, as well as able to be used for image-guided biopsies and drainages. Limitations of US are recognized, not least are the requirement for operator experience, insufficient assessment of deep lobe masses, and suboptimal accuracy and incomplete evaluation of malignancies.

ACKNOWLEDGMENTS

The authors would like to thank Professor Anil Ahuja (The Chinese University of Hong Kong) for kindly providing many images for this article.

SUPPLEMENTARY DATA

Supplementary data related to this article can be found online at https://doi.org/10.1016/j.nic.2018.01.007.

REFERENCES

1. Bialek EJ, Jakubowski W, Zajkowski P, et al. US of the major salivary glands: anatomy and spatial relationships, pathologic conditions, and pitfalls. Radiographics 2006;26(3):745–63.

2. Brown RE, Harave S. Diagnostic imaging of benign and malignant neck masses in children-a pictorial review. Quant Imaging Med Surg 2016;6(5):591–604.

3. Inancli HM, Kanmaz MA, Ural A, et al. Fine needle aspiration biopsy: in the diagnosis of salivary gland neoplasms compared with histopathology. Indian J Otolaryngol Head Neck Surg 2013;65(Suppl 1):121–5.

4. Seethala RR, LiVolsi VA, Baloch ZW. Relative accuracy of fine-needle aspiration and frozen section in the diagnosis of lesions of the parotid gland. Head Neck 2005;27(3):217–23.

5. Song IH, Song JS, Sung CO, et al. Accuracy of core needle biopsy versus fine needle aspiration cytology for diagnosing salivary gland tumors. J Pathol Transl Med 2015;49(2):136–43.

6. Kim HJ, Kim JS. Ultrasound-guided core needle biopsy in salivary glands: a meta-analysis. Laryngoscope 2018;128(1):118–25.

7. Toure G, Vacher C. Relations of the facial nerve with the retromandibular vein: anatomic study of 132 parotid glands. Surg Radiol Anat 2010;32(10):957–61.

8. Ying M, Ahuja A. Sonography of neck lymph nodes. Part I: normal lymph nodes. Clin Radiol 2003;58(5):351–8.

9. Hughes GK, Miszkiel KA. Imaging of the lacrimal gland. Semin Ultrasound CT MR 2006;27(6):476–91.

10. Madani G, Beale T. Tumors of the salivary glands. Semin Ultrasound CT MR 2006;27(6):452–64.

11. Higashino M, Kawata R, Haginomori S, et al. Novel differential diagnostic method for superficial/deep tumor of the parotid gland using ultrasonography. Head Neck 2013;35(8):1153–7.

12. Abdel Razek AAK, Mukherji S. Imaging of sialadenitis. Neuroradiol J 2017;30(3):205–15.

13. Lustmann J, Regev E, Melamed Y. Sialolithiasis. A survey on 245 patients and a review of the literature. Int J Oral Maxillofac Surg 1990;19(3):135–8.

14. Ngu RK, Brown JE, Whaites EJ, et al. Salivary duct strictures: nature and incidence in benign salivary obstruction. Dentomaxillofac Radiol 2007;36(2):63–7.

15. Ying M, Wu VW, Kwong DL. Comparison of sonographic appearance of normal and postradiotherapy parotid glands: a preliminary study. Ultrasound Med Biol 2007;33(8):1244–50.

16. Abdel Razek AA. Imaging of connective tissue diseases of the head and neck. Neuroradiol J 2016;29(3):222–30.

17. Cho HW, Kim J, Choi J, et al. Sonographically guided fine-needle aspiration biopsy of major salivary gland masses: a review of 245 cases. AJR Am J Roentgenol 2011;196(5):1160–3.

18. Cornec D, Jousse-Joulin S, Pers JO, et al. Contribution of salivary gland ultrasonography to the diagnosis of Sjogren's syndrome: toward new diagnostic criteria? Arthritis Rheum 2013;65(1):216–25.

19. Grevers G, Ihrler S, Vogl TJ, et al. A comparison of clinical, pathological and radiological findings with magnetic resonance imaging studies of lymphomas in patients with Sjogren's syndrome. Eur Arch Otorhinolaryngol 1994;251(4):214–7.

20. Gritzmann N, Rettenbacher T, Hollerweger A, et al. Sonography of the salivary glands. Eur Radiol 2003;13(5):964–75.

21. Ahuja AT, Richards PS, Wong KT, et al. Kuttner tumour (chronic sclerosing sialadenitis) of the submandibular gland: sonographic appearances. Ultrasound Med Biol 2003;29(7):913–9.

22. Fujita A, Sakai O, Chapman MN, et al. IgG4-related disease of the head and neck: CT and MR imaging manifestations. Radiographics 2012;32(7):1945–58.

23. Asai S, Okami K, Nakamura N, et al. Sonographic appearance of the submandibular glands in patients with immunoglobulin G4-related disease. J Ultrasound Med 2012;31(3):489–93.

24. Cho CC. Benign lymphoepithelial lesions-HIV. In: Ahuja A, editor. Diagnostic uitrasound: head and neck. 1st edition. Manitoba (Canada): Amirsys; 2014. p. 50–3.

25. Madani G, Beale T. Inflammatory conditions of the salivary glands. Semin Ultrasound CT MR 2006; 27(6):440–51.

26. Razek AA, Castillo M. Imaging appearance of granulomatous lesions of head and neck. Eur J Radiol 2010;76(1):52–60.

27. Cho CM, Tong SL, Bhatia KS, et al. Unusual parotid gland lesions: a pictorial review. J Clin Ultrasound 2013;41(8):501–8.

28. Lee YY, Wong KT, King AD, et al. Imaging of salivary gland tumours. Eur J Radiol 2008;66(3): 419–36.

29. Wu S, Liu G, Chen R, et al. Role of ultrasound in the assessment of benignity and malignancy of parotid masses. Dentomaxillofac Radiol 2012;41(2):131–5.

30. Abdel Razek AA, Ashmalla GA, Gaballa G, et al. Pilot study of ultrasound parotid imaging reporting and data system (PIRADS): inter-observer agreement. Eur J Radiol 2015;84(12):2533–8.

31. Rong X, Zhu Q, Ji H, et al. Differentiation of pleomorphic adenoma and Warthin's tumor of the parotid gland: ultrasonographic features. Acta Radiol 2014;55(10):1203–9.

32. Yasumoto M, Yoshimura R, Sunaba K, et al. Sonographic appearances of malignant lymphoma of the salivary glands. J Clin Ultrasound 2001;29(9):491–8.

33. Cho CC. Submandibular metasasis. In: Ahuja A, editor. Diagnostic uitrasound: head and neck. 1st edition. Manitoba (Canada): Amirsys; 2014. p. 66–7.

34. Bamber J, Cosgrove D, Dietrich C, et al. EFSUMB guidelines and recommendations on the clinical use of ultrasound elastography. Part 1: basic principles and technology. Ultraschall Med 2013;34(02): 169–84.

35. Wierzbicka M, Kaluzny J, Szczepanek-Parulska E, et al. Is sonoelastography a helpful method for evaluation of parotid tumors? Eur Arch Otorhinolaryngol 2013;270(7):2101–7.

36. Bhatia KS, Lee YY, Yuen EH, et al. Ultrasound elastography in the head and neck. Part II. Accuracy for malignancy. Cancer Imaging 2013;13(2):260–76.

37. Ghajarzadeh M, Mohammadifar M, Emami-Razavi SH. Role of sonoelastography in differentiating benign and malignant salivary gland tumors: a systematic review and meta analysis. Austin J Radiol 2016;3(2):1047.

38. Bhatia KSS, Cho CCM, Tong CSL, et al. Shear wave elastography of focal salivary gland lesions: preliminary experience in a routine head and neck US clinic. Eur Radiol 2012;22(5):957–65.

39. Dumitriu D, Dudea S, Botar-Jid C, et al. Real-time sonoelastography of major salivary gland tumors. AJR Am J Roentgenol 2011;197(5):W924–30.

40. Cantisani V, David E, De Virgilio A, et al. Prospective evaluation of Quasistatic Ultrasound Elastography (USE) compared with Baseline US for parotid gland lesions: preliminary results of elasticity contrast index (ECI) evaluation. Med Ultrason 2017;19(1):32–8.

41. Klintworth N, Mantsopoulos K, Zenk J, et al. Sonoelastography of parotid gland tumours: initial experience and identification of characteristic patterns. Eur Radiol 2012;22(5):947–56.

42. Samier-Guerin A, Saraux A, Gestin S, et al. Can ARFI elastometry of the salivary glands contribute to the diagnosis of Sjogren's syndrome? Joint Bone Spine 2016;83(3):301–6.

43. Hofauer B, Mansour N, Heiser C, et al. Sonoelastographic modalities in the evaluation of salivary gland characteristics in Sjogren's syndrome. Ultrasound Med Biol 2016;42(9):2130–9.

44. Knopf A, Hofauer B, Thurmel K, et al. Diagnostic utility of Acoustic Radiation Force Impulse (ARFI) imaging in primary Sjoegren's syndrome. Eur Radiol 2015;25(10):3027–34.

45. Kaluzny J, Kopec T, Szczepanek-Parulska E, et al. Shear wave elastography: a new noninvasive tool to assess the intensity of fibrosis of irradiated salivary glands in head and neck cancer patients. Biomed Res Int 2014;2014:157809.

46. Mansour N, Hofauer B, Knopf A. Ultrasound elastography in diffuse and focal parotid gland lesions. ORL J Otorhinolaryngol Relat Spec 2017;79(1–2):54–64.

47. David E, Cantisani V, De Vincentiis M, et al. Contrast-enhanced ultrasound in the evaluation of parotid gland lesions: an update of the literature. Ultrasound 2016;24(2):104–10.

48. Wei X, Li Y, Zhang S, et al. Evaluation of microvascularization in focal salivary gland lesions by contrast-enhanced ultrasonography (CEUS) and Color Doppler sonography. Clin Hemorheol Microcirc 2013;54(3):259–71.

49. Knopf A, Mansour N, Chaker A, et al. Multimodal ultrasonographic characterisation of parotid gland
lesions–a pilot study. Eur J Radiol 2012;81(11):
3300–5.

50. Klotz LV, Gurkov R, Eichhorn ME, et al. Perfusion
characteristics of parotid gland tumors evaluated
by contrast-enhanced ultrasound. Eur J Radiol
2013;82(12):2227–32.

51. Mansour N, Bas M, Stock KF, et al. Multimodal ultrasonographic pathway of parotid gland lesions. Ultraschall Med 2017;38(2):166–73.

52. Zengel P, Berghaus A, Weiler C, et al. Intraductally
applied contrast-enhanced ultrasound (IA-CEUS)
for evaluating obstructive disease and secretory
dysfunction of the salivary glands. Eur Radiol
2011;21(6):1339–48.

Imaging of Minor Salivary Glands

Ahmed Abdel Khalek Abdel Razek, MD[a],*, Suresh K. Mukherji, MD, MBA[b]

KEYWORDS

• Minor • Salivary gland • Malignant • Benign • Tumor

KEY POINTS

- The most common malignant tumors of minor salivary glands are adenoid cystic carcinoma and mucoepidermoid carcinoma, and the most common benign tumor is pleomorphic adenoma.
- Routine postcontrast MR imaging helps in detection and extension of minor salivary gland tumors.
- Advanced MR imaging as diffusion MR imaging and dynamic contrast MR imaging may help in characterization of some minor salivary gland tumors.
- Non-neoplastic lesions may involve minor salivary glands such as Sjogrene disease, immunoglobulin G4-related disease, stones, necrotizing sialometaplasia, and subacute necrotizing sialadenitis.
- Computed tomography scan helps in diagnosis of non-neoplastic lesions of minor salivary glands.

INTRODUCTION

The number of minor salivary glands is 450 to 1000, and they are widely distributed in the head and neck region. Most (70%–90%) are located in the oral cavity and oropharynx, including the palate, the tongue, the lips and the buccal mucosa, and the retro-molar trigone. The remainders are located in the nose, paranasal sinuses, pharynx, and the larynx. These salivary glands, as compared with the major salivary glands, are more numerous and have a reduced volume, an abbreviated ductal system, and a paucity of capsular tissue. They contribute 8% to 10% of the saliva.[1–8]

METHODS OF EXAMINATION

MR imaging is best imaging modality for evaluation of minor salivary gland tumors. Routine precontrast imaging and postcontrast imaging accurately localize the tumor and its extension into the adjacent soft tissue and perineural extension. Malignant palatal tumors may demonstrate perineural spread along the greater and lesser palatine nerves, followed by extension to the pterygopalatine fossa and cavernous sinus.[9–11] Diffusion-weighted MR imaging with calculation of apparent diffusion coefficient value (ADC)[12–15] and dynamic contrast-enhanced MR imaging with analysis of time intensity curve may be helpful in characterization of minor salivary gland tumors, but there is overlap in their results.[16–20] Malignant tumors of the minor salivary glands tend to have an irregular tumor margin, signal heterogeneity, tumor infiltration into the surrounding tissue, low signal on T2-weighted images, and restricted diffusion at diffusion-weighted MR imaging. The benign minor salivary gland tumors tend to have a well-defined margin with high signal intensity, and unrestricted diffusion at diffusion-weighted MR imaging.[9–11] Routine computed tomography (CT) scan localizes minor salivary gland tumors, detects associated bony changes, and helps in diagnosis of non-neoplastic lesions of minor salivary glands. Advanced CT such as CT perfusion and dual-energy CT scan, as well as positron emission tomography

[a] Department of Diagnostic Radiology, Mansoura University, Elgomheryia Street, Mansoura 35512, Egypt;
[b] Department of Radiology, Michigan State University, Michigan State University Health Team, 846 Service Road, East Lansing, MI 48824, USA
* Corresponding author.
E-mail address: arazek@mans.edu.eg

Neuroimag Clin N Am 28 (2018) 295–302
https://doi.org/10.1016/j.nic.2018.01.008
1052-5149/18/© 2018 Elsevier Inc. All rights reserved.

(PET-CT), has a limited role in characterization of minor salivary gland, and these methods are associated with radiation exposure and contrast medium injection.[21–23] Ultrasound is of limited value in evaluation of minor salivary gland lesions, although it has a role in guidance for biopsy.[24,25]

Neoplastic Lesions

Minor salivary gland tumors account for 10% to 15% of all salivary gland tumors and 2% to 4% of head and neck cancers. The proportions of benign to malignant tumors ranged from 20% to 50% benign to 50% to 80% malignant.[1–4] The incidence of malignancy varies according to the site of occurrence, with 40% to 60% malignancy in palatal tumors, but, as one goes from the tongue to the floor of the mouth, the incidence increases up to 90%.[2–5] Most minor salivary gland tumors are located in the oral cavity (70%); other locations include the nasal cavity/sinuses/nasopharynx (25%) and the larynx (3%). The most common location in the oral cavity is the hard palate (50%), mostly at the junction of the hard and soft palate.[3–8]

Most patients are in the sixth decade, and incidence is more common in women (66%) and in black people. Most patients present with a painless nonulcerative, submucosal swelling associated with metastatic cervical lymph nodes in 15% of patients.[3–5] Tumors arising in the oropharyngeal area can cause a painless lump. Minor salivary gland tumors of the nasopharynx and the nasal cavity may cause facial pain, nasal obstruction, or bleeding. If the tumor occurs in the larynx, it can cause hoarseness, voice change, or dyspnea.[4,8] Surgery is the treatment of choice of minor salivary gland tumors that may be followed by radiotherapy in some patients.[7]

The most common malignant tumors of minor salivary gland are adenoid cystic carcinoma (40%–50%) and mucoepidermoid carcinoma (30%–40%). Less frequent tumors are acinic cell carcinoma, polymorphous adenocarcinoma, secretory carcinoma, adenocarcinoma not otherwise specified (NOS), carcinoma ex pleomorphic adenoma, and lymphomas. The most common benign tumors of minor salivary gland are pleomorphic adenoma, followed with myoepithelioma and canalicular adenoma. Other benign tumors include Warthin tumors and basal cell adenomas, which have been reported in minor salivary glands.[4–8]

Malignant tumors
Adenoid cystic carcinoma Adenoid cystic carcinoma is the most common malignancy of minor salivary gland tumors (60%) and occurs most frequently in the oral cavity (palate) (**Figs. 1 and 2**) followed by the paranasal sinuses. The pathologic subtypes of adenoid cystic carcinomas are tubular, cribriform, and solid subtypes, and malignancy is graded as cribriform or tubular (grade I), less than 30% solid (grade II), or greater than 30% solid (grade III).[26,27] The characteristic feature of this tumor is perineural spread, and it may be associated with cervical nodal metastasis. At imaging, high-grade tumors show a destructive pattern and invasion of the underlying bone and surrounding structures. On T2-weighted images, high-grade tumors show hypointensity because of high cellularity, and low-grade tumors show hyperintensity caused by low cellularity (**Fig. 3**).

Mucoepidermoid carcinoma Mucoepidermoid carcinoma is the second common malignant tumor of minor salivary glands. In the oral cavity, these tumors can also be found in the retromolar region, palate, the floor of the mouth, lips, and buccal mucosa. These tumors are pathologically classified as low-, intermediate-, and high-grade subtypes. Mucoepidermoid carcinoma is the most frequent malignant tumor arising from intraoral minor salivary glands, representing about 36% to 59% of all malignant intraoral salivary gland tumors.[28,29] CT and MR images vary according to the pathologic tumor grade. Low-grade tumors have smooth margins and are characterized by mucin-containing cystic components, which appear as hyperintense spots on T1- and T2-weighted images. High-grade tumors tend to be rather solid with poorly defined margins, and they extend into the adjacent structures. High-grade tumors often present as hypo- or isointense lesions on T2-weighted images, indicating their high cellularity (**Fig. 4**).[9–11]

Polymorphous low-grade adenocarcinoma Polymorphous low-grade adenocarcinoma is a rare type of salivary gland malignancy found almost exclusively in the minor salivary glands. The most common site is the hard or soft palate.[8,30] This tumor can potentially cause bone resorption, medullary infiltration, and invasion of nearby nerves. Advanced tumors often extend to the maxillary sinus, nasal cavity, and oropharynx and are accompanied by extensive hard palate bone destruction. CT and MR imaging may be helpful in determining the extent of the tumor (**Fig. 5**).[9–11]

Acinic cell carcinoma Acinic cell carcinoma is an uncommon low-grade malignancy that rarely affects the minor salivary glands. The pathologic subtypes of this tumor are solid, microcystic, papillary-cystic, and follicular types.[4,31] The imaging findings are nonspecific, and most acinic cell

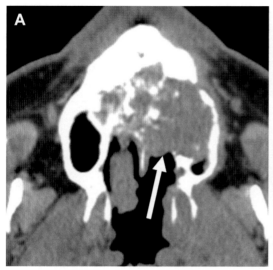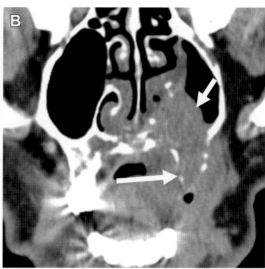

Fig. 1. Adenoid cystic carcinoma. Axial (*A*) and coronal (*B*) CT through the hard palate shows a destructive mass involving the left side of the hard palate (*arrow*). The coronal image shows the mass extending laterally to involve the left maxillary alveolar ridge (*long arrow*) and extending into the alveolar recess of the adjacent maxillary sinus (*short arrow*).

carcinomas have a generally benign appearance. Intratumoral cystic components are occasionally observed on contrast-enhanced CT Images. Therefore, CT findings are classified into 3 patterns: solid mass, cystic mass with mural nodule, and cystic mass (**Fig. 6**).[10,11]

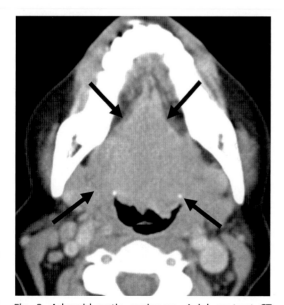

Fig. 2. Adenoid cystic carcinoma. Axial contrast CT shows an aggressive soft tissue mass (*arrows*) replacing the tongue base. These imaging findings are nonspecific and can also be seen in squamous cell carcinoma and other epithelial and mesenchymal neoplasms (benign and malignant).

Myoepetholial carcinoma Myoepithelial carcinoma is a rare tumor, in which tumor cells manifest almost exclusively myoepithelial differentiation that may arise from minor salivary gland tumors. It arises either de novo or as a carcinoma arising from a pre-existing pleomorphic adenoma or myoepithelioma. This tumor has various morphologic tumor cell types, as epithelioid, spindle, hyaline, or clear cell.[32] The imaging appearance of myoepithelial carcinoma is nonspecific. Imaging is important for accurate localization of the tumor with its extension (**Fig. 7**).

Malignant lymphoma Lymphoma of minor salivary glands is more commonly seen in elderly patients as nonulcerated soft, submucosal swelling. The most common histologic subtype is diffuse large B-cell lymphoma (70%). On MR imaging, lymphoma is often of homogeneous intermediate signal intensity at T2-weighted images with homogeneous enhancement and restricted diffusion at diffusion-weighted MR imaging because of its high cellularity. It is often associated with enlarged cervical lymph nodes that tend to display signal intensity similar to primary tumor and may be associated with permeative bone destruction.[33]

Benign tumors
Pleomorphic adenoma Pleomorphic adenoma is the most common benign tumor of minor salivary glands (50%). The most common site for pleomorphic adenoma is the hard palate, followed by the upper lip, and it may be reported in tongue, nasal cavity, and larynx.[34] On T2-weighted MR images,

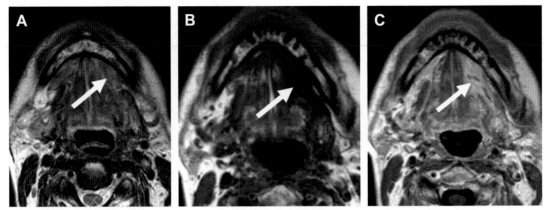

Fig. 3. Adenoid cystic carcinoma. (*A*) Axial T2-weighted image obtained through the floor of the mouth (FOM) show a subtle abnormality involving the anterior left FOM (*arrow*). The lesion is easily detected on noncontrast T1-weighted image and has low signal (*B*) (*arrow*). The mass avidly enhances (*arrow*) following administration of intravenous gadolinium (*C*).

the tumor shows characteristic high signal intensity because of extensive hyalinization components of the tumor and presence of low-intensity rim reflecting the fibrous capsule surrounding the tumor.[9–11] The tumor shows characteristic unrestricted diffusion at diffusion-weighted MR imaging.[12,13] Rarely, this tumor may be massive and undergo malignant degeneration before presentation (**Fig. 8**).[1–5]

Myoepithelioma Myoepithelioma is a rare tumor of myoepithelial differentiation that accounts for 1.5% of all salivary gland tumors. The patterns of this tumor are non-myxoid (solid), myxoid (pleomorphic adenoma-like), reticular (canalicular-like), and mixed. Palatal lesions present as well-demarcated masses, and adjacent bone erosion may be observed. Palatal lesions show hypointensity on T1-weighted images and hyperintensity on T2-weighted images (**Fig. 9**). The tumor shows various degrees of enhancement according to its histologic components.[35]

Warthin tumor Warthin tumor is more commonly seen in the parotid tail and rarely reported in minor

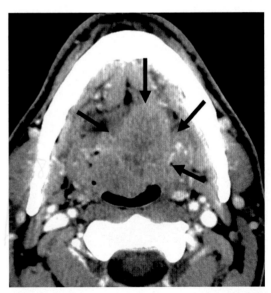

Fig. 5. Polymorphous adenocarcinoma base of tongue. Axial contrast CT shows an aggressive soft tissue mass (*arrows*) replacing the tongue base and extending into the posterior aspect of the floor of mouth. These nonspecific imaging findings can also be seen in squamous cell carcinoma and other benign and malignant epithelial and mesenchymal neoplasms.

Fig. 4. Mucoepidermoid carcinoma. Coronal CT scan shows an ill-defined destructive permeative mass seen in the left side of the hard plate with extension into the adjacent maxillary sinus.

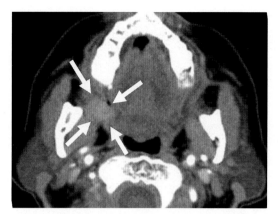

Fig. 6. Acinic cell carcinoma. Axial contrast CT shows a soft tissue mass (*arrows*) located in the right retromolar trigone. The CT imaging findings of this acinic cell carcinoma are nonspecific.

salivary gland as hard palate. Ninety percent are found in smokers. Twenty percent are bilateral, and 30% are cystic; 2.7% to 12% may arise in extraparotid tissue such as periparotid lymph nodes. On MR imaging, they are well-defined lesions, with variable enhancement. They demonstrate intermediate-to-high T2 signal, restricted diffusion, and rapid contrast uptake with rapid contrast washout as compared with pleomorphic adenoma. Unlike pleomorphic adenomas, Warthin tumors demonstrate increased uptake on Tc99m-pertechnetate scans and PET scan.[36]

Oncocytoma Oncocytoma is uncommon benign parotid tumor (1%) that occurs in women more than in men (2:1). Patients are usually older than 50 years. It arises from the oncoystes. It generally

presents as a single nodule that demonstrates decreased signal intensity on both T1- and T2-weighted images, attributed to the high cellularity and low free water content. This tumor shows restricted diffusion on diffusion-weighted MR images, and early enhancement with early washout on dynamic contrast MR images.[37]

Ductal papilloma Ductal papilloma is a benign epithelial tumor composed of fingerlike projections of squamous epithelium, and it commonly occurs in the oral cavity and oropharynx. The soft palate is the most common site for oral cavity lesions. Human papilloma virus (HPV) subtypes 6 and 11 have been identified in up to 50% of oral papilomas. At imaging, papilloma appears as polypoid lesions that may have stalks.[10,38]

Non-neoplastic Lesions

Sjogrene syndrome
Sjogrene syndrome is a relatively common systemic autoimmune disease that characterized by lymphocytic infiltration and destruction of the salivary glands leading to secretory dysfunction. It is characterized by bilateral symmetrically enlarged major salivary glands with honey comb appearance that may involve the minor salivary glands.[39,40]

Immunoglobulin G4-related disease
Immunoglobulin G4 (IgG4)-related disease is a chronic disorder characterized by elevated serum IgG4 levels and infiltration of IgG4-positive plasma cells into the tissue. This disorder commonly affects the submandibular glands, but may affect labial minor salivary glands. The affected glands are diffusely enlarged with homogenous contrast

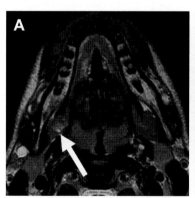
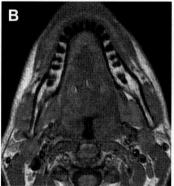
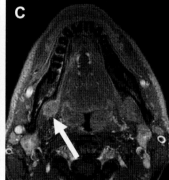

Fig. 7. Myoepithelial cell carcinoma. (*A*) Axial T2-weighted image obtained through the floor of the mouth (FOM) demonstrates a heterogeneous mass (*arrow*) located in the right posterolateral aspect of the FOM. The lesion is isointense to muscle on T1-weighted images and difficult to identify (*B*). However, the mass avidly enhances with contrast (*arrow*) and can be easily identified on the fat-suppressed contrast-enhanced T1W sequences (*C*). These findings are nonspecific and can be associated with various malignancies of the FOM including squamous cell carcinoma and other minor salivary neoplasms.

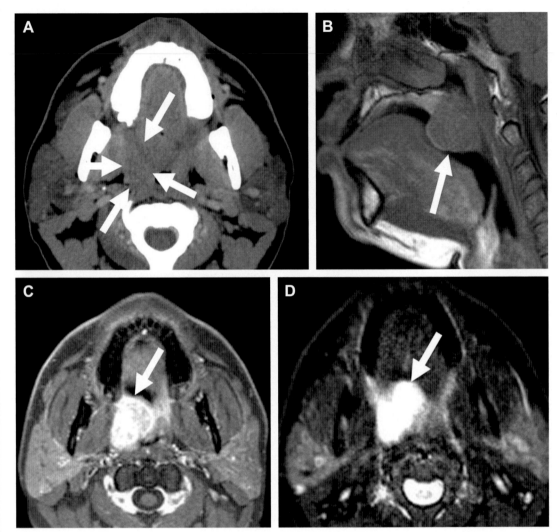

Fig. 8. Pleomorphic adenoma of soft palate. (*A*) Axial CT shows a soft mass (*arrows*) involving the right side of the soft palate. (*B*) Sagittal noncontrast T1-weighted MR imaging shows an intermediate signal mass expanding the soft palate (*arrow*). (*C*) Axial fat-suppressed T1-weighted image sequence shows the mass (*arrow*) to homogeneously enhance with contrast. The mass (*arrow*) has increased signal on the T2-weighted images (*D*), which is consistent with pleomorphic adenoma.

enhancement and restricted diffusion on diffusion-weighted MR imaging.[39,40]

Sarcoidosis

Sarcoidosis is a rare autoimmune disorder characterized by noncaseating epitheloid granuloma that is most commonly seen in second to fourth decade of life. It is 10 to 20 times more common in black people than white people. The disorder commonly affects parotid gland and may the submandibular and minor salivary gland. On imaging, there are bilateral multiple, noncavitating masses with foamy appearance that are seen in both parotid glands and may in minor salivary gland be associated with cervical lymphadenopathy.[41,42]

Necrotizing sialometaplasia

Necrotizing sialometaplasia is a rare, self-limited, necrotizing process of minor salivary glands, mainly located in the hard palate. It may relate to ischemic event of the vasculature supplying the salivary gland lobules. The predisposing factors are smoking, alcohol use, denture wearing, surgery, trauma, and anorexia. At imaging, it appears as a focal mass mostly at the posterior part of hard palate with no bony erosion.[42,43]

Subacute necrotizing sialadenitis

Subacute necrotizing sialadenitis is a self-limited, inflammatory condition of the minor salivary glands of unknown etiology. The lesion typically

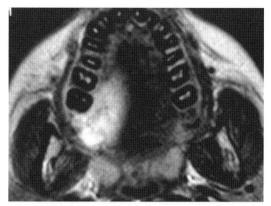

Fig. 9. Myoepithelioma of hard palate. Axial T2-weighted image shows hyperintense mass of the hard palate.

presents as a localized, palatal lesion with abrupt onset of pain. The etiology of subacute necrotizing sialadenitis is unknown, but traumatic, infectious, and allergic etiologies have been suggested. It appears as mass in the hard palate or may be in the floor of the mouth simulating malignancy.[42,43]

Stones

Stones are rarely reported in minor salivary glands, mostly in the fifth to sixth decade of life, and occur mainly in male patients, most frequently in the buccal mucosa and upper lip. CT scan is sensitive for detection of stones of minor salivary glands.[16]

Mucocele

Mucocele is the most common cystic lesion of the salivary glands. Extravasation mucocele (90%) is most frequently encountered in children in the lower lip. Retention mucocele is rarer, but is most often seen in older patients in the floor of the mouth, palate, or buccal mucosa.[44]

SUMMARY

The authors concluded that contrast MR imaging and CT are adequate for accurate localization and extension of neoplastic and non-neoplastic lesions of minor salivary glands.

REFERENCES

1. Wang XD, Meng LJ, Hou TT, et al. Frequency and distribution pattern of minor salivary gland tumors in a northeastern Chinese population: a retrospective study of 485 patients. J Oral Maxillofac Surg 2015; 73:81–91.

2. Vander Poorten V, Hunt J, Bradley PJ, et al. Recent trends in the management of minor salivary gland carcinoma. Head Neck 2014;36:444–55.

3. Abrahão AC, Santos Netto Jde N, Pires F, et al. Clinicopathological characteristics of tumors of the intraoral minor salivary glands in 170 Brazilian patients. Br J Oral Maxillofac Surg 2016;54: 30–4.

4. Bradley PJ. Tumors of minor salivary gland origin. Chapter 20. In: Myers EN, Ferris RL, editors. Salivary gland disorders. Springer; 2007. p. 323–37.

5. Baddour HM Jr, Fedewa SA, Chen AY. Five- and 10-year cause-specific survival rates in carcinoma of the minor salivary gland. JAMA Otolaryngol Head Neck Surg 2016;142:67–73.

6. Haymerle G, Schneider S, Harris L, et al. Minor salivary gland carcinoma: a review of 35 cases. Eur Arch Otorhinolaryngol 2016;273:2717–26.

7. Abdel Razek AAK, Mukherji SK. Imaging of post-treatment salivary gland tumors. Neuroimag Clin N Am 2018;28(2):199–208.

8. Khurram SA, Barrett AW, Speight PM. Diagnostic difficulties in lesions of the minor salivary glands. Diagn Histopathol 2017;23:250–9.

9. Abdel Razek AAK, Mukherji SK. State-of-the-art imaging of salivary gland tumors. Neuroimag Clin N Am 2018;28(2):303–17.

10. von Stempel C, Morley S, Beale T, et al. Imaging of palatal lumps. Clin Radiol 2017;72:97–107.

11. Kato H, Kanematsu M, Makita H, et al. CT and MR imaging findings of palatal tumors. Eur J Radiol 2014;83:e137–46.

12. Razek AA. Diffusion-weighted magnetic resonance imaging of head and neck. J Comput Assist Tomogr 2010;34:808–15.

13. Abdel Razek A. Prediction of malignancy of submandibular gland tumors with apparent diffusion coefficient. Oral Radiol, in press.

14. Abdel Razek AA. Assessment of solid lesions of the temporal fossa with diffusion-weighted magnetic resonance imaging. Int J Oral Maxillofac Surg 2015;44:1081–5.

15. Li S, Cheng J, Zhang Y, et al. Differentiation of benign and malignant lesions of the tongue by using diffusion-weighted MRI at 3.0 T. Dentomaxillofac Radiol 2015;44:20140325.

16. Razek AA, Elsorogy LG, Soliman NY, et al. Dynamic susceptibility contrast perfusion MR imaging in distinguishing malignant from benign head and neck tumors: a pilot study. Eur J Radiol 2011;77:73–9.

17. Matsuzaki H, Yanagi Y, Hara M, et al. Minor salivary gland tumors in the oral cavity: diagnostic value of dynamic contrast-enhanced MRI. Eur J Radiol 2012;81:2684–91.

18. Abdel Razek AA, Gaballa G. Role of perfusion magnetic resonance imaging in cervical lymphadenopathy. J Comput Assist Tomogr 2011;35:21–5.

19. Gaddikeri S, Gaddikeri RS, Tailor T, et al. Dynamic contrast-enhanced MR imaging in head and neck cancer: techniques and clinical applications. AJNR Am J Neuroradiol 2016;37:588–95.

20. Abdel Razek AA, Samir S, Ashmalla GA. Character-ization of parotid tumors with dynamic susceptibility contrast perfusion-weighted magnetic resonance imaging and diffusion-weighted MR imaging. J Comput Assist Tomogr 2017;41:131–6.

21. Thorawat A, Shetty PK, Tarakji B. Minor salivary gland carcinoma of hard palate with CT findings- report of a case. J Clin Diagn Res 2016;10:ZJ10–Z11.

22. Razek AA, Tawfik AM, Elsorogy LG, et al. Perfusion CT of head and neck cancer. Eur J Radiol 2014;83:537–44.

23. Tawfik AM, Razek AA, Kerl JM, et al. Comparison of dual-energy CT-derived iodine content and iodine overlay of normal, inflammatory and metastatic squamous cell carcinoma cervical lymph nodes. Eur Radiol 2014;24:574–80.

24. Sengupta A, Brown J, Rudralingam M. The use of in-traoral ultrasound in the characterization of minor salivary gland malignancy: report of two cases. Den-tomaxillofac Radiol 2016;45:20150354.

25. Abdel Razek AA, Ashmalla GA, Gaballa G, et al. Pi-lot study of ultrasound parotid imaging reporting and data system (PIRADS): inter-observer agree-ment. Eur J Radiol 2015;85:2533–8.

26. Shum JW, Chatzistefanou I, Qaisi M, et al. Adenoid cystic carcinoma of the minor salivary glands: a retrospective series of 29 cases and review of the literature. Oral Surg Oral Med Oral Pathol Oral Ra-diol 2016;121:210–4.

27. Jaiswara C, Dhiman NK, Singh AK, et al. Adenoid cystic carcinoma of the floor of the mouth - a rare presentation. J Oral Biol Craniofac Res 2016;6:S65–9.

28. Dossani R, Akbarian-Tefaghi H, Lemonnier L, et al. Mucoepidermoid carcinoma of palatal minor salivary glands with intracranial extension: a case report and literature review. J Neurol Surg Rep 2016;77:e156–9.

29. Mesolella M, Iengo M, Testa D, et al. Mucoepider-moid carcinoma of the base of tongue. Acta Otorhi-nolaryngol Ital 2015;35:58–61.

30. Sathyanarayanan R, Suresh V, Therese Thomas BA. Polymorphous low-grade adenocarcinoma of the palate: a rare case report. Iran J Cancer Prev 2015;9:e3447.

31. Erpek G, Günel C, Meteoğlu I. Acinic cell carcinoma of the posterior wall of the pharynx. Ear Nose Throat J 2015;94:E30–1.

32. Yang S, Zeng M, Zhang J, et al. Clear cell myoe-pithelial carcinoma of minor salivary gland: a case report. Int J Oral Maxillofac Surg 2010;39:297–300.

33. Celenk C, Celenk P. Palate lymphoma: CT findings. AJR Am J Roentgenol 2016;207:628–30.

34. Qureshi MY, Khan TA, Dhurjati VN, et al. Pleomor-phic adenoma in retromolar area: a very rare case report and review of literature. J Clin Diagn Res 2016;10:ZD03–5.

35. Policarpo M, Longoni V, Garofalo P, et al. Voluminous myoepithelioma of the minor salivary glands involving the base of the tongue. Case Rep Otolar-yngol 2016;2016:3785979.

36. Iwai T, Baba J, Murata S, et al. Warthin tumor arising from the minor salivary gland. J Craniofac Surg 2012;23:e374–6.

37. Motallebnejad M, Seyedmajidi M, Khakbaz Baboli O, et al. Oncocytoma of palatal minor salivary gland. Arch Iran Med 2015;18:320–1.

38. Ramaswamy P, Khaitan T, Anuradha A, et al. Intra-ductal papilloma: atypical presentation. Case Rep Dent 2013;2013:652728.

39. Abdel Razek AA. Imaging of connective tissue dis-eases of the head and neck. Neuroradiol J 2016;29:222–30.

40. Andrew N, Kearney D, Sladden N, et al. Immuno-globulin G4-related disease of the hard palate. J Oral Maxillofac Surg 2014;72:717–23.

41. Razek AA, Castillo M. Imaging appearance of gran-ulomatous lesions of head and neck. Eur J Radiol 2010;76:52–60.

42. Abdel Razek AAK, Mukherji S. Imaging of sialadeni-tis. Neuroradiol J 2017;30:205–15.

43. Tsuji T, Nishide Y, Nakano H, et al. Imaging findings of necrotizing sialometaplasia of the parotid gland: case report and literature review. Dentomaxillofac Radiol 2014;43(6):20140127.

44. Abdel-Aziz M, Khalifa B, Nassar A, et al. Mucocele of the hard palate in children. Int J Pediatr Otorhino-laryngol 2016;85:46–9.

State-of-the-Art Imaging of Salivary Gland Tumors

Ahmed Abdel Khalek Abdel Razek, MD[a],*, Suresh K. Mukherji, MD, MBA[b]

KEYWORDS

• Parotid • Salivary • Benign • Malignant • Spread • Staging

KEY POINTS

- MR imaging is the state-of-the-art imaging modality of choice in the evaluation of salivary gland tumors.
- Routine postcontrast MR imaging is important for accurate localization, locoregional extension of salivary gland tumors.
- Contrast MR imaging is excellent for detection of perineural spread of salivary malignancy, which is commonly reported in patients in adenoid cystic carcinoma.
- Multiparametric imaging of advanced MR imaging, such as diffusion-weighted MR imaging and dynamic contrast-enhanced (DCE) MR imaging, may help in characterization of some salivary gland tumors.
- Diffusion-weighted MR imaging can be used to differentiate recurrence from post-treatment changes and monitor patients with malignant salivary gland tumors after therapy.

INTRODUCTION
Epidemiology

Salivary gland tumors are rare, accounting for about 2% to 6.5% of all head and neck tumors and about 0.5% of all malignancies.[1,2] The most common location of salivary tumors is the parotid gland (70%), followed by the submandibular gland, the minor salivary glands, and the sublingual gland in descending order. Most tumors are benign pleomorphic adenomas (65% of parotid tumors), followed by Warthin tumor (15%–20% of parotid tumors). The most common malignant tumor is mucoepidermoid carcinoma, which forms 10% of salivary tumors and 30% of malignancies; approximately half of these occur in the parotid glands.[3–5] Salivary gland tumors are classified according to the World Health Organization histologic classification into 20 malignant epithelial salivary gland tumors and 11 benign epithelial salivary gland tumors.[6]

Methods of Examination

MR imaging is the modality of choice in patients with salivary gland tumors. Routine precontrast and postcontrast MR imaging is commonly used for assessment of salivary gland tumors.[7–15] Multiparametric imaging of diffusion-weighted MR imaging and dynamic contrast-enhanced (DCE) MR imaging are incorporated into routine imaging in evaluation of salivary gland tumors in our center.[16–20] Other recent sequences of MR imaging, such as diffusion tensor imaging, intravoxel incoherent motion diffusion MR imaging, proton MR spectroscopy, and dynamic susceptibility contrast MR imaging have recently been used to characterize salivary gland tumors but they are not validated and need further studies for their clinical application.[21–24] Routine postcontrast computed tomography (CT) scan may be used to better evaluate cortical invasion of the skull base.[25,26] Advanced CT techniques, such

[a] Department of Diagnostic Radiology, Mansoura University, Elgomheryia Street, Mansoura 35512, Egypt;
[b] Department of Radiology, Michigan State University, Michigan State University Health Team, 846 Service Road, East Lansing, MI 48824, USA
* Corresponding author.
E-mail address: arazek@mans.edu.eg

Neuroimag Clin N Am 28 (2018) 303–317
https://doi.org/10.1016/j.nic.2018.01.009
1052-5149/18/

as CT perfusion and dual-energy CT, have limited role in evaluation of salivary gland tumors and need further studies.[27–32] PET-CT is helpful for detection of distant metastasis from salivary gland cancer.[33] The details and protocols of these techniques are discussed in Christopher Atkinson and colleagues' article, "Cross-Sectional Imaging Techniques and Normal Anatomy of the Salivary Glands," in this issue.

ROLE OF IMAGING IN SALIVARY GLAND TUMORS

Imaging provides information about accurate localization of salivary gland tumors either in superficial or deep lobe, identification of the intraparotid course of facial nerve, differentiation of malignancy from benignity, characterization of some benign and malignant salivary gland tumors, and staging of salivary cancer. In addition, imaging helps in differentiating between recurrent malignant salivary gland tumors from post-treatment changes, monitoring patients after therapy, and may help in differentiation of salivary gland tumors from simulating lesions.[7–15]

Localization of Salivary Gland Tumors

It is important to identify whether a mass arises from the deep lobe or superficial lobe of the parotid gland, because the surgical approach for these tumors differs. A mass that arises from the deep lobe of the parotid is centered lateral to the parapharyngeal space and invades the parapharyngeal space from the lateral to medial direction (**Fig. 1**). The mass also widens the interval between the styloid process and the mandible known as the stylomandibular tunnel.[8,11,34]

Identification of Intraparotid Course of Facial Nerve

Differentiation of deep and superficial lobe parotid tumors hinges on the identification of the intraparotid course of the facial nerve. When evaluating most parotid tumors, it is usually sufficient to map the expected course of the nerve using anatomic landmarks (eg, stylomastoid foramen, retromandibular vein, and posterior belly of digastric and the mandibular ramus) (see **Fig. 1**). Three-dimensional FIESTA sequence was described in Christopher Atkinson and colleagues' article, "Cross-Sectional Imaging Techniques and Normal Anatomy of the Salivary Glands," in this issue and can help demonstrate the facial nerve. This T2-weighted sequence has the advantage of distinguishing duct (high signal) from the low-signal-intensity nerve.[2–10]

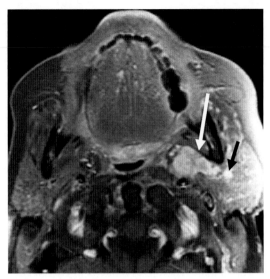

Fig. 1. Localization of salivary gland deep lobe of pleomorphic adenoma. Axial contrast-enhanced T1W image with fat-suppression shows an enhancing mass (*white arrow*) located in the left parotid gland. The mass is deep to the retromandibular vein (*black arrow*). Because the facial nerve is located lateral to the retromandibular vein, the mass is localized to the deep lobe of the parotid gland.

Malignancy Versus Benignity

Presence of certain MR imaging findings at routine postcontrast MR imaging may help distinguish between malignant and benign salivary tumors. However, the imaging findings are often nonspecific.[7–15] Multiparametric MR imaging of diffusion-weighted MR and dynamic contrast MR imaging has a role in differentiation of malignant salivary gland tumors from benign tumors.[10–17] Recently, advanced MR imaging sequences were used for characterization of salivary gland tumors, but they need further study for clinical applications.[21–24]

Routine MR imaging

Benign salivary gland tumors typically have smooth and well-defined borders, hyperintense signal on T2-weighted images, and are often superficially located. The MR imaging findings suggestive of high-grade malignant salivary gland tumors are ill-defined borders, invasion into adjacent tissues, low T2 signal, heterogeneous enhancement, cystic changes, and central necrosis.[7,9,35] Cystic components are seen in 50% of benign and 78% of malignant tumors. Eccentric location of the cystic areas is seen in 90% of benign tumors and 50% of malignant salivary tumors and central cystic areas are seen only in malignant tumors.[36] Rim enhancement is present in approximately 77% of benign and 67% of malignant salivary tumors. The presence of irregular thickening and peripheral nodules within the wall are seen more commonly in malignant tumors.[37] Bilateral and multifocal tumors are most commonly reported in Warthin tumor and lymphoma. Other causes of multifocal tumors include acinic cell carcinoma, oncocytoma, and intraparotid metastatic lymph nodes in patients with head and neck melanoma or squamous cell carcinoma.[7–15]

Diffusion-weighted MR imaging

Diffusion-weighted MR imaging with calculation of apparent diffusion coefficient (ADC) is used to differentiate benign and malignant salivary gland tumors. Tumors with high ADC value are more likely to be benign (Fig. 2). Most malignant tumors had low or very low ADC areas constituting more than 60% of the tumor area (Fig. 3). The challenge is that the low ADC threshold does not reliably distinguish between malignancies and Warthin tumors.[14–18]

Dynamic contrast-enhanced MR imaging

DCE MR imaging helps in characterization of salivary gland tumors. Following contrast administration, multiple T1-weighted images of the salivary tumor are obtained for several minutes to monitor the uptake and washout of contrast. The time of peak enhancement correlates with the microvessel count and tends to be short when the microvessel count is high. Washout depends on the cellularity-stromal grade, with cellular tumors having faster washout. Pleomorphic adenomas tend to demonstrate progressive enhancement (low

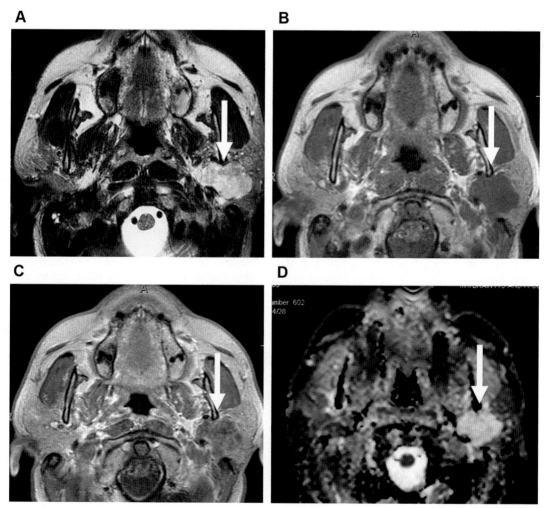

Fig. 2. Pleomorphic adenoma. (*A*) Axial T2W image shows a well-circumscribed lobulated high T2 signal mass that involved the superficial and deep lobes (*arrow*). The mass is low signal on T1W images (*B*) and homogeneously enhances with contrast (*C*). The mass has high ADC (*D*), which supports the diagnosis of a benign lesion.

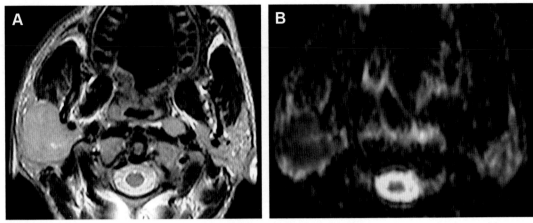

Fig. 3. Mucoepidermoid carcinoma. (*A*) Axial T2W image shows an ill-defined hypointense mass in the right parotid. (*B*) Axial ADC map shows restricted diffusion with low ADC value of the mass.

microvessel count and cellularity-stromal grade) (**Fig. 4**). Warthin tumors demonstrate rapid enhancement and washout (high microvessel count and cellularity-stromal grade). Malignant tumors demonstrate rapid enhancement, but washout tends to be slower than in Warthin tumors (high microvessel count and lower cellularity-stromal grade). Multiparametric approach using DCE and ADC may improve the accuracy of distinguishing between benign and malignant salivary gland tumors.[14–20]

Advanced MR imaging

Proton MR spectroscopy of the salivary glands shows differences between salivary gland tumors with significantly different choline/creatine ratios of Warthin tumors compared with pleomorphic adenomas and malignant salivary gland tumors. Ratios of greater than 2.4 were predictive of a benign tumor.[21,22] The mean percentage of dynamic contrast enhancement of malignant parotid tumors (33.53% ± 3.99%) is significantly different (P = .001) from that of benign parotid tumors (22.29% ± 4.13%). There is a significant difference in mean percentage of dynamic contrast enhancement and ADC values between pleomorphic adenomas and Warthin tumors (P = .001).[23] The fractional anisotropy and mean diffusivity of malignant salivary gland tumors shows a significant difference (P = .001) than benign tumors (**Fig. 5**). There is significant difference in fractional anisotropy between Warthin tumors and malignant tumors (P = .001).[24]

Computed tomography

CT perfusion has potential to differentiate benign and malignant salivary gland tumors by demonstrating higher blood flow and volume in benign tumors (**Fig. 6**) than malignancy because of abundant microscopic areas of necrosis in malignancies. Warthin tumors have higher tumor blood flow and volume than malignancy, and

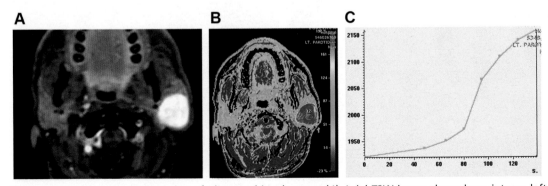

Fig. 4. Dynamic contrast MR imaging of pleomorphic adenoma. (*A*) Axial T2W image shows hyperintense left parotid mass. (*B*) Tumor blood flow map shows increased flow of left parotid tumor with region of interest localization. (*C*) Time intensity curve shows progressive enhancement of the tumor.

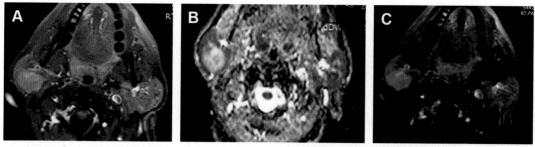

Fig. 5. Diffusion tensor imaging of pleomorphic adenoma. (*A*) Axial contrast T1W image shows mildly enhanced mass in the right parotid gland. (*B*) ADC map shows unrestricted diffusion of the mass. (*C*) Mean diffusivity map shows the tumor with low diffusivity.

pleomorphic adenomas have significantly lower blood flow and blood volume.[27–30] 18-Fluorodeoxyglucose-PET/CT imaging has had little role in initial work-up of parotid tumors. The normal activity in the parotid gland may mask an underlying lesion. Both malignant and benign parotid tumors (**Fig. 7**) have increased glucose metabolism and even some inflammatory processes can demonstrate increased uptake. There is a role for PET surveillance for recurrent disease or for assessing distant metastases.[14,33]

Characterization of Benign Salivary Gland Tumors

Pleomorphic adenomas versus Warthin tumors
Pleomorphic adenomas classically contain a significant proportion of myxomatous tissue, which causes less restriction of water diffusion, high ADCs, and very high signal intensity on the ADC map when compared with salivary cancer.[8–13]

Warthin tumors may contain abundant densely packed lymphoid cells, which accounts for their lower ADCs (**Fig. 8**), which overlap with those of malignancy; however, Warthin tumors are usually highly vascular compared with pleomorphic adenomas and malignant salivary gland tumors. Therefore, intravoxel incoherent motion may help to distinguish benign from malignant tumors by using high D* to reflect higher pseudodiffusion in the microcirculation in Warthin tumors and high D to reflect less restricted pure diffusion in pleomorphic adenomas.[38–41]

Other epithelial and mesenchymal benign salivary gland tumors
Myoepitheliomas appear as small, unilocular, round tumors with smooth contours that are located in the superficial lobe and abut the capsule of the parotid gland, display the capsule on T2-weighted and contrast-enhanced T1-weighted imaging, and exhibit homogeneous signal intensities or densities

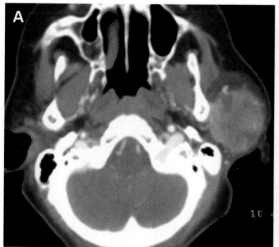
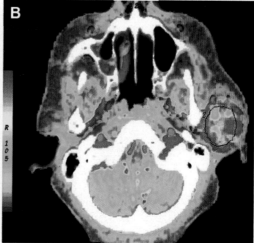

Fig. 6. Perfusion CT of pleomorphic adenoma. (*A*) Axial contrast T1W image shows mildly enhanced mass involving most of the left parotid gland. (*B*) Tumor blood flow map shows increased blood flow in the left parotid tumor.

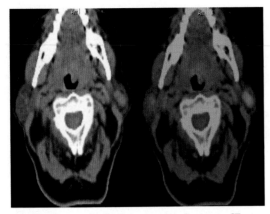

Fig. 7. PET-CT of Warthin tumor. Contrast CT scan shows mass in left parotid gland that shows increased fluorodeoxyglucose uptake at PET-CT image.

based on MR imaging and CT.[42] Oncocytomas seem to share unique imaging characteristics of hypointense, well-demarcated lesions on T1-weighted images that become isointense ("vanish") to parotid tissue contrast T1-weighted images. These lesions are hyperintense to isointense to the parotid gland on T2-weighted images (Fig. 9).[43] Basal cell adenomas tend to be small and show early intense enhancement. The solid tumor is common in the superficial region of the parotid gland, and cystic lesions occur mostly in the deeper parts of the superficial lobe or in the deep lobe (Fig. 10).[44] Hemangiomas are more common in children and show homogenous intense contrast enhancement that may shows areas of signal void regions (Fig. 11). Lipoma shows characteristic high signal intensity of T1-weighted images of fatty tissue (Fig. 12).[45]

Characterization of Malignant Salivary Tumors

Malignant epithelial salivary tumors were categorized into 20 histologies at the World Health Organization in 2017, but the most common four are adenoid cystic carcinoma (26%), mucoepidermoid carcinoma (17%), acinic cell carcinoma (14%), and adenocarcinoma not otherwise specified (11%). Characterization of salivary gland malignancy is important for prognosis. The CT (Fig. 13) and MR imaging (Fig. 14) findings of malignant salivary gland tumors are nonspecific. Perineural spread is commonly seen in adenoid cystic carcinoma but may be seen in other pathologic subtypes of salivary malignancy.[46–48]

Nonepithelial malignant tumors represent a minority of malignant salivary gland tumors. Extranodal primary lymphoma of the salivary glands is rare, accounting for only 5% of all extranodal non-Hodgkin lymphoma, 2% of all salivary gland tumors, and 16% of all malignant salivary gland tumors. Eighty percent are located in the parotid gland with bilateral disease in most of cases (Fig. 15). Mucosa-associated lymphoma type is the most prevalent histologic subtype. Metastasis into intraparotid lymph nodes (Fig. 16) has been reported from squamous cell carcinoma of head and neck.[1–8]

Grading of Malignant Salivary Gland Tumors

The most common low-grade malignant salivary gland tumors are mucoepidermoid carcinoma, adenocarcinoma not otherwise specified, and acinic cell carcinoma. The high-grade malignant

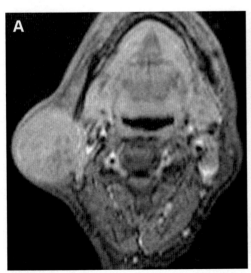
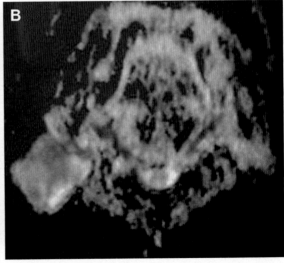

Fig. 8. Warthin tumor. (A) Axial contrast T1W image shows enhanced mass is seen involving the right parotid gland. (B) ADC map shows restricted diffusion with low ADC value confusing with malignancy.

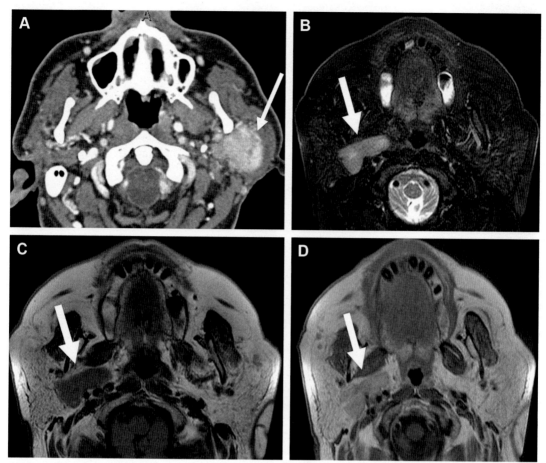

Fig. 9. Oncocytoma. (*A*) Axial contrast-enhanced CT shows a densely enhancing well-circumscribed mass (*arrow*) located in the left parotid gland. (*B–D*) Axial images obtained in a different patient demonstrate a lobulated right parotid lesion predominately located in the deep lobe (*arrows*). The lesion has high signal on the T2W image (*A*). The oncocytoma has low T1 signal (*B*) and homogeneously enhances with contrast (*C*).

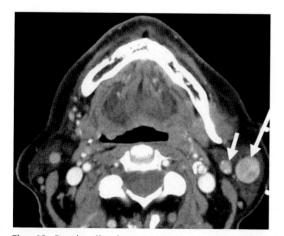

Fig. 10. Basal cell adenoma. Contrast-enhanced CT shows an intensely enhancing solid mass (*large arrow*) with well-defined margins located in the superficial lobe of the left parotid gland. Note that the retromandibular vein (*small arrow*) is deep to the lesion.

salivary gland tumors include adenoid cystic carcinoma, carcinoma ex pleomorphic adenoma, myoepithelial carcinoma, carcinosarcoma, large cell undifferentiated carcinoma, small cell undifferentiated carcinoma, and salivary duct carcinoma.[3–6] Low-grade malignant tumors may resemble benign lesions at routine MR imaging. The size of a malignant tumor is correlated with grade of malignancy; tumors less than 4 cm have a better prognosis than tumors greater than 4 cm. The high-risk salivary gland cancer shows lower ADC value compared with high-risk malignancy salivary gland tumors. Nodal and distant metastases are more commonly seen in high-grade than in low-grade salivary gland cancer.[7–15] Diffusion-weighted MR imaging can differentiate high-risk from low-risk malignancy[18] and helps to select the best biopsy with areas of lowest ADC value selected for biopsy that represent the most cellular area of the tumor.[17]

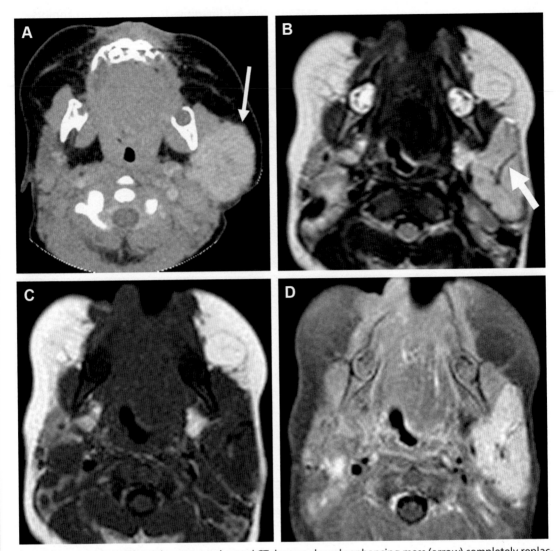

Fig. 11. Hemangioma. (*A*) Axial contrast-enhanced CT shows a densely enhancing mass (*arrow*) completely replacing the left parotid gland in a 1-year-old child. (*B*) Axial T2W sequence shows the mass has a high T2 signal that contains a flow void (*arrow*). This finding indicates the mass is hypervascular and suggests a benign process in a child. (*C*) Axial T1WI sequence shows diffusely low signal. (*D*) Axial fat-suppressed post contrast T1W sequence shows intensely enhances the mass.

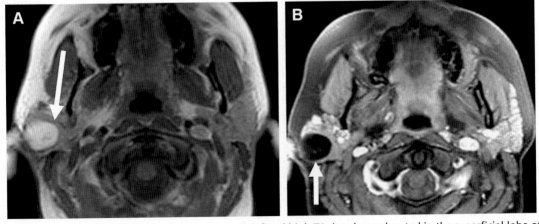

Fig. 12. Lipoma. (*A*) Axial T1W image shows a well-defined high T1 signal mass located in the superficial lobe of the right parotid gland (*arrow*). The homogeneously high T1 signal is suggestive of fat. (*B*) The T1W fat-suppressed image shows complete loss of the high T1 signal confirming the diagnosis of parotid lipoma.

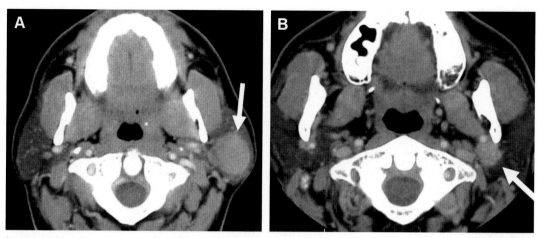

Fig. 13. Malignant tumors, nonspecific CT appearance. (*A, B*) Axial contrast CT performed in two different patients. Both patients have well-defined soft tissue mass (*arrows*) in the left parotid gland with similar degrees to enhancement. The pathology in A was adenoid cystic carcinoma and the pathology in B was mucoepidermoid carcinoma.

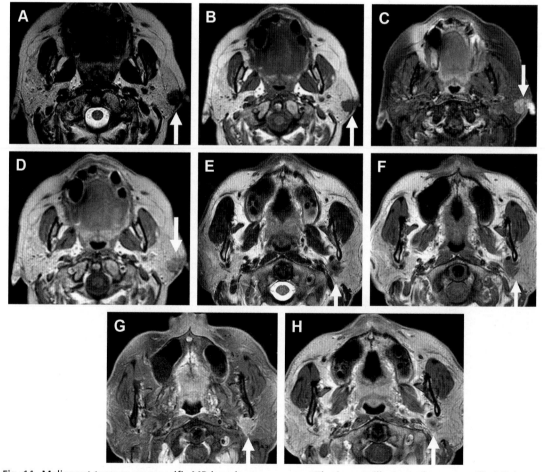

Fig. 14. Malignant tumors, nonspecific MR imaging appearance. The images illustrate the nonspecific MR imaging appearance of adenoid cystic (*A–D*) and mucoepidermoid carcinomas (*E–G*). Both lesions (*arrows*) have low T2 (*A, E*) and T1 signal (*B, F*) with ill-defined margins. Both lesions enhance on the following contrast (*C, G*) and are easily detected on the fat-suppressed contrast-enhanced T1W sequences (*D, H*).

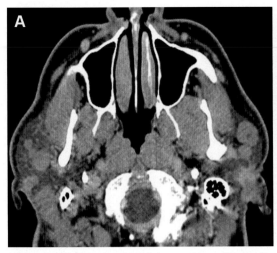
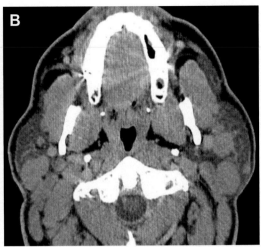

Fig. 15. Parotid lymphoma. Axial noncontrast CT obtained at the level of the midportion of the maxillary sinuses (*A*) and maxillary alveolar ridge (*B*) shows multiple bilateral large intraparotid masses in a patient with non-Hodgkin lymphoma. The masses are caused by lymphomatous involvement of the intraparotid lymph nodes.

Spread (Staging) of Salivary Gland Cancer

Salivary gland malignant tumors spread by direct invasion, metastases, and perineural spread. Local extension and invasion, the presence of perineural spread, and nodal and/or distant metastases affect surgical management decision.[46–48]

Locoregional staging

Staging of salivary gland malignancy is based on tumor size, extraglandular spread, and local extent. A T1 tumor measures less than 2 cm, and a T2 tumor measures between 2 and 4 cm. T3 lesions measure more than 4 cm or demonstrate

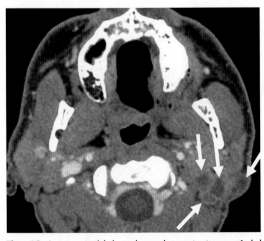

Fig. 16. Intraparotid lymph node metastases. Axial contrast CT shows multiple low-attenuation masses (*arrows*) in the left parotid gland that are caused by intraparotid lymph node metastases from a left tonsillar carcinoma.

extraglandular spread. T4a lesions include tumors with skin, mandible, external auditory canal, and/or facial nerve invasion. T4b lesions invade the skull base and/or the pterygoid plates and/or encase the internal carotid artery.[47] Routine postcontrast MR imaging can detect glandular and extraglandular extension of tumor. Diffusion-weighted MR imaging can detect the extent of the tumor. Contrast-enhanced CT can detect cortical invasion and extension into adjacent bony structures of the skull base or mandible.[25,26] Permeative invasion into bone marrow of the skull base and mandible appears as replacement of the medullary bone marrow with abnormal signal intensity at routine T1-weighted MR imaging. CT is superior to MR imaging in detection of cortical invasion.[46,47]

Perineural spread

Perineural spread of salivary gland cancer predicts worse prognosis. The commonly involved nerves in perineural spread of salivary gland cancer are the facial (VII) and trigeminal (V) nerves, which are closest to the major salivary glands, with the auriculotemporal nerve serving as an important connection.[7–10] The auriculotemporal nerve connects the facial nerve to the mandibular branch of the trigeminal nerve that runs parallel to the superficial temporal artery and vein and extends posteriorly around the mandibular condyle and laterally toward the periauricular area. Perineural spread of parotid malignancy can extend along the course of the nerve to mandibular branch of trigeminal nerve and then travel intracranially through foramen ovale.[10–15] In minor salivary gland malignant tumors of the palate and in sublingual

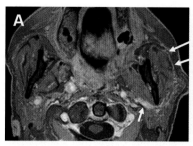
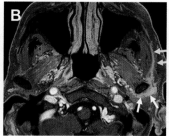
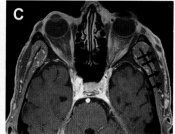

Fig. 17. Perineural spread involving multiple branches of the facial nerve from adenoid cystic carcinoma. (*A–C*) Multiple fat-suppressed contrast-enhanced T1W images obtained in a patient with recurrent adenoid cystic carcinoma shows perineural spread along multiple peripheral branches of the facial nerve. The facial nerve branches that are involved are the following: buccal branch, long white arrows; auriculotemporal nerve, short white arrows; zygomatic branch, yellow arrows; temporal branch, black arrows.

and submandibular gland tumors, the palatine nerves and the inferior alveolar nerve, respectively, are primarily involved. The perineural spread appears on contrast MR imaging as enlargement or abnormal enhancement of the nerve, obliteration of the neural fat pads adjacent to the neurovascular foramina, or neuroforaminal enlargement (**Fig. 17**).[49,50] Further data about perineural spread are provided in Christopher Atkinson and colleagues' article, "Cross-Sectional Imaging Techniques and Normal Anatomy of the Salivary Glands," in this issue.

Nodal staging
Nodal metastases from malignant salivary gland tumors are seen in 10% to 15% of patients at presentation but are more common (>30%) in high-grade than in low-grade salivary gland malignancy.[51] Nodal spread of salivary cancer is more likely to occur with high-grade salivary cancer. The rate of lymph node metastasis is directly correlated with the extension of the primary tumor. The incidence of lymph node metastasis is approximately 7% to 16% in T1 and T2 tumors. Clinically occult nodal metastases occur in approximately 8% to 19% of cases. Lymphatic spread tends to occur to intraparotid and periparotid lymph nodes, with further dissemination to the upper and midjugular chain nodes (levels II and III), followed by high posterior triangle nodes (level VA). Retropharyngeal spread uncommonly occurs.[51–56]

Distant metastases
Distant metastases most commonly involve the lungs, followed by bones and liver. Salivary ductal carcinoma and adenoid cystic carcinoma are the most common histologic types associated with

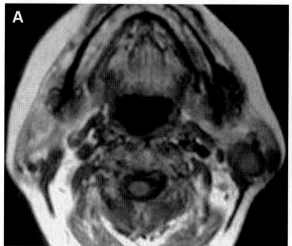
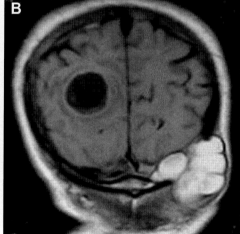

Fig. 18. Distant metastasis from adenoid cystic carcinoma. (*A*) Axial contrast T1W image shows enhanced mass is seen in the right parotid lobe. (*B*) Coronal contrast T1W image of the same patient shows expansile lytic lesion of the skull vault and cystic brain metastasis.

distant metastases. The rate of distant metastases was 11% at 15 years and 24% at 40-year follow-up; 25% of patients developed distant metastases despite apparent local cure. Distant metastases occur in about 10% to 50% of patients at first presentation and may be seen in low and in high T stages during follow-up. Distant metastases to lung, bone, and soft tissues occur in 20% of salivary malignancies overall (**Fig. 18**).[57–59]

Prediction of Malignant Transformation

Malignant transformation of pleomorphic adenomas

Pleomorphic adenomas have the potential to undergo malignant transformation into carcinoma ex pleomorphic adenoma (**Fig. 19**). The development of this malignancy has a direct relationship with duration of pleomorphic adenoma, with rates being 9.4% at 15 years. Untreated pleomorphic adenomas eventually undergo malignant transformation in 25% of patients. The incidence of malignant transformation is even higher in recurrent pleomorphic adenomas. The ADC values are used to evaluate for areas of malignant change within a pleomorphic adenoma, with low ADC values correlating with the hypercellular carcinomatous portions of the tumor that selected for biopsy site. The perfusion property may be effective for predicting carcinoma ex pleomorphic adenoma of pleomorphic adenomas.[60–62]

Lymphomas of Sjögren syndrome

Sjögren syndrome is considered a risk factor for the development of malignant lymphoma (**Fig. 20**).

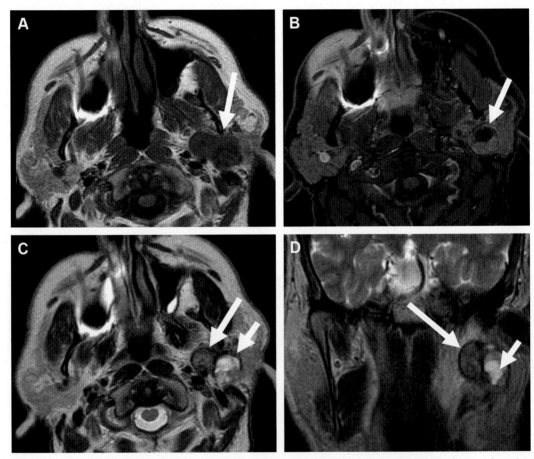

Fig. 19. Pleomorphic adenoma ex carcinoma. (*A*) Axial non-contrast-enhanced T1W image shows a low-signal mass located in the left parotid gland (*arrow*). (*B*) The mass heterogeneously enhances following contrast on the fat-suppressed T1W sequence with a focal area of nonenhancement (*arrow*). Pathology revealed pleomorphic adenoma ex carcinoma. (*C, D*) The axial and coronal T2W sequences demonstrate a heterogeneous mass that contains a medial low-signal solid component (*large arrow*) and a portion that has high T2 signal (*small arrow*) that correlates with the region of nonenhancement. Because pleomorphic adenomas are characterized by increased T2 signal, these findings suggest that this pleomorphic adenoma ex carcinoma arose from an underlying pleomorphic adenoma.

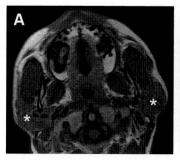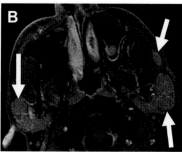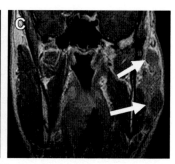

Fig. 20. Lymphoma associated with Sjögren syndrome. Axial T1W image (*A*) in a patient with Sjögren syndrome shows loss of the normal high T1 signal in both parotid glands (*asterisks*). Axial contrast-enhanced fat-suppressed T1W image (*B*) and coronal postcontrast enhanced T1W (*C*) shows multiple bilateral masses (*arrows*). Biopsy of one of the masses revealed lymphoma.

Salivary glands and ocular adnexa are the most common sites for secondary lymphoma with Sjögren syndrome. Various histologic subtypes of lymphoma have been described in patients with Sjögren syndrome, but mucoid-associated lymphoid tissue lymphoma is the most common. Lymphomas revealed restricted diffusion with low ADC value caused by high cellularity of the tumor (see **Fig. 14**).[63,64]

Differentiation of Neoplastic from Simulating Lesions

Inflammatory lesions
Inflammatory lesions are more common in submandibular glands than tumors. Sialadenitis is usually diffuse and is differentiated from tumor on ultrasound. Sialadenitis may be focal lesion and simulate tumor. Intralesional duct dilatation is suggestive of an inflammatory mass, whereas distortion of the vascular anatomy is suggestive of neoplasia.[65,66]

Autoimmune disorders
The autoimmune disorders of the salivary gland include Sjögren syndrome and immunolgbulin-IgG4 sialadenitis. Sjögren syndrome is characterized by bilateral salivary gland involvement and multiple cystic lesions scattered in salivary parenchyma. Immunoglobulin-IgG4 shows bilateral salivary gland involvement; however, the involvement tends to be unilateral when the disease involves the submandibular gland, which may simulate tumor.[66,67]

Post-treatment of Salivary Tumors

Diffusion-weighted MR imaging has shown promising results in differentiating post-treatment changes from recurrent head and neck squamous cell carcinoma. Diffusion-weighted MR imaging has a role in predication of salivary tumor recurrence and surveillance of salivary gland malignant

tumor after treatment and is an area of active investigation.[68–70] This topic is covered in Akifumi Fujita's article, "Imaging of Sjögren Syndrome and Immunoglobulin G4-Related Disease of the Salivary Glands," in this issue.

SUMMARY

Routine precontrast and postcontrast MR imaging is essential for initial diagnosis and accurate localization and locoregional extension of salivary gland tumors. Advanced MR imaging, such as diffusion and dynamic contrast MR imaging, provides additional tissue characterization when combined with standard MR imaging.

REFERENCES

1. Gao M, Hao Y, Huang MX, et al. Salivary gland tumours in a northern Chinese population: a 50-year retrospective study of 7190 cases. Int J Oral Maxillofac Surg 2017;46:343–9.
2. Del Signore AG, Megwalu UC. The rising incidence of major salivary gland cancer in the United States. Ear Nose Throat J 2017;96:E13–6.
3. Carlson ER. Management of parotid tumors. J Oral Maxillofac Surg 2017;75:247–8.
4. Kuan EC, Mallen-St Clair J, St John MA. Evaluation of parotid lesions. Otolaryngol Clin North Am 2016; 49:313–25.
5. Seethala RR. Salivary gland tumors: current concepts and controversies. Surg Pathol Clin 2017;10: 155–76.
6. Seethala RR, Stenman G. Update from the 4th Edition of the World Health Organization classification of head and neck tumours: tumors of the salivary gland. Head Neck Pathol 2017;11:55–67.
7. Dai YL, King AD. State of the art MRI in head and neck cancer. Clin Radiol 2018;73(1):45–59.
8. Abraham J. Imaging for head and neck cancer. Surg Oncol Clin N Am 2015;24:455–71.

9. Madani G. Imaging of salivary glands. In: Brennan PA, Schliephake H, Ghali GE, et al, editors. Maxillofacial surgery, vol. 1, 3rd edition. Italy: Churchill Livingstone; 2017. p. 668–85.

10. Prasad RS. Parotid gland imaging. Otolaryngol Clin North Am 2016;49:285–312.

11. Abdel Razek AA, Ashmalla GA, Gaballa G, et al. Pilot study of Ultrasound Parotid Imaging Reporting and Data System (PIRADS): inter-observer agreement. Eur J Radiol 2015;85:2533–8.

12. Kontzialis M, Glastonbury CM, Aygun N. Evaluation: imaging studies. In: Bradley PJ, Eisele DW, editors. Salivary gland neoplasms. Adv otorhinolaryngol, vol. 78. Basel (Switzerland): Karger; 2016. p. 25–33.

13. Abdel Razek AAK, Mukherji SK. Imaging of minor salivary glands. Neuroimag Clin N Am 2018;28(2):295–302.

14. Bag AK, Curé JK, Chapman PR, et al. Practical imaging of the parotid gland. Curr Probl Diagn Radiol 2015;44:167–92.

15. Afzelius P, Nielsen MY, Ewertsen C, et al. Imaging of the major salivary glands. Clin Physiol Funct Imaging 2016;36:1–10.

16. Attyé A, Troprès I, Rouchy RC, et al. Diffusion MRI: literature review in salivary gland tumors. Oral Dis 2017;23:572–5.

17. Razek AA. Diffusion-weighted magnetic resonance imaging of head and neck. J Comput Assist Tomogr 2010;34:808–15.

18. Abdel Razek A. Prediction of malignancy of submandibular gland tumors with apparent diffusion coefficient. Oral Radiol, in press.

19. Stefanovic X, Al Tabaa Y, Gascou G, et al. Magnetic resonance imaging of parotid gland tumors: dynamic contrast-enhanced sequence evaluation. J Comput Assist Tomogr 2017;41:541–6.

20. Lam PD, Kuribayashi A, Imaizumi A, et al. Differentiating benign and malignant salivary gland tumours: diagnostic criteria and the accuracy of dynamic contrast-enhanced MRI with high temporal resolution. Br J Radiol 2015;88:20140685.

21. Abdel Razek AA, Poptani H. MR spectroscopy of head and neck cancer. Eur J Radiol 2013;82:982–9.

22. King A, Yeung D, Ahuja A, et al. Salivary gland tumors at in vivo proton MR spectroscopy. Radiology 2005;237:563–9.

23. Razek AA, Elsorogy LG, Soliman NY, et al. Dynamic susceptibility contrast perfusion MR imaging in distinguishing malignant from benign head and neck tumors: a pilot study. Eur J Radiol 2011;77:73–9.

24. Abdel Razek A, Nada N. Characterization of salivary gland tumors with diffusion tensor imaging, in press.

25. Jin G, Su D, Xie D, et al. Distinguishing benign from malignant parotid gland tumours: low-dose multiphasic CT protocol with 5-minute delay. Eur Radiol 2011;21:1692–8.

26. Yerli H, Aydin E, Coskun M, et al. Dynamic multislice computed tomography findings for parotid gland tumors. J Comput Assist Tomogr 2007;31:309–16.

27. Razek AA, Tawfik AM, Elsorogy LG, et al. Perfusion CT of head and neck cancer. Eur J Radiol 2014;83:537–44.

28. Dong Y, Lei GW, Wang SW, et al. Diagnostic value of CT perfusion imaging for parotid neoplasms. Dentomaxillofac Radiol 2013;43:20130237.

29. Bisdas S, Baghi M, Wagenblast J, et al. Differentiation of benign and malignant parotid tumors using deconvolution-based perfusion CT imaging: feasibility of the method and initial results. Eur J Radiol 2007;64:258–65.

30. Tawfik AM, Razek AA, Elsorogy LG, et al. Perfusion CT of head and neck cancer: effect of arterial input selection. AJR Am J Roentgenol 2011;196:1374–80.

31. Chawla A, Srinivasan S, Lim TC, et al. Dual-energy CT applications in salivary gland lesions. Br J Radiol 2017;90(1074):20160859.

32. Tawfik AM, Kerl JM, Razek AA, et al. Image quality and radiation dose of dual-energy CT of the head and neck compared with a standard 120-kVp acquisition. AJNR Am J Neuroradiol 2011;32:1994–9.

33. Hadiprodjo D, Ryan T, Truong MT, et al. Parotid gland tumors: preliminary data for the value of FDG PET/CT diagnostic parameters. AJR Am J Roentgenol 2012;198:W185–90.

34. Attyé A, Karkas A, Troprès I, et al. Parotid gland tumours: MR tractography to assess contact with the facial nerve. Eur Radiol 2016;26:2233–41.

35. Christe A, Waldherr C, Hallett R, et al. MR imaging of parotid tumors: typical lesion characteristics in MR imaging improve discrimination between benign and malignant disease. AJNR Am J Neuroradiol 2011;32:1202–7.

36. Kato H, Kanematsu M, Watanabe H, et al. Salivary gland tumors of the parotid gland: CT and MR imaging findings with emphasis on intratumoral cystic components. Neuroradiology 2014;56:789–95.

37. Sakamoto M, Iikubo M, Kojima I, et al. Diagnostic value of capsule-like rim enhancement on magnetic resonance imaging for distinguishing malignant from benign parotid tumours. Int J Oral Maxillofac Surg 2014;43:1035–41.

38. Espinoza S, Felter A, Malinvaud D, et al. Warthin's tumor of parotid gland: surgery or follow-up? Diagnostic value of a decisional algorithm with functional MRI. Diagn Interv Imaging 2016;97:37–43.

39. Miao LY, Xue H, Ge HY, et al. Differentiation of pleomorphic adenoma and Warthin's tumour of the salivary gland: is long-to-short diameter ratio a useful parameter? Clin Radiol 2015;70:1212–9.

40. Abdel Razek AA, Samir S, Ashmalla GA. Characterization of parotid tumors with dynamic susceptibility contrast perfusion-weighted magnetic resonance

imaging and diffusion-weighted MR imaging. J Comput Assist Tomogr 2017;41:131–6.

41. Kato H, Kanematsu M, Watanabe H, et al. Perfusion imaging of parotid gland tumours: usefulness of arterial spin labeling for differentiating Warthin's tumours. Eur Radiol 2015;25:3247–54.

42. Ding J, Wang W, Peng W, et al. MRI and CT imaging characteristics of myoepithelioma of the parotid gland. Acta Radiol 2016;57:837–43.

43. Patel ND, van Zante A, Eisele DW, et al. Oncocytoma: the vanishing parotid mass. AJNR Am J Neuroradiol 2011;32:1703–6.

44. Shi L, Wang YX, Yu C, et al. CT and ultrasound features of basal cell adenoma of the parotid gland: a report of 22 cases with pathologic correlation. AJNR Am J Neuroradiol 2012;33:434–8.

45. Razek AA, Huang BY. Soft tissue tumors of the head and neck: imaging-based review of the WHO classification. Radiographics 2011;31:1923–54.

46. Freling N, Crippa F, Maroldi R. Staging and follow-up of high-grade malignant salivary gland tumours: the role of traditional versus functional imaging approaches - a review. Oral Oncol 2016;60:157–66.

47. Adelstein D, Gillison ML, Pfister DG, et al. NCCN guidelines insights: head and neck cancers, version 2.2017. J Natl Compr Canc Netw 2017;15:761–70.

48. Friedman ER, Saindane AM. Pitfalls in the staging of cancer of the major salivary gland neoplasms. Neuroimag Clin North Am 2013;23:107–22.

49. Badger D, Aygun N. Imaging of perineural spread in head and neck cancer. Radiol Clin North Am 2017; 55:139–49.

50. Abdel Khalek Abdel Razek A, King A. MRI and CT of nasopharyngeal carcinoma. AJR Am J Roentgenol 2012;198:11–8.

51. Lim CM, Gilbert MR, Johnson JT, et al. Clinical significance of intraparotid lymph node metastasis in primary parotid cancer. Head Neck 2014;36:1634–7.

52. Abdel Razek AA, Soliman NY, Elkhamary S, et al. Role of diffusion-weighted MR imaging in cervical lymphadenopathy. Eur Radiol 2006;16:1468–77.

53. Megwalu UC, Sirjani D. Risk of nodal metastasis in major salivary gland adenoid cystic carcinoma. Otolaryngol Head Neck Surg 2017;156:660–4.

54. Abdel Razek AA, Gaballa G. Role of perfusion magnetic resonance imaging in cervical lymphadenopathy. J Comput Assist Tomogr 2011;35:21–5.

55. Bradley PJ. Primary malignant parotid epithelial neoplasm: nodal metastases and management. Curr Opin Otolaryngol Head Neck Surg 2015;23: 91–8.

56. Tawfik AM, Razek AA, Kerl JM, et al. Comparison of dual-energy CT-derived iodine content and iodine overlay of normal, inflammatory and metastatic squamous cell carcinoma cervical lymph nodes. Eur Radiol 2014;24:574–80.

57. Sheedy S, Welker K, DeLone D, et al. CNS metastases of carcinoma ex pleomorphic adenoma of the parotid gland. AJNR Am J Neuroradiol 2006;27:1483–5.

58. Lau R, Fernández-Coello A, Vidal-Sarró N, et al. Brain metastasis of carcinoma ex pleomorphic adenoma of the parotid gland: case report and review of the literature. Acta Neurochir 2017;159:459–63.

59. Lecouvet FE. Whole-body MR imaging: musculoskeletal applications. Radiology 2016;279:345–65.

60. Kato H, Kanematsu M, Mizuta K, et al. Carcinoma ex pleomorphic adenoma of the parotid gland: radiologic-pathologic correlation with MR imaging including diffusion-weighted imaging. AJNR Am J Neuroradiol 2008;29:865–7.

61. Razek AA, Megahed AS, Denewer A, et al. Role of diffusion-weighted magnetic resonance imaging in differentiation between the viable and necrotic parts of head and neck tumors. Acta Radiol 2008;49:364–70.

62. Katayama I, Eida S, Fujita S, et al. Perfusion MR imaging detection of carcinoma arising from preexisting salivary gland pleomorphic adenoma by computer-assisted analysis of time-signal intensity maps. PLoS One 2017;12:e0178002.

63. Abdel Razek AA. Imaging of connective tissue diseases of the head and neck. Neuroradiol J 2016; 29:222–30.

64. Kojima I, Sakamoto M, Iikubo M, et al. Diagnostic performance of MR imaging of three major salivary glands for Sjögren's syndrome. Oral Dis 2017;23:84–90.

65. Abdel Razek AA, Nada N. Role of diffusion-weighted MRI in differentiation of masticator space malignancy from infection. Dentomaxillofac Radiol 2013; 42(4):20120183.

66. Abdel Razek AAK, Mukherji S. Imaging of sialadenitis. Neuroradiol J 2017;30:205–15.

67. Razek AA, Castillo M. Imaging appearance of granulomatous lesions of head and neck. Eur J Radiol 2010;76:52–60.

68. Abdel Razek AAK, Mukherji SK. Imaging of posttreatment salivary gland tumors. Neuroimag Clin N Am 2018;28(2):199–208.

69. Abdel Razek AA, Kandeel AY, Soliman N, et al. Role of diffusion-weighted echo-planar MR imaging in differentiation of residual or recurrent head and neck tumors and posttreatment changes. AJNR Am J Neuroradiol 2007;28:1146–52.

70. Abdel Razek AA, Gaballa G, Ashamalla G, et al. Dynamic susceptibility contrast perfusion-weighted MR imaging and diffusion-weighted MR imaging in differentiating recurrent head and neck cancer from post-radiation changes. J Comput Assist Tomogr 2015;39:849–54.

Moving?

Make sure your subscription moves with you!

To notify us of your new address, find your **Clinics Account Number** (located on your mailing label above your name), and contact customer service at:

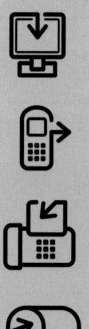

Email: journalscustomerservice-usa@elsevier.com

800-654-2452 (subscribers in the U.S. & Canada)
314-447-8871 (subscribers outside of the U.S. & Canada)

Fax number: 314-447-8029

Elsevier Health Sciences Division
Subscription Customer Service
3251 Riverport Lane
Maryland Heights, MO 63043

*To ensure uninterrupted delivery of your subscription, please notify us at least 4 weeks in advance of move.

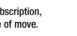

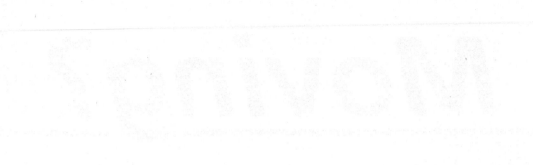